DIAGNOSIS
AND
TREATMENT
OF THE
UPPER EXTREMITIES

NONOPERATIVE ORTHOPAEDIC MEDICINE AND MANUAL THERAPY

DOS WINKEL, PT

Instructor, Scientific Society of Flemish General Practitioners
Antwerp, Belgium
Director, Dutch and German Academy of Orthopaedic Medicine
Delft, the Netherlands and Göttingen, Germany
President, International Academy of Orthopaedic Medicine

OMER MATTHIJS, PT

Instructor, International Academy of
  Orthopaedic Medicine
Instructor, American Academy of
  Orthopedic Medicine, Inc.
Tucson, Arizona

VALERIE PHELPS, PT

Instructor, International Academy of
  Orthopaedic Medicine
Director and Instructor, American
  Academy of Orthopedic Medicine, Inc.
Tucson, Arizona

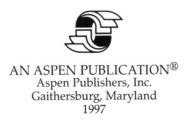

AN ASPEN PUBLICATION®
Aspen Publishers, Inc.
Gaithersburg, Maryland
1997

Library of Congress Cataloging-in-Publication Data

Winkel, Dos.
Diagnosis and treatment of the upper extremities: nonoperative
orthopaedic medicine and manual therapy / Dos Winkel with Omer
Matthijs, Valerie Phelps.
p. cm.
"Translation and adaptation of material previously published in
Dutch under the titles: Orthopedische geneeskunde en manuele
therapie, Diagnostiek extremiteiten (deel 2b) and Orthopedische
geneeskunde en manuele therapie, Therapie extremiteiten (deel 3b) by
Dos Winkel with Geert Aufdemkampe and Onno G. Meijer; Weke delen
aandoeningen van het bewegingsapparaat, Anatomie in vivo (deel 1) by
Andry Vleeming, Dos Winkel, and Onno G. Meijer"—T.p. verso.
Includes bibliographical references and index.
ISBN 0-8342-0901-2
1. Shoulder joint—Wounds and injuries. 2. Elbow—Wounds and
injuries. 3. Shoulder joint—Diseases. 4. Elbow—Diseases.
5. Shoulder joint—Pathophysiology. 6. Elbow—Pathophysiology.
I. Matthijs, Omer. II. Phelps, Valerie. III. Winkel, Dos.
Orthopedische geneeskunde en manuele therapie. IV. Vleeming, Andry.
Weke delen aandoeningen van het bewegingsapparaat. V. Title.
[DNLM: 1. Shoulder Joint—pathology. 2. Arm—pathology. 3. Joint
Diseases—diagnosis. 4. Joint Diseases—therapy. WE 810 W773d 1997]
RD557.W56 1997
617.5'7044—dc21
DNLM/DLC
for Library of Congress
96-46879
CIP

Orders: (800) 638-8437
Customer Service: (800) 234-1660

About Aspen Publishers • For more than 35 years, Aspen has been a leading professional publisher in a variety of disciplines. Aspen's vast information resources are available in both print and electronic formats. We are committed to providing the highest quality information available in the most appropriate format for our customers. Visit Aspen's Internet site for more information resources, directories, articles, and a searchable version of Aspen's full catalog, including the most recent publications: http://www.aspenpub.com
Aspen Publishers, Inc. • The hallmark of quality in publishing
Member of the worldwide Wolters Kluwer group.

The authors have made every effort to ensure the accuracy of the information herein. However, appropriate information sources should be consulted, especially for new or unfamiliar procedures. It is the responsibility of every practitioner to evaluate the appropriateness of a particular opinion in the context of actual clinical situations and with due consideration to new developments. Authors, editors, and the publisher cannot be held responsible for any typographical or other errors found in this book.

Editorial Resources: Ruth Bloom

Library of Congress Catalog Card Number: 96-46879
ISBN: 0-8342-0901-2

Printed in the United States of America

1 2 3 4 5

Table of Contents

Contributors

Geert Aufdemkampe, PT
Physical Therapist
Central Netherlands School of Higher
  Professional Education
Faculty of Health Care Education
Academy for Physical Therapy
Utrecht, The Netherlands

Gaby M. van Meerwijk, PT
Physical Therapist
St. Lucas Hospital
Instructor
Stichting Academy of Physical Therapy
Amsterdam, The Netherlands

Omer Matthijs, PT
Physical Therapist/Manipulative Therapist
Instructor, International Academy of
  Orthopaedic Medicine
Instructor, Academy for Orthopaedic
  Medicine
Göttingen, Germany
Instructor, Association for Physical Therapy
Stuttgart, Germany
Instructor, American Academy of Orthope-
  dic Medicine, Inc.
Tucson, Arizona

Onno G. Meijer, PhD, MD
Movement Scientist
Study Group for the Theory and History of
  Movement Science
Free University of Amsterdam
Amsterdam, The Netherlands

Didi G.H. van Paridon-Edauw, PT
Physical Therapist/Manipulative Therapist
Instructor, International Academy of
  Orthopaedic Medicine
Instructor, Academy for Orthopaedic
  Medicine
Göttingen, Germany
Instructor, Association for Physical Therapy
Stuttgart, Germany
Instructor, American Academy of Orthope-
  dic Medicine, Inc.
Tucson, Arizona

Valerie Phelps, PT
Physical Therapist/Manipulative Therapist
Instructor, International Academy of
  Orthopaedic Medicine
Instructor, Academy for Orthopaedic
  Medicine
Göttingen, Germany
Instructor, Association for Physical Therapy
Stuttgart, Germany
Director and Instructor, American Academy
  of Orthopedic Medicine, Inc.
Tucson, Arizona

Dos Winkel, PT
Instructor, Scientific Society of Flemish
  General Practitioners
Antwerp, Belgium
Director, Dutch and German Academy of
  Orthopaedic Medicine
Delft, the Netherlands and Göttingen,
  Germany
President, International Academy of Ortho-
  paedic Medicine

Foreword

Once again I am pleasantly surprised by the several volume series *Diagnosis and Treatment of the Spine, Diagnosis and Treatment of the Lower Extremities*, and *Diagnosis and Treatment of the Upper Extremities* by Dos Winkel. Practical information has been assembled for the health care professional in an ideal combination of extensive but conveniently organized subject matter and thorough but easy-to-read discussion of various topics. Basic data regarding functional anatomy and biomechanics, followed by thorough descriptions of the clinical examination and thorough discussions of pathology and treatment, make these volumes essential reference books that deserve a place in every medical library. Moreover, the most recent diagnostic techniques are illustrated in every volume.

During our many years of working together, I have gotten to know and appreciate Dos Winkel as an extremely qualified clinician with an analytical mind, which is evident in his approach to clinical problems, during his frequent seminars, and from his many publications and books. I also recognize a friend in Dos Winkel, for whom the writing of this preface is an expression of thanks for our fascinating, cooperative working relationship with the orthopedic patient.

Marc Martens, MD, PhD
Professor and Chief of Orthopedics
O.L.V. Middelares Hospital
Deurne, Belgium
Consultant Orthopedist
University Hospital
Antwerp, Belgium

Preface

Orthopedic medicine is a medical specialty that has gone through enormous changes during past decades. Research is being conducted worldwide in the various fields of movement science. This research includes arthrokinematics and dynamic electromyography, often with the aid of motion pictures. Because of such research, the causes of many disorders have become increasingly apparent, thus facilitating a more causal approach in the treatment of patients. A direct consequence of this is the decrease in the use of injection therapy, arthroscopy, and other surgical procedures. The opposite impression is gained, however, when one is dealing with patients' histories.

I am very grateful to **Valerie Phelps, PT**, Director of the American Academy of Orthopedic Medicine, for the translation of this series of books. This was a monumental task, which she performed with excellence. I am grateful to her as well, and to Omer Matthijs, for having updated this series of books from both the Dutch and German versions. Omer Matthijs has for years been one of my closest coworkers and collaborators, as well as a most excellent practitioner and teacher.

In recognition of the fact that improvements in the field are constantly being made, it is necessary to provide updated information as well as hands-on practice via a series of instructional courses designed around the techniques described in these books. Therefore, in addition to individual use, this series of books supports and provides source material for instructional courses organized by the American Academy of Orthopedic Medicine, Inc. For information about these courses, call 1-800-AAOM-305 (1-800-226-6305).

I hope that this series of books will improve the effectiveness of practitioners in diagnoses and providing the appropriate treatment techniques. To everyone who will use these books, I hope you enjoy great success in using this knowledge and these techniques to the benefit of your patients. We look forward to hearing all remarks and considerations that could lead to further improvement of the text.

Dos Winkel
Bonaire (Dutch Antilles)

Acknowledgments

This book would never have come into existence without the help of many experts who have made specific contributions. Didi van Paridon-Edauw and Omer Matthijs, who have been instructors at seminars in orthopedic medicine and manual therapy both nationally and internationally, have had a continuous significant influence on the ultimate contents of this book. I would also like to express my gratitude to Dr. Marc Martens, Dr. Geert DeClercq, and Dr. Peter Hirshfeld for the many illustrations they so willingly contributed. I would also like to thank Aspen Publishers, whose staff again patiently followed and adapted to the process of writing this book.

I would like to acknowledge the contributions of Onno G. Meijer and Geert Aufdemkampe, whose work influenced *Nonoperative Orthopaedic Medicine and Manual Therapy*. In addition, the contribution of Gaby M. van Meerwijk for the thoracic outlet compression syndrome is also gratefully acknowledged.

Introduction

Every day, physicians and physiotherapists see a number of patients disabled by a lesion in the sphere of orthopedic medicine. Sooner or later, in the course of our lives, all of us suffer from nonsurgical disorders of the moving parts, be it, for example, a stiff shoulder or neck, lumbago, or a sprained knee. In these cases an exact diagnosis may be difficult to reach because referred pain and referred tenderness divert attention from the actual site of the lesion. The absence of objective signs puts physicians off, and misleading radiographic appearances add to the confusion.

What the clinician needs is a quick and simple way to examine patients whereby the tissue at fault can be identified with precision. This is exactly what this book offers. The method that it advocates is selective tension. Tension is applied in different ways to each separate structure from which the symptom could originate. After such an examination is adequately performed and correlated with a full and accurate history, exact localization is seldom difficult. The pattern of movements elicited by this means is interpreted on the basis of functional anatomy, and the site of the lesion is singled out.

Dos Winkle has pioneered this work in Holland. His summary of the theory of this approach to pain and the discussions of possible findings in this book greatly facilitate one's arrival at a precise diagnosis. Treatment can now be formulated on factual grounds, often with rapid success, even in cases hitherto regarded as intractable. This method of diagnosis also identifies patients with emotional problems that have been projected to their moving parts. This detection avoids waste of their own and physiotherapists' time in treating the wrong tissue.

All Dos Winkel's colleagues will be grateful to him for publishing this concise account of the fundamental approach to diagnosis. I recommend this book to all professionals facing problems in orthopedic medicine. He imparts, to physicians no less than to physiotherapists, new, essential knowledge—for which no substitute exists—about the proper attitude to the many soft tissue lesions that they encounter so often.

James Cyriax

Editor's Note: This originally appeared as the Foreword in *Soft Tissue Affections of the Musculature System, Part 2, Diagnostic*, in 1984.

Part I

The Shoulder

1

Functional Anatomy of the Shoulder

In orthopaedic medicine, the term *shoulder* refers to the glenohumeral joint and surrounding structures. When describing shoulder pain, patients usually refer to the deltoid region (the upper part of the C5 dermatome). Pain in the upper trapezius area is generally caused by problems in the cervical spine or acromioclavicular joint.

The shoulder itself is part of a kinematic chain, that is, the shoulder girdle. Three joints—the glenohumeral, acromioclavicular, and sternoclavicular—play a central role in the functional anatomy of the shoulder girdle. For optimal function of the shoulder girdle, corresponding movements also have to occur in three other places: the scapulothoracic and cervicothoracic junctions and the connections of the first three ribs with the spine and sternum.

This chapter describes the joints comprising the shoulder girdle and their functional dependence on other parts of the body. Normal movement ranges and the influence of variables, such as gender and body weight, are also discussed.

JOINTS

Glenohumeral Joint (Articulatio Glenohumeralis)

The glenohumeral joint is a ball and socket joint. The "ball" (head of the humerus) and "socket" (glenoid cavity of the scapula) contribute little to the stability of the joint.

The glenoid cavity is enlarged slightly by the glenoid labrum, a fibrocartilaginous structure. Functionally, the socket is also enlarged by the acromion (the massive lateral part of the scapular spine) and the coracoacromial ligament, which runs between the acromion and the coracoid process (a bony protrusion from the anterior aspect of the scapula) (Figure 1–1).

The glenohumeral joint capsule is very lax, allowing for virtually unrestricted movement. However, within the (outer) fibrous capsule, there are three thick collagenous bands that strengthen the capsule: the superior, middle, and inferior glenohumeral ligaments. All three ligaments restrict motion and are located within the anterior part of the capsule. Often, the medial ligament is poorly developed; sometimes it is absent entirely. The coracohumeral ligament, which runs from the coracoid process to the greater tubercle of the humerus, strengthens the superioanterior aspect of the capsule.

In the fibrous membrane, there are two (and sometimes more) openings: one under the coracoid process (connecting the suprascapular bursa to the joint cavity) and one that allows passage of the biceps tendon.

Although the glenohumeral joint capsule is not very strong, it is strengthened by the insertion of the so-called rotator cuff muscles. The long head of the triceps is also connected to the capsule (as well as to the glenoid labrum).

An inner (synovial) membrane lines the fibrous capsule and secretes synovial fluid into the joint cavity. It extends from the glenoid labrum down to the neck of the humerus (Figure 1–2). At the inferior aspect of the joint,

6

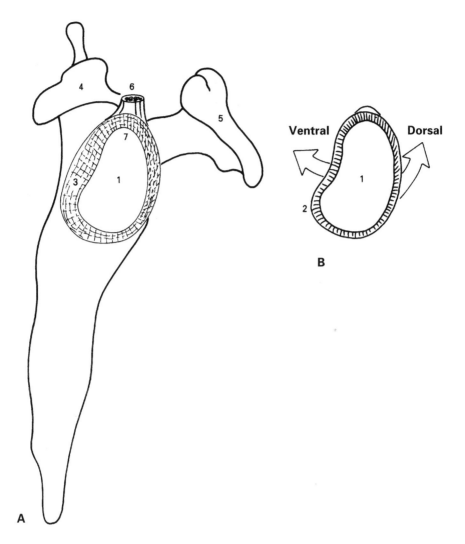

Figure 1–1 A, Lateral view of the scapula. **1,** Glenoid cavity; **3,** glenoid labrum; **4,** coracoid process; **5,** acromion; **6,** tendon of the long head of the biceps brachii; **7,** supraglenoid tubercle. **B,** Aspects of the bony edge of the glenoid cavity (**2**).

the fibrous capsule forms a pocket, the articular recess (or axillary pouch), which is also covered with synovial membrane.

Acromioclavicular Joint (Articulatio Acromioclavicularis)

The acromioclavicular joint is formed by the acromion and the lateral end of the clavicle. Its joint surfaces are covered by fi-

brous cartilage. Sometimes an articular disc is found in the joint cavity.

The acromioclavicular joint capsule can be seen as a continuation of the fasciae from both the deltoid and trapezius muscles. It is strengthened by the inferior and superior acromioclavicular ligaments. These ligaments provide joint stability, particularly in a ventral-dorsal direction. Two of the most important stabilizers, the coracoclavicular liga-

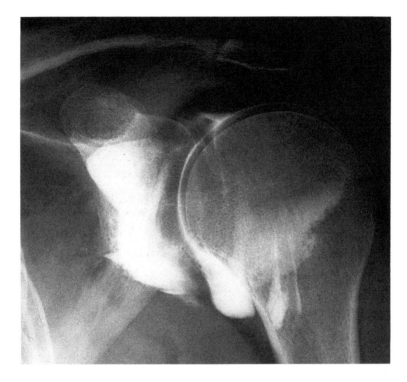

Figure 1–2 Arthrogram of a healthy shoulder. Note the contour of the joint cavity.

ments, are located some distance from the joint. These ligaments are the lateral trapezoid (quadrangular) and the medial conoid (triangular) ligaments. The coracoclavicular ligaments stabilize the joint in a cranial-caudal direction. In other words, they prevent the scapula from moving downward in relation to the clavicle.

Sternoclavicular Joint (Articulatio Sternoclavicularis)

Anatomically, the sternoclavicular joint is a saddle joint, located between the sternal manubrium and the medial end of the clavicle. Here, too, the joint surfaces are covered with fibrous cartilage. An articular disc completely divides the joint cavity into two compartments.

The rather thin capsule is strengthened both ventrally and dorsally by ligaments. There is also an interclavicular ligament, which connects both clavicles. In addition, at the level of the sternoclavicular joint, the clavicle is connected to the first rib by the costoclavicular ligament. Because of the articular disc and lax capsule, the sternoclavicular joint is functionally a ball and socket joint with a wide range of motion.

Disturbances in sternoclavicular joint function lead immediately to limited range of motion of the shoulder girdle. Arm elevation is the first motion to manifest this dysfunction.

Scapulothoracic Junction

The scapulothoracic junction plays a significant role in every movement of the shoulder girdle. Although anatomically this junction is not a joint, functionally it is. The scapulothoracic gliding surfaces are formed by the subscapularis fascia and serratus anterior fascia.

Movements of the scapula in relation to the trunk are mainly controlled by the rhomboid, trapezius, and serratus anterior muscles.

MUSCLES

In 1974, Sugahara[1] published an extensive electromyographic (EMG) study of muscle activity in the shoulder region during active movements.

From anterior to posterior, the rotator cuff is formed by the subscapular, supraspinatus, infraspinatus, and teres minor muscles. Because of its optimal location in relation to the axes of movement and its insertion into the glenohumeral joint capsule, the rotator cuff has a stabilizing influence on the glenohumeral joint.

Because of the large range of motion in the shoulder, functions of the muscles can change. For instance, De Luca and Forest[2] registered EMG activity in the subscapularis muscle during active abduction from specific positions. When abduction was resisted, activity of even the teres major was seen.

Glousman et al.[3] compared the muscle activity of patients with shoulder instability with that of a control group. Compared with the control group, the patients demonstrated increased activity of the biceps and triceps during throwing motions. In contrast, the pectoralis major, latissimus dorsi, and serratus anterior muscles of the patients showed significantly less activity.

Thus, muscle function depends on the dynamic parameters of the situation, and attempts to define function are further complicated by the fact that most muscles are polyarticular.

OTHER STRUCTURES

Subacromial-Subdeltoid Bursa

The subacromial-subdeltoid bursa is very large and is connected to several structures: the greater tubercle of the humerus, the tendons of the supra- and infraspinatus, acromion, and the coracoacromial ligament (Figure 1–3).

In the past, anatomical literature differentiated the subacromial from the subdeltoid bursa. However, recent radiographic contrast studies have demonstrated that the two are usually one continuous bursa.

The subacromial-subdeltoid bursa is a very sensitive structure. Because of its connection with the rotator cuff muscles, the acromion, and the acromioclavicular joint, inflammation of the bursa often occurs when there is pathology of one or more of these bordering structures. For instance, if a rotator cuff lesion causes a bursitis, the bursitis can cause pain long after the rotator cuff has healed. However, by means of a thorough functional examination, it can actually be quite simple to differentiate between the various structures.

Vascularization of the Rotator Cuff Muscles

Branches from the posterior humeral circumflex artery and the suprascapular artery supply the posterior aspect of the rotator cuff muscles (Figure 1–4). The anterior aspect is vascularized by the anterior humeral circumflex artery. Other arteries, such as the thoracoacromial and subscapularis, contribute in varying degrees to the vascularization of the rotator cuff muscles.

Pressure from the acromion can cut off or diminish blood flow in branches from the above-mentioned arteries that lie underneath the acromion. This can lead to ischemia of the rotator cuff insertions, particularly the supraspinatus.

BIOMECHANICS

Because of the complexity of movements in the shoulder girdle, it is difficult to analyze and describe the range of motion in each separate joint. For example, when elevating the arm, approximately 50% of the total mo-

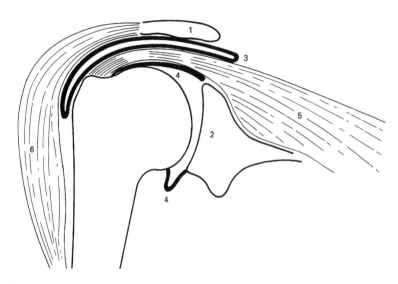

Figure 1–3 Structures in the area of the "roof" of the shoulder. **1**, Acromion; **2**, glenoid cavity; **3**, subacromial-subdeltoid bursa; **4**, joint capsule; **5**, supraspinatus muscle; **6**, deltoid muscle.

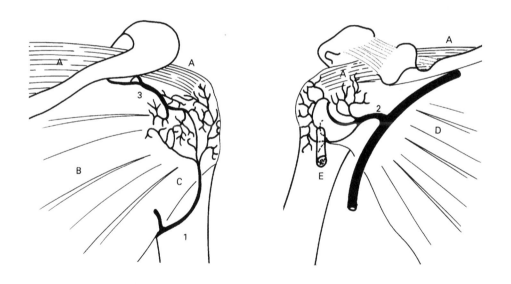

Figure 1–4 Vascularization of the rotator cuff muscles. **Left**, Posterior view; **Right**, anterior view. **1**, Posterior circumflex humeral artery; **2**, anterior circumflex humeral artery; **3**, suprascapular artery; **A**, supraspinatus muscle; **B**, infraspinatus muscle; **C**, teres minor muscle; **D**, subscapularis muscle; **E**, tendon of the long head of the biceps brachii muscle.

tion takes place in the glenohumeral joint. However, motion also occurs in every other joint (and junction) of the shoulder girdle.

Generally defined, *elevation* is an upward movement of the arm. It can occur in a number of different planes, including the sagittal or frontal planes. Individual differences exist in the maximal range of motion for *elevation through flexion* (forward movement of the arm in the sagittal plane). Research has shown the range of motion to be slightly more extensive in women than in men. On the average, elevation through flexion can be performed to a maximum of 180°.[4] *Elevation though extension* (backward movement of the arm in the sagittal plane) is possible to approximately 60°. Maximal *elevation through abduction* (upward movement of the arm in the frontal plane) averages 100° to 120°.[5]

Adduction is restricted by the thorax. Further movement is possible when adduction is performed in combination with flexion or extension.

Measuring from the zero position, where the subject is standing with arm relaxed and flexed to 90° in the elbow (see Chapter 3), internal and external shoulder rotation can usually be performed to approximately 90° in each direction.

Inman et al.[5] found a maximum of 20° possible motion in the acromioclavicular joint. Motion in this joint occurs particularly during the first 30° and last 45° of glenohumeral abduction.

In the sternoclavicular joint, 4° of elevation was observed for every 10° of arm elevation. This ratio of motion was noted during the first 90° of glenohumeral abduction, after which almost no sternoclavicular elevation occurred. In addition, approximately 50° of backward spin (rotation around the clavicle's longitudinal axis) occurs in the sternoclavicular joint during arm elevation.

Besides the dynamics of a joint, forces exerted *on* the joint as well as reactive forces *within* the joint can also be analyzed. Calcu-lating reactive forces in the shoulder is very complicated. The contribution of forces from various muscles depends on the amount of arm elevation, as well as the plane in which the elevation takes place.

Poppen and Walker[6] assume that all muscles are active during 90° abduction of the arm. Muscle force is determined by dividing an integrated EMG signal by the surface area of that muscle. Calculated in this way, glenohumeral reactive forces can be up to a maximum of 90% of the body weight. To simplify the situation, suppose that only the deltoid muscle is active during arm abduction. Assuming that the weight of the arm is 5% of the body weight, and the lever arm of the deltoid is 3 cm, Poppen and Walker calculate a reactive force equal to approximately half the total body weight.

Much has been written about the relationship between glenohumeral elevation and scapulothoracic movement.[4,5,7] Motions in the scapulothoracic junction include protraction and retraction, elevation and depression, and medial and lateral rotation.

In determining the relationship between glenohumeral elevation and scapulothoracic movement, a number of factors have to be considered: position of the glenoid fossa, form of the thorax, muscle force, and so forth. Furthermore, the round form of the humeral head in relation to the glenoid fossa allows for elevation—in principle—in an infinite number of planes. Roughly speaking, during arm elevation there is a 3:2 ratio: for every 3° of abduction in the glenohumeral joint, 2° of scapulothoracic lateral rotation occurs.

In Chapter 2, we describe how many of the structures discussed here in functional anatomy can be localized and palpated on the human body.

2

Surface Anatomy of the Shoulder Region

Palpation of the shoulder girdle and arm is performed with the subject in a sitting or standing position and is directed at localizing specific structures. The structures to be localized are sequenced in a way that is best for the practical study of surface anatomy. Thus, the following method of classification deviates from the usual systematic or topographic anatomical descriptions. First, the palpable bony and ligamentous structures, organized per region, are discussed, followed by the palpable muscles and other soft tissue structures. An overview is provided to describe the blood vessels and neurological structures of the shoulder girdle and arm, emphasizing their topographic relationships (see Appendix A).

Because of the emphasis on *surface* anatomy, the relevant structures are classified and sequenced based on two main considerations: (1) the ability to palpate the structure and (2) its practical application in the clinic. Thus, if some structures are not mentioned, they either are not easily palpable (usually they are located too deeply or are covered by other structures) or palpation of the structures is not clinically significant. The sequence in which the various structures are discussed is based on orientation. For instance, during examination of a certain region, characteristic structures ("reference points" or "landmarks") are found before more specific palpations are performed.

Every palpation is preceded by inspection of the region. If the inspection is not performed, an "anatomy book knowledge" is often projected onto the body without having established a basis in fact. After the inspection, palpation of the relaxed structures follows. *For the purpose of study, as well as in the clinic, it is advisable to outline the palpated structures with a marker or skin pencil.* In this way, the examiner is forced to see the results of the palpation and can avoid gross mistakes.

In the framework of joint examination, every inspection and palpation at rest is followed by inspection and palpation during motion. When examining muscles, inspection and palpation during contraction are also desirable. (This contraction can be static or dynamic.) Thus, the following sequence is applied during a session of surface anatomy:

- specific inspection at rest
- palpation at rest
- inspection during movement/contraction
- palpation during movement/contraction

Of course, the entire sequence does not have to be followed when palpating every structure, but in evaluating joints and muscles it can be very helpful. Phenomena such as "misleading tenderness" and "referred pain" confuse every examiner who does not follow a logical palpation sequence.

PALPATION OF BONY AND LIGAMENTOUS STRUCTURES

Initial Position: Sitting

To identify anomalies of bony and ligamentous structures, one has to be familiar with the characteristic palpation of normal bony

12

and ligamentous structures. For instance, a bony structure feels hard on palpation. Uncovered bony structures are not encountered in surface anatomy; bones and their prominences are surrounded by periosteum and usually by muscles. In addition, palpation is always made through subcutaneous and cutaneous layers. Ligamentous structures generally feel firm. Joint lines also tend to be firm on palpation and lie between two structures that are hard on palpation.

Sternoclavicular Joint

The connections between sternum and clavicles are normally located at the level of the T3 spinous process. The sternoclavicular joint and its surrounding structures are easy to palpate.

Between both sternoclavicular joints, at the cranial border of the sternal manubrium an indentation can be found, the jugular (or suprasternal) notch. This notch serves as an important reference point for localizing several structures. The caudal border of the larynx is located approximately 3 cm above the notch. (The larynx and jugular notch are used as reference points when performing a tracheotomy. The tracheotomy is performed between these two structures; further cranially there is risk of damaging the thyroid gland; further away from the midline, vascular structures can be damaged.) The jugular notch also serves as a reference point when counting the ribs. However, the sternal angle, which is at the level of the second rib, is more often used in localizing ribs at the ventral aspect of the thorax.

The interclavicular ligament is palpable within the jugular notch. The sternal bellies of the sternocleidomastoid muscles, which are a mixture of muscle and tendinous tissue, form the flanks of the notch on both sides, and are easy to palpate. The sternal ends of the clavicle, which are covered by the sternocleidomastoid, project cranially over the border of the manubrium.

During movements of the shoulder girdle, movement of the sternal end of the clavicle in relation to the sternal manubrium can be palpated. In a dislocation of the sternoclavicular joint, the end of the clavicle usually shifts cranially and medially, and the normal contours of the notch disappear.

Between the incongruent joint surfaces of the sternoclavicular joint lies an articular disc. Palpation of this disc is difficult because of the overlying sternoclavicular ligament and tendon of the sternocleidomastoid muscle. Active protraction and retraction of the shoulder girdle help to confirm the site of the joint.

Arthrotic changes of the sternoclavicular joint lead to palpable mild crepitation during internal or external rotation of the shoulder when the upper arm is positioned in 90° abduction. Arthrotic processes in these joints usually have a mild course and are accompanied by only small functional losses.

Clavicle

Further laterally, the ventral and cranial aspects of the clavicle are easy to palpate. These aspects are covered only by the platysma, the superficial throat muscle.

The medial two thirds of the clavicle has an almost round cross-section. Its ventrocaudal border and caudal aspect are difficult to palpate because of muscle insertions.

The concave lateral third of the clavicle is less round and demonstrates flattened ventrocranial and dorsocranial surfaces. The true dimensions of the clavicle's ventrodorsal diameter are generally underestimated; at its lateral end, the clavicle is wider than expected. Surface indentations at both the cranial and caudal aspects of the lateral end of the clavicle are visible as well as palpable. These indentations are (1) the greater supraclavicular fossa, bordered medially by the clavicular part of the sternocleidomastoid and laterally by the inferior belly of the omohyoid muscle (this fossa forms the lower part of the lateral region of the throat), and (2) the infraclavicular fossa between pectoralis major, deltoid, and clavicle. The infraclavicular fossa is more obvious during flexion or abduction of the shoulder (Figures 2–1 and 2–2).

Coracoid Process

In the infraclavicular fossa, or directly lateral to it, the coracoid process is sometimes visible and always easily palpable. Its tip and medial aspect are best felt with the shoulder positioned in extension.

Several palpable ligaments and muscles are connected to the coracoid process: the coracoclavicular ligaments, coracoacromial ligament, pectoralis minor, coracobrachial muscle, and short head of the biceps (Figures 2–1, 2–2, and 2–10).

Coracoclavicular Ligaments

In thin or nonmuscular persons, a prominence (the coracoclavicular ligaments) running vertically between the coracoid process and the clavicle can often be observed. Palpation of the coracoclavicular ligaments is performed by placing the finger on this prominence and moving back and forth transversely over the structure. Only the anterior part of the coracoclavicular ligaments is accessible to palpation.

Acromioclavicular Joint

Lesions of the acromioclavicular joint cause local pain that can include the entire C4 dermatome (there are no radiating symptoms into the arm). This dermatome is localized between the clavicle (ventrally), acromion (laterally), scapular spine (dorsally), and halfway up the lateral aspect of the neck (medially).

When injecting the acromioclavicular joint, the physician often encounters difficulties inserting the needle into the joint. Nonspecific palpation before the injection is often the cause.

Generally a prominence is visible at the lateral (acromial) end of the clavicle. Although this prominence may not be obvious, it is always palpable. Too often, the middle of this prominence is mistakenly thought to be the joint line of the acromioclavicular joint. How-

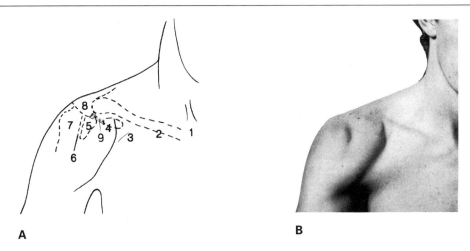

A   **B**

Figure 2–1 Right shoulder, anterior view. **1**, Sternocleidomastoid muscle, pars sternalis; **2**, clavicle; **3**, infraclavicular fossa; **4**, coracoid process; **5**, lesser tubercle; **6**, deltoid, groove between clavicular and acromial heads (reference point for the localization of the intertubercular sulcus, with the shoulder in the zero position); **7**, greater tubercle; **8**, acromion; **9**, coracoacromial ligament.

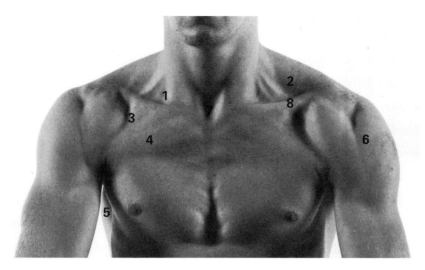

Figure 2–2 1, Platysma; **2**, trapezius; **3**, Infraclavicular fossa; **4**, pectoralis major, clavicular part; **5**, latissimus dorsi; **6**, deltoid, groove between clavicular and acromial heads (in here the tendon of the long head of the biceps is palpable); **7**, jugular (suprasternal) notch; **8**, greater supraclavicular fossa.

ever, the joint line is usually located somewhat laterally to the prominence. Occasionally the joint line is obvious during inspection, but palpation of the joint line during translatory anteroposterior movements should always be performed to confirm the site. The following procedure is the best to apply in localizing the joint:

Standing behind the patient, the examiner palpates the lateral border of the acromion with the tip of the index finger of the ipsilateral hand. The border is followed in a ventral direction until reaching a ventral corner, formed by the acromion as it meets the clavicle medially at an almost perpendicular angle. Approximately 1.5 to 2 cm medial to this corner, a small indentation in the form of a V is encountered; its apex points in a dorsal direction (Figure 2–8). This is the ventral part of the acromioclavicular joint. Next, the cranial border of the scapular spine is palpated from

a medial to lateral direction until it is impossible to proceed further laterally. At this point the scapular spine meets the dorsal aspect of the clavicle (Figures 2–3 and 2–4). Here too, an indentation in the form of a V is palpable; its apex points in a lateral direction.

By connecting the apexes of both ventral and dorsal V's with an imaginary laterally convex line, an impression of the lateral end of the clavicle and the joint line is obtained. (The joint line lies along the ventral part of this line.) Specific palpation for the joint line is performed by continuing to palpate from the dorsal V, perpendicularly against the lateral end of the clavicle, in a ventral direction. Along the dorsal half of the imaginary line, a bony step is usually palpated. At the ventral half of the imaginary line, a smooth incline is felt instead of the bony step; this is the superior acromioclavicular ligament, which

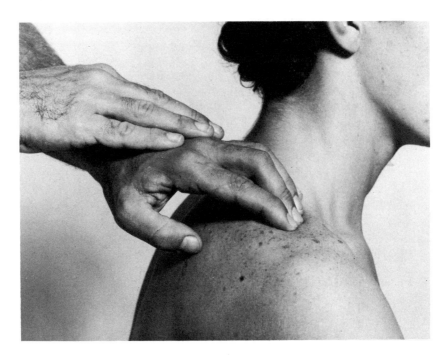

Figure 2–3 Palpation of the space between clavicle and spine of the scapula.

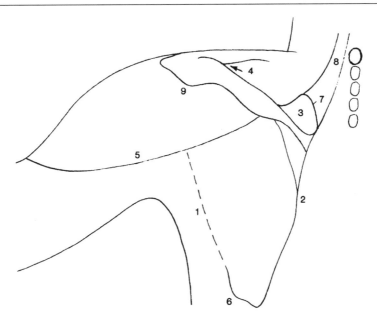

Figure 2–4 Left shoulder, dorsal view. **1**, Lateral border of the scapula, covered by a thick muscular layer; **2**, medial border of the scapula, easy to palpate; **3**, scapular spine, flat triangle at its medial aspect; **4**, palpable landmark in localizing the acromioclavicular joint, posterior V; **5**, deltoid, running of the spinal part; **6**, inferior angle, palpable, covered only by the latissimus dorsi; **7**, superior angle, palpable; **8**, levator scapulae; **9**, prominent dorsal corner of the acromion.

reinforces the acromioclavicular joint capsule.

Coracoacromial Ligament

The coracoacromial ligament, running between the coracoid process and the ventral corner of the acromion, is often easy to palpate (Figure 2–1). Because palpation takes place through the deltoid muscle, moderate pressure is required while palpating transversely over the fibers of the ligament.

Acromion

The acromion is found at the lateral end of the scapular spine; the spine of the scapula starts at the medial border of the scapula and is well palpable along its entire length (Figures 2–4 to 2–8). Along with the greater tubercle of the humerus and the overlying acromial part of the deltoid muscle, the acromion is also responsible for the round contour of the shoulder. When determining arm length, correct palpation of the groove between the acromion and greater tubercle is imperative; measurements are made from this reference point (Figure 2–7).

QUICK AND SYSTEMATIC PALPATION OF THE ACROMIOCLAVICULAR JOINT, CORACOID PROCESS, CORACOCLAVICULAR LIGAMENT, LESSER TUBERCLE, INTERTUBERCULAR GROOVE, AND GREATER TUBERCLE

In a thin subject, palpation of the acromioclavicular joint, coracoid process, lesser tubercle, and greater tubercle can usually be performed without difficulty. This situation is optimal in order to get to know these structures through palpation.

Whatever the situation, it is of utmost importance that the examiner palpate these bony structures in a systematic manner. This apparently simple localization process can become very difficult and disorienting when examining persons with joint diseases, thicker subcutaneous tissue, and/or possible bursitides.

While standing behind the subject, palpate the dorsal border of the clavicle up to the V-shaped indentation between the lateral end of the scapular spine's cranial aspect and the clavicle (Figures 2–3 and 2–4).

Palpate the caudal border of the scapular spine until the spine turns into the laterocaudal border of the acromion, marked by a drastic change in direction (Figure 2–5). This junction is an important reference point when administering intra-articular shoulder injections, as well as in treatment (transverse friction or injection) of the infraspinatus insertion (Figure 2–6). With the index finger, follow the caudolateral border of the acromion to the ventral, less obvious, smooth, round corner (in contrast to the perpendicularly angled dorsal corner) (Figure 2–7).

Place the index finger of the ipsilateral hand on the lateral border of the acromion and, with the tip of the other index finger, follow the ventral border of the acromion in a medial direction. Approximately 1.5 cm medial to the lateral border of the acromion, a small but obvious V-shaped indentation is found. This is the ventral opening of the acromioclavicular joint (Figure 2–8). After marking the joint (a line connecting the tips of both dorsal and ventral indentations), the examiner has the subject abduct or flex the arm in order to demonstrate the infraclavicular fossa (Figure 2–9).

The infraclavicular fossa serves as a starting point in searching for the coracoid process. Its medial tip is palpable directly lateral to the fossa and is covered by the clavicular head of the deltoid (variations exist among individuals). The palpation can be made more obvious by keeping the subject's arm in a position between internal and external rotation and simultaneously bringing the shoulder into extension (Figure 2–10).

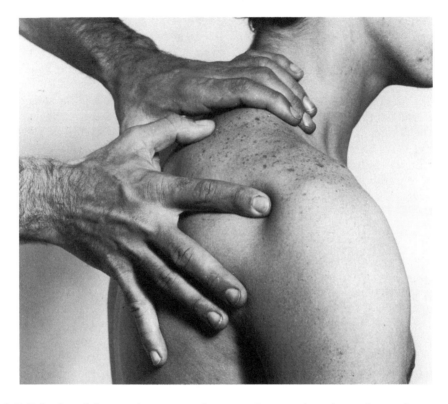

Figure 2–5 Palpation of the prominent corner between the scapular spine and acromion.

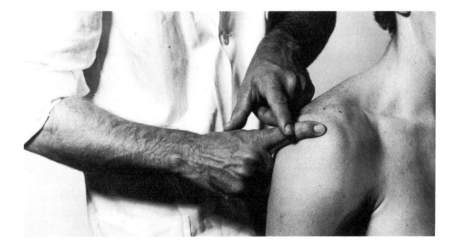

Figure 2–6 Demonstration of the almost perpendicular transition between the scapular spine and laterocaudal border of the acromion.

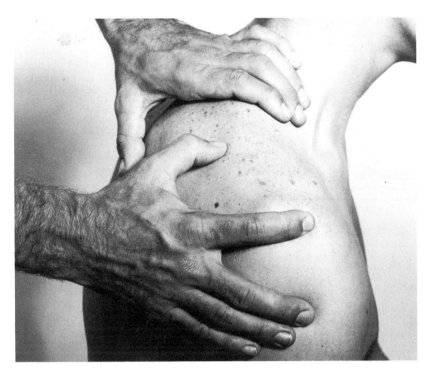

Figure 2–7 Palpation of the flat, round, ventral corner of the acromion.

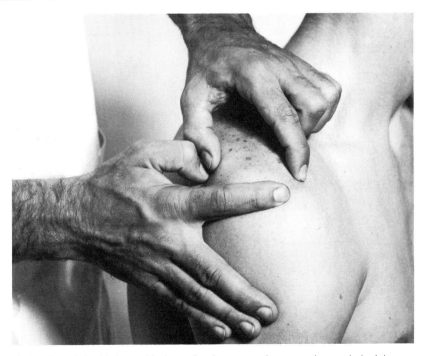

Figure 2–8 Palpation of the V-shaped indentation between the acromion and clavicle.

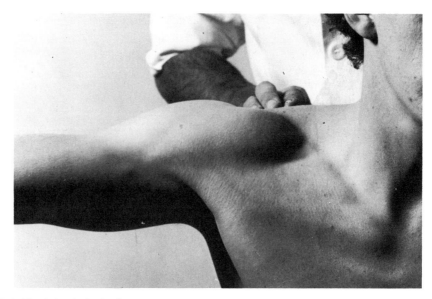

Figure 2–9 The infraclavicular fossa.

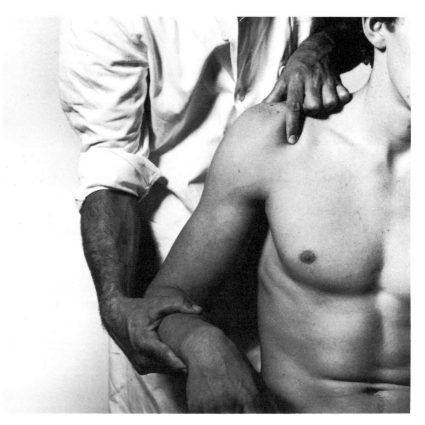

Figure 2–10 Palpation of the coracoid process.

During passive internal and external rotation of the shoulder, the lesser tubercle is easily palpable approximately one fingerwidth lateral to the coracoid process. In contrast to the almost immobile coracoid process, it moves back and forth underneath the palpating index finger (Figure 2–11). The lesser tubercle is shaped like an inverted teardrop or pear; its proximal part is wide and has an obvious prominence, while the distal part is narrower.

After marking the lesser tubercle, the subject is instructed to move the arm actively into flexion. In so doing, an obvious groove appears within the deltoid muscle (Figure 2–12). This groove forms the border between the clavicular and acromial heads of the deltoid and, when the arm is in the anatomical zero position, the groove is located directly lateral to the lesser tubercle. (This groove is usually not recognizable at dissection.)

Now place the index finger in the groove formed by the clavicular and acromial heads of the deltoid, and with the arm in the anatomical zero position, alternately rotate the upper arm passively into internal and external directions (for just a few degrees in each direction). Usually, in this position, the index finger rests in the intertubercular sulcus, and the edges of the lesser tubercle and greater tubercle can be palpated during external and internal rotation, respectively.

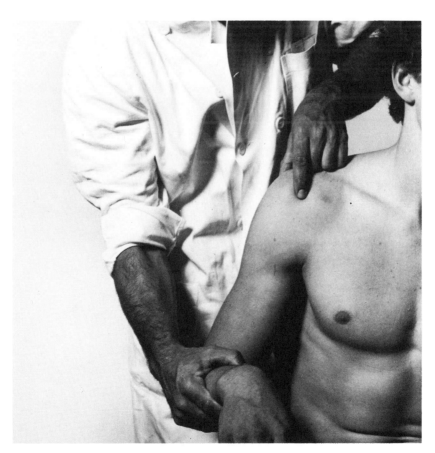

Figure 2–11 Palpation of the lesser tubercle.

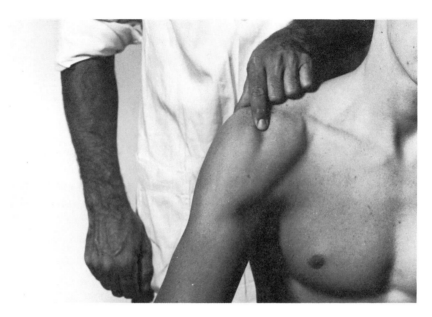

Figure 2–12 Palpation of the groove between the clavicular and acromial heads of the deltoid.

In this way the borders of the intertubercular sulcus* are palpated, as well as sometimes the tendon of the long head of the biceps. This palpation cannot be performed at dissection because of the absence of muscle tone.

The tendon of the long head of the biceps has its own tendon sheath, which originates intracapsularly at the supraglenoid tubercle. To a certain extent, the transverse humeral ligament, a retinacular structure, ensures the position of the tendon and its sheath within the groove. Patients with shoulder complaints often indicate their pain and tenderness in the region of this tendon within the sulcus. Not only do patients localize their pain at the "wrong" site (referred pain), but these sites, which are not affected, often demonstrate misleading tenderness (referred tenderness). Treatment based only on palpation is usually ineffective. Therefore, the examiner should palpate the suspected injured

*Not to be confused with the medial/lateral bicipital sulcus, which is formed by the soft tissue structures of the upper arm.

structure only *after* performing the functional examination.

From the intertubercular sulcus, the greater tubercle (which builds its lateral border) can be palpated. The thickness of the deltoid makes further palpation in a dorsolateral direction rather difficult. The greater tubercle can be best palpated directly ventral from the acromion in an internally rotated shoulder (Figure 2–13).

Scapula

Medial Border and Inferior Angle

Palpation of the medial border of the scapula starts at the medial (vertebral) end of the scapular spine (at the level of the T3 spinous process) and is performed from cranial to caudal (Figure 2–4). For the most part, palpation takes place through the trapezius muscle. The inferior angle of the scapula is found at the lower border; it is usually located approximately at the level of the T7 spinous process and is not covered by the trapezius.

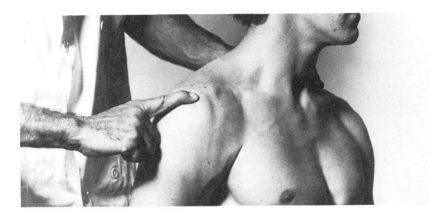

Figure 2–13 Palpation of the greater tubercle with an internally rotated upper arm.

In upright posture, with the arms hanging alongside the body (forearms in supination), the medial border of the scapula lies flat against the rib cage, approximately 6 cm lateral to the thoracic spinous processes. Muscles responsible for this fixation are the serratus anterior, trapezius, and the rhomboids. Winging of the scapula (scapula alata from Latin *ala* [wing], a deformity in which both scapulae project conspicuously), is usually caused by paralysis of the serratus anterior. However, it can also be the result of cranial pressure from the ribs in a scoliotic spine.

Superior Angle and Superior Border

Generally, the superior angle of the scapula is more difficult to locate than the inferior angle because the cranial part of the scapula's medial border is covered by the trapezius and the superior angle points in a cranioventral direction (Figure 2–4). Thus, it disappears somewhat underneath the palpating fingers. In addition, it is covered by the origin of the levator scapulae.

Because of the thick layer of muscle, palpation of the superior border of the scapula has to be performed with considerable pressure and is sometimes uncomfortable. Therefore, general indirect palpation is encouraged.

When using a marker or skin pencil, especially in this region, outline all indirectly palpated structures with a broken line (Figure 2–14).

In patients who complain of pain specifically at the level of the superior angle of the scapula, disorders of the cervical spine should be considered. Pain in this area is most often referred from the cervical spine.

Lateral Border

Palpation here is very difficult, due to the teres major (Figure 2–4). Because the palpation is indirect, indicate this border with a broken line.

Scapular Spine

The scapular spine has a wide, almost triangular base starting at the vertebral border of the scapula (Figure 2–4). Its cranial border can be followed to where it meets the clavicle. Standing behind the subject, palpate the V-shaped space between the lateral end of the upper border of the scapular spine and the dorsal border of the lateral end of the clavicle (Figure 2–3). Then, with the index finger, palpate the caudal edge of the scapular spine until reaching the abrupt, obvious corner, where the scapular spine makes the transition into the acromion (Figure 2–6).

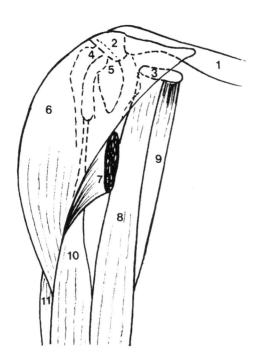

Figure 2–14 Right shoulder, ventral view; tubercles, coracoid process, and intertubercular sulcus. **1**, Clavicle; **2**, acromion; **3**, coracoid process; **4**, greater tubercle; **5**, lesser tubercle; **6**, deltoid muscle; **7**, pectoralis major muscle, cut; **8**, biceps muscle, short head; **9**, coracobrachialis muscle; **10**, biceps muscle, long head; **11**, brachialis muscle.

The laterocaudal border of the acromion can be followed up to the ventral, less obvious, smooth round corner (in contrast to the perpendicularly angled dorsal corner).

Ventrally Located Bony Prominences of the Scapula

The ventrally localized coracoid process has already been discussed. The infraglenoid tubercle is the only scapular structure remaining that is palpable. This palpation is painful for the subject because of the presence of the axillary nerve, and therefore should be performed only when specifically indicated.

The infraglenoid tubercle and the glenoid labrum can be palpated deep within the axillary fossa: the palpating fingers slide into the

axilla from dorsal, directly ventral to the dorsal axillary wall and subscapularis muscle.

PALPATION OF MUSCLES AND OTHER SOFT TISSUE STRUCTURES IN THE SHOULDER REGION

Sternocleidomastoid

The sternocleidomastoid (*sterno-claviculo-mastoideus*, terminology according to origin and insertion) muscle is located in the superficial layer of the cervical fascia and is an important reference point for orientation (Figures 2–15 and 2–16).

Rotating the head gives a clear view of both the tendinous sternal and the muscular clavicular bellies. The rotational relationship is contralateral; in other words, contraction of the right muscle rotates the head to the left, and vice versa. The entire muscle surface is palpable, even though its caudal part is covered by the platysma. (The platysma is a superficial throat muscle, important for facial expressions, and is occasionally palpable as a collection of fine rolling muscle fibers underneath the clavicle.)

At the common origin of both sternocleidomastoid bellies on the mastoid process, the muscle lies very close to the retromandibular part of the parotid gland. From there to its sternal insertion, it runs over the sternohyoid and sternothyroid muscles, as well as the sternoclavicular joint.

The lower fourth of the sternocleidomastoid crosses over the omohyoid muscle, where the latter makes a curve and can be palpated lateral to the sternocleidomastoid as an oblique, rolling muscle "cord" bordering the greater supraclavicular fossa. Medially and cranially to it, pulsation from the common carotid artery can be felt. This structure should be palpated with careful pressure* at both sides (but not simultaneously) and com-

---

*Pressure on the carotid sinus can cause dangerous, severe, vegetative reactions, such as loss of consciousness.

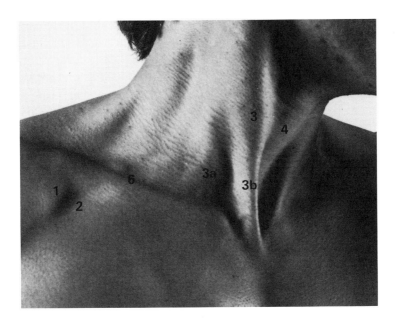

Figure 2–15 Sternocleidomastoid muscle. **1**, Coracoid process; **2**, infraclavicular fossa; **3**, sterno-cleidomastoid muscle; **3a**, sternocleidomastoid muscle, clavicular part; **3b**, sternocleidomastoid muscle, sternal part; **4**, sternohyoid muscle; **5**, sternal notch; **6**, clavicle.

pared with the arteries in the groin. If the pulsations at the throat are more forceful than the ones at the groin, this could be an indication of an aortic narrowing somewhere between the aortic arch and the aortic bifurcation.

The branches of the brachial plexus pass through the posterior scalenic triangle* and run in a laterocaudal direction, further in the lateral region of the neck. Deep within this region, they are often palpable. Dorsolateral to the midpoint of the sternocleidomastoid, the supraclavicular nerves, transverse nerve of the neck, greater auricular nerve, and lesser occipital nerve emerge.

Hypertonic muscles in this region can lead to compression, particularly of the lesser occipital nerve, which emerges between the sternocleidomastoid and the levator scapulae.

Both the sternocleidomastoid and the trapezius muscles developed embryologically from pharyngeal arch material, which explains their innervation by the 11th cranial nerve (accessory nerve, XI). In paresis, paralysis, or spasticity of both muscles, pathology in the upper spinal cord or somewhere along the course of the nerve as it exits the jugular foramen should be suspected. Its superficial track over the levator scapulae offers the opportunity to palpate it (sometimes as a rolling structure under the finger) in this area.

Advanced spasticity or contracture of the sternocleidomastoid can lead to a so-called torticollis. In this instance, the head is sidebent ipsilateral to the affected muscle and rotated contralaterally.

Car accidents, especially rear-end collisions, often result in a whiplash trauma. The sudden effect of the collision can lead to pain in the sternocleidomastoid, which subsequently hinders translation of the vertebrae.

---

*Posterior scalenic triangle = opening between anterior and middle scalene muscles.

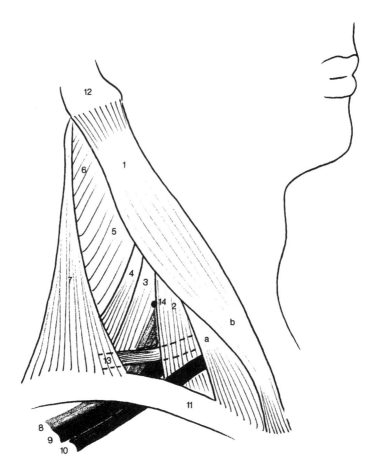

Figure 2–16 Throat region, lateral view of the right side: relationship between muscles and neurovascular structures. **1**, Sternocleidomastoid muscle; **a**, clavicular part; **b**, sternal part; **2**, anterior scalene muscle; **3**, middle scalene muscle; **4**, posterior scalene muscle; **5**, levator scapulae muscle; **6**, splenius capitis muscle; **7**, trapezius muscle; **8**, cords of the brachial plexus; **9**, subclavian artery; **10**, subclavian vein; **11**, clavicle; **12**, mastoid process; **13**, omohyoid muscle; **14**, punctum nervosum.

One can check for swollen lymph nodes by palpating the ventral (medial) and dorsal (lateral) aspects of the muscle, as well as along the caudal border of the mandible.

Topography of the Scalene Triangles

Between the posterior border of the sternocleidomastoid, the anterior border of the trapezius, and the upper border of the clavicle, a more or less triangular area is located, the lateral region of the neck (Figure 2–16).

In the more anterior part of this region the scalene muscles can be palpated. They originate at the transverse processes of the cervical spine and have their insertion at the ribs (the anterior and middle scalene to the first rib, the posterior scalene to the second rib). The fasciae of these muscles are interwoven with the pleural membrane at the deep aspect of the throat.

Between the middle and anterior scalenes, the so-called *posterior scalenic triangle* is located. The *anterior scalenic triangle* lies between the anterior scalene muscle and the clavicular insertion of the sternocleidomastoid. The omohyoid muscle runs anterior to the lower aspect of the posterior scalenic triangle.

The posterior scalenic triangle is an important site in regard to the brachial plexus. The nerve fibers of the brachial plexus reorganize after leaving the cervical spine and run in a laterocaudal direction through the posterior scalenic triangle and underneath the omohyoid. After passing through the lateral throat region, they dive behind the clavicle into the axilla.

At the craniodorsal aspect of the posterior scalenic triangle, the *punctum nervosum* (part of the cervical plexus) can be palpated.

From its exit at the thorax, the subclavian artery runs in a lateral direction over the first rib and then through the posterior scalenic triangle. From a topographic point of view, the brachial plexus first runs above the artery, and later surrounds it with its branches. At the level of the posterior scalenic triangle, the subclavian artery gives rise to numerous branches, some of which already originate at the deep aspect of the throat and emerge through the anterior scalenic triangle. The subclavian artery can be felt on deep palpation.

The course of the brachial plexus and subclavian artery through the posterior scalenic triangle sometimes has important clinical consequences. Narrowing of the triangle (due to a cervical rib or accessory insertion of the serratus anterior) can lead to entrapment of the nerves or artery with all the possible consequences.

The most important structure that runs through the anterior scalenic triangle is the subclavian vein, which is not palpable.

Trapezius

In order to contract the trapezius muscle, the arms are abducted to 90° and the hands clasp each other and pull laterally (Jendrassik* maneuver). The course of the entire muscle is now visible in a thin, muscular subject. The ascending part runs in the direction of the scapular spine, the transverse part runs laterally, and the descending part runs in an oblique craniomedial to caudolateral direction (Figure 2–17).

The trapezius origin is palpable at the medial aspect of the superior nuchal line at the occipital bone, the external occipital protuberance, and the nuchal ligament.

Starting at the origin, the descending part can be followed to its insertion at the acromion and lateral end of the clavicle. The easily palpable anterior border of this part of the muscle is both the ventral border of the muscle and the posterior border of the lateral region of the neck.

The fibers of the transverse part can be palpated to their insertion on the spine. The ascending part can also be palpated; the flat index finger is placed at the level of T8 to T12 in order to follow the suspected course of the muscle's border up to the scapular spine. Confusion with the fiber direction of the more deeply located erector spinae is possible, however not likely, when palpation is performed superficially.

Sometimes patients complain of considerable pain at the origin of the trapezius at the nuchal line or in its descending part directly above the midpoint of the scapular spine. The former structure can be painful because of impingement of the sensory greater occipital nerve against the skull; often this results in a migraine at the back of the head. Pain occurring in the latter area of the trapezius is re-

---

*Ernö Jendrassik, 1858–1921, internist in Budapest.

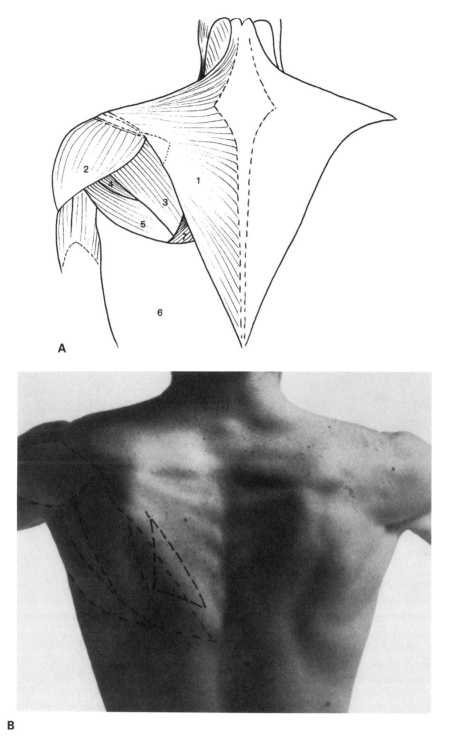

Figure 2–17 A, Triangle of auscultation, dorsal view. **1**, Trapezius muscle; **2**, deltoid muscle; **3**, infraspinatus muscle; **4**, teres minor muscle; **5**, teres major muscle; **6**, latissimus dorsi muscle; **7**, triangle of auscultation (rhomboid muscle). **B**, Increase of the triangle through abduction of the arm.

ferred from the cervical spine (for instance, disc or zygapophyseal joint problems).

Triangle of Auscultation

The medial border of the scapula, the ascending part of the trapezius, and the border of the latissimus dorsi form an area called the triangle of auscultation (Figure 2–17). This is the ideal location at which to listen for sounds from the thorax (for instance, breathing) because of the thin muscle layer covering the ribs. In the upper part of the triangle, the fibers of the greater rhomboid can be palpated, running from mediocranial to laterocaudal.

Rhomboids

The rhomboids (divided into the lesser, which is cranial, and greater, which is caudal) run in an oblique direction from craniomedial (spinous processes) to caudolateral (medial border of the scapula).

The caudal border is made visible by performing the following maneuver:

> The subject, standing upright, places the dorsal aspect of the hands on the lower thoracic (upper lumbar) part of the spine. The upper arms are in extension and internal rotation, the forearms in flexion and pronation. Now the examiner pulls the arms backward (away from the trunk) with a small jerk.

With this movement, the internal rotators of the scapula contract and the lower edge of the rhomboids become visible. (During the same maneuver, the pectoralis minor and levator scapulae are also activated.) The caudal edge of the rhomboid can be palpated at rest and on contraction.

Palpation of the cranial edge is seldom possible. It runs parallel to the lower border and inserts at the superior angle of the scapula (the lower border inserts near the inferior angle of the scapula). In this area, palpation of muscle fibers running in the characteristic direction of the rhomboid fibers can still be part of the more superficial trapezius muscle.

Serratus Anterior

The serratus anterior, with its characteristic form, is often very easy to see in men (Figure 2–18). It can be palpated at the medial border of the axilla. Its muscle bellies can be palpated laterocaudal to the pectoralis major, where they originate between the muscle bellies of the external oblique abdominal muscle. The palpation takes place by laying the entire hand flat on the ribs and following the convexity of the thorax within and underneath the axilla.

Deep within the axilla, the ventral border of the latissimus is found. With an elevated arm, part of the subscapularis can be palpated between the serratus anterior and the latissimus dorsi muscles. Paralysis of the serratus anterior leads to winging of the scapula (scapula alata).

Pectoralis Major

In men, the pectoralis major is usually palpable along its entire surface and also to its tendinous insertion (Figures 2–19 and 2–20). In women, this muscle is not palpable to the same extent, because the central part of the muscle is covered by the breast.

The sternocostal part of the muscle can be palpated at its origin, which covers a large part of the sternum. Sometimes differentiation can be made between the tendinous cords running over the sternum and the muscle fibers originating from them.

The clavicular part can be palpated at the craniolateral aspect of the muscle. Between this part and the clavicular part of the deltoid, a triangular indentation is both visible and palpable. This indentation is the infraclavicular fossa, which becomes a groove more distally where both muscles join. This groove is termed the deltoid-pectoral triangle, or Mohrenheim's groove.* In this groove lies the cephalic vein, which flows into the subclavian

---

*Baron Joseph Jacob Freiherr von Mohrenheim, Austrian physician in Petersburg; died in 1799.

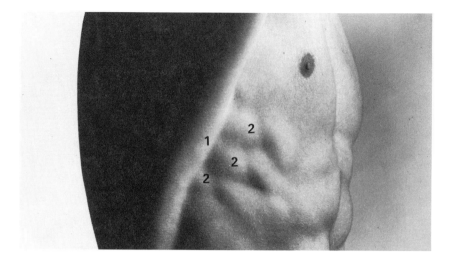

Figure 2–18 Lateral view, right side. **1**, Latissimus dorsi muscle; **2**, muscle bellies of the serratus anterior.

vein and sometimes also into the axillary vein, deep in the infraclavicular fossa.

The caudal border of the abdominal part varies between individuals and can be palpated at its origin in the fascia of the rectus abdominis. A distinct muscle border cannot be palpated in any of the above-mentioned palpations of the origin of the pectoralis major. Only near the insertion of the muscle does the caudal border become palpable.

By grasping around the caudal border of the pectoralis major in the region of the axilla, occasional deviations can be seen. Significant interindividual and sometimes intraindividual differences are found.

On palpation, the tendinous insertion of the pectoralis major muscle consists of two layers. The superficial layer is the thickest. The crossing of these layers can also be palpated (Figure 2–20A). The dorsal (deeper) layer, called the posterior lamina, inserts more proximal on the humerus and covers the intertubercular sulcus. The different layers can be observed by performing adduction and internal rotation against isometric resistance. A pull-up on a bar or rings best shows the function of the pectoralis major.

The rarely seen (4%) sternal muscle is a superficial cord running from the fascia of the rectus abdominis to the sternal manubrium, usually asymmetrically, or it can be connected to one or both of the sternocleidomastoid muscles.

Pectoralis Minor

The pectoralis minor runs from the coracoid process obliquely in a caudomedial direction, and is completely covered by the pectoralis major. The easiest way to observe the pectoralis minor is by performing the maneuver mentioned for the rhomboids. With a medially rotated scapula, sometimes a cord running from the coracoid process in an oblique caudomedial direction can be palpated through the pectoralis major.

Latissimus Dorsi

The large superficial latissimus dorsi is palpable between the iliac crest and the diamond-shaped thoracolumbar fascia (Figures 2–17, 2–18, 2–20B, and 2–21). Above T11-T12 (interindividual variance), its origin can

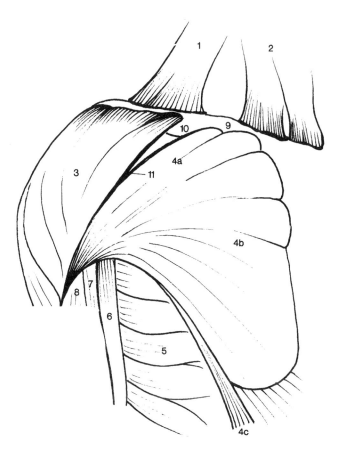

Figure 2–19 Ventral view, right side. **1**, Trapezius muscle; **2**, sternocleidomastoid muscle; **3**, deltoid muscle; **4**, pectoralis major muscle; **4a**, clavicular part; **4b**, sternocostal part; **4c**, abdominal part; **5**, serratus anterior muscle; **6**, latissimus dorsi muscle; **7**, biceps muscle, short head; **8**, biceps muscle, long head; **9**, clavicle; **10**, infraclavicular fossa; **11**, Mohrenheim's groove.

no longer be followed because it is covered by the trapezius. The edge of the muscle can be palpated at the posterior wall in the axillary region and can be followed in a mediocaudal direction. Palpation of this muscle at rest is almost impossible.

The cranial border of the latissimus dorsi runs over the inferior border of the scapula, after which it turns in a laterocranial and ventral direction (almost parallel to the lateral border of the scapula). A horizontal edge of the muscle can be palpated by sliding a finger positioned horizontally from just underneath the scapular spine downward along the back.

If locating the passive muscle is impossible, contraction helps the palpation.

The muscle ends ventrally in a flat tendon that inserts at the crest of the lesser tubercle. Sometimes accessory fibers of the latissimus dorsi are found, which cross the axilla as a kind of flap and end at the tendon of the pectoralis major.

In the lumbar region, the lumbar trigone (Petit's triangle*) can be found between the external oblique muscle of the abdomen, iliac

---

*Jean Louis Petit, 1674–1760, French anatomist and surgeon, Paris.

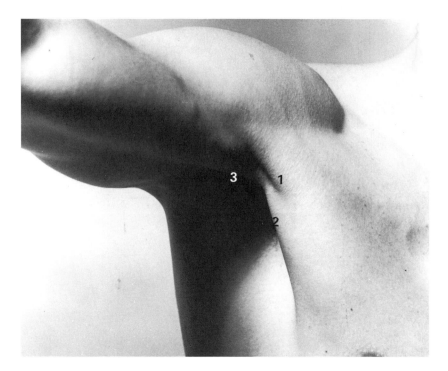

Figure 2–20A Ventral view, right side. **1**, Pectoralis major muscle, lower inserting ventral layer; **2**, pectoralis major muscle, upper inserting dorsal layer; **3**, coracobrachialis muscle.

crest, and the latissimus dorsi. The floor of the triangle is composed of the internal oblique muscle of the abdomen. Ask the subject to blow out against the forearm in order to make palpation easier. The function of this muscle becomes very obvious during pull-ups.

Teres Major

The teres major can be palpated between the cranial part of the latissimus dorsi, the spinal part of the deltoid, and the teres minor (Figures 2–17 and 2–21). The muscle, which is sometimes visible during internal rotatory motions of the shoulder, originates close to the inferior angle of the scapula. It can be observed as a round muscle belly adjacent to the cranial border of the latissimus dorsi. In the axilla, the tendinous insertion of the latissimus turns underneath the teres major from caudal to ventral. The muscle can be ob-

served in the axilla; it is differentiated from the latissimus dorsi during isometrically resisted internal rotation and adduction, with the shoulder in 90° abduction and maximal external rotation.

Deltoid

Observed from above, the deltoid muscle forms a U shape. The clavicular part originates at the lateral third of the clavicle and the spinal part at the spine of the scapula. The apex of the U is formed by the acromial part at its lateral origin at the acromion (Figures 2–17, 2–19, 2–21, and 2–22).

The clavicular part borders the infraclavicular fossa laterally and covers the coracoid process as well as the lesser tubercle. Between the clavicular and acromial heads, a groove is visible and palpable when the shoulder is actively flexed to 90°. This groove allows for palpation of the tendon of the long

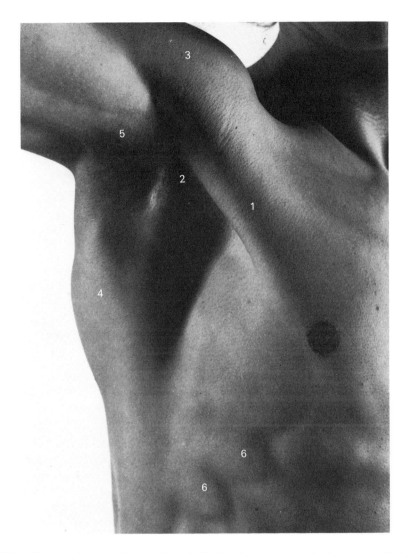

Figure 2–20B Axillary cavity, right frontal view. **1**, Pectoralis major muscle; **2**, subscapularis muscle; **3**, deltoid muscle; **4**, latissimus dorsi muscle; **5**, coracobrachialis and neurovascular bundle; **6**, serratus anterior muscle.

head of the biceps (located at the floor of the groove), when the shoulder is in the zero position (Figures 2–1 and 2–12).

Directly lateral to the groove, muscle fibers of the acromial head are palpated. This part of the deltoid muscle is multipenniform. Its fibers run in the form of a feather from proximal to distal. They end in a common tendinous insertion just above the midpoint of the humerus, between the long head of the bi-

ceps, the origin of the brachialis muscle, and the lateral head of the triceps. The greater tubercle can be palpated through the deltoid muscle, ventrolaterally just underneath the acromion.

In 90° abduction, a groove is visible at the caudal aspect of the deltoid's spinal head, indicating the border at the medial aspect of the scapular spine. The spinal part of the deltoid is often underestimated (drawn too

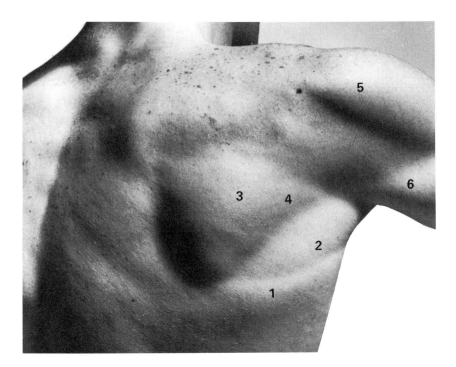

Figure 2–21 Dorsal view, right side. **1**, Latissimus dorsi; **2**, teres major; **3**, infraspinatus; **4**, teres minor; **5**, deltoid, spinal part; **6**, triceps, long head.

small) when outlining the structure with a marker.

In prolonged use of axillary crutches, entrapment of the motor nerve in the axilla can occur. Quickly progressing atrophy of the deltoid is observed, along with decreased strength in abduction and a tendency for the humerus to dislocate. On the other hand, a dislocation of the humerus can cause a lesion of the axillary nerve.

Often, patients with shoulder complaints indicate their pain and tenderness in the deltoid region, and sometimes even more precisely at the insertion of the deltoid. This does not mean that the muscle itself is affected, however. This is almost always an area of referred pain within the C5 dermatome (the shoulder developed from the C5 segment). In general, the amount of distal pain radiation correlates to the degree of the lesion. In severe shoulder problems, pain can be felt down to the base of the first metacarpal, which is the most distal part of the C5 dermatome.

Subscapularis

The insertion of the subscapularis muscle at the lesser tubercle is not directly palpable. However, the proximal part of the lesser tubercle is easy to localize and can be used as a reference point for treatment techniques such as transverse friction (Figure 2–14).

The lateral part of the subscapularis is partly reachable in the axilla, and is visible with the arm abducted (located between the posterior wall of the latissimus dorsi and the anterior wall of the pectoralis major) (Figure 2–20B). In the axilla two structures running longitudinally can be observed. The anterior structure is the short head of the biceps and the coracobrachialis; the posterior structure is the neurovascular bundle. Further dorsally,

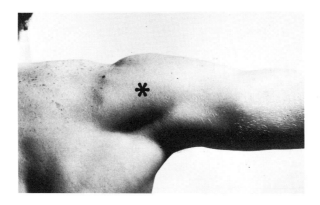

Figure 2-22A Deltoid muscle, spinal part, dorsal view, right side.

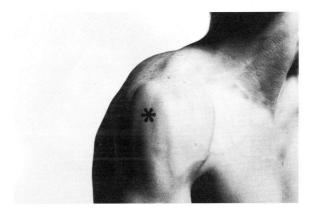

Figure 2–22B Deltoid muscle, acromial part, lateral view, right side.

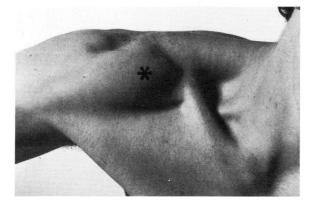

Figure 2–22C Deltoid muscle, clavicular part, ventral view, right side.

and deep within the axilla, the lateral part of the subscapularis can be palpated. The medial part of the muscle covers the scapula, and as part of the posterior axillary wall it inserts ventrally on the humerus. With isometrically resisted internal rotation of the shoulder, the subscapularis is easy to palpate in the axilla.

Supraspinatus

Palpation of the origin and muscle belly of the supraspinatus in the supraspinous fossa is possible only indirectly through the trapezius. The easiest way to perform the palpation is by adducting the relaxed hanging arm with a short jerk. The muscle's tendinous insertion runs to the cranial facet of the greater tubercle and is palpable only with an internally rotated arm (Figure 2–23A). In this position, the insertion is located in front of, and slightly caudal to, the acromion (Figure 2–23B); it is palpated indirectly through the deltoid.

Of all the muscle insertions around the shoulder, the supraspinatus is the most often affected. Palpation of its tendinous insertion through the deltoid requires a lot of experience. The subject sits inclined at approximately 120°, with the hand resting on the lower back; thus, the shoulder is internally rotated, slightly extended and slightly abducted. First the ventral corner of the acromion is palpated, and the tip of the index finger is placed directly distal to it. The index finger now lies horizontally on the plateau of the greater tubercle and points in a medial direction.

The palpating finger repeatedly gives pressure caudally while slowly sliding in a medial direction. After approximately 1 inch (interindividual variance) the lateral border of the intertubercular sulcus is palpated, which at the same time is the medial border of the insertion of the tendon. The lateral border of the insertion, located approximately 1 cm more lateral, is not palpable. Its distal end lies approximately 1 cm from the acromion.

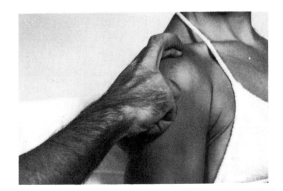

A

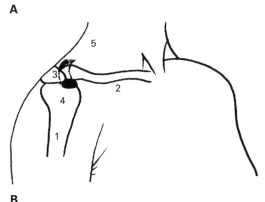

B

Figure 2–23 A, Palpation of the teno-osseous insertion of the supraspinatus takes place with an internally rotated and adducted (right) arm. **B,** Insertion of the supraspinatus in the (right) arm. **1,** Humerus; **2,** clavicle; **3,** acromion; **4,** insertion of the supraspinatus; **5,** acromioclavicular joint.

Infraspinatus and Teres Minor

The long head of the triceps is often clearly recognizable when the arm is brought backward in the transverse plane from a position of 90° abduction. This structure can be used as a reference point while searching for the teres major and teres minor. The long head of the triceps runs between both muscles, whereby the teres minor is located cranial to the teres major. The two spaces that occur between the three muscles and the shaft of the humerus are called the triangular space (medial) and the quadrangular space (located laterally).

Counting from the border of latissimus dorsi, the teres minor is the second muscle belly. It can be followed for just a short distance because it is covered by the deltoid. The same may be said for the infraspinatus, which also is covered by a thick fascia and is located between the borders of the ascending part of the trapezius and the spinal part of the deltoid. This makes only a small part of the infraspinatus accessible to direct palpation.

The border between the teres minor and the teres major cannot be found precisely through palpation. In general, the cranial part of the teres major and the caudal part of the teres minor can be palpated, while the subject alternately internally and externally rotates the arm. If the middle finger is placed on the expected location of the teres minor and the index finger on the expected location of the teres major, contraction is felt underneath the middle finger during external rotation and under the index finger during internal rotation.

Lesions of the infraspinatus are usually localized at the tendon or at its insertion. However, neither structure is palpable with the arm resting alongside the body. In order to make these sites accessible, the subject leans on the elbows in a prone position with the upper arms vertical and approximately 20° externally rotated (Figures 2–24A and 2–24B). In this way, the greater tubercle is brought dorsally out from under the acromion. Adducting the upper arm brings the tendon and its insertion even more accessible to (indirect) palpation (Figure 2–24C).

The tendon is palpable approximately 2 cm distal to the dorsal corner of the acromion. The best way to perform the palpation is by adducting the thumb in the direction of the acromion. The insertion is found by following the tendon in a lateral direction until a bony ridge is felt (greater tubercle) (Figures 2–24D to 2–24F). Lesions of the infraspinatus are seen more often than those of the teres minor.

Surface Anatomy of the Axilla

Every palpation of the axilla requires thorough knowledge of the complex topographic relationships in this area (Figure 2–20B). For this purpose the axilla can be seen as a three-dimensional space bordered by the following structures:

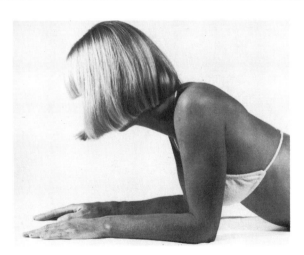

Figure 2–24A Initial position: prone leaning on the elbows. Elbows approximately 4 inches from the edge of the table, shoulder and elbow are vertically aligned.

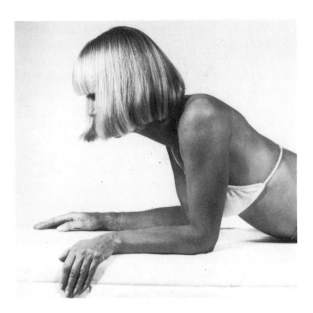

Figure 2–24B The arm is externally rotated and the subject grasps the edge of the table; the elbow remains in place. In so doing, the insertion of the infraspinatus muscle at the greater tubercle is brought approximately 20° dorsal.

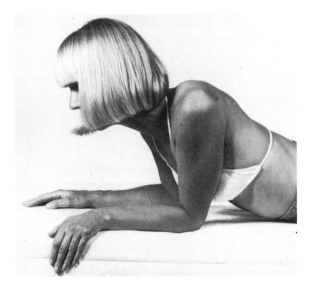

Figure 2–24C Now the shoulder is brought toward the edge of the table. In this position, the greater tubercle is brought dorsally out from under the acromion.

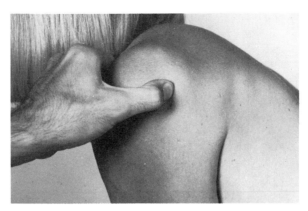

Figure 2–24D With the thumb, the tendon of the infraspinatus is palpated 2 cm caudal to the prominent dorsal corner of the acromion. By adducting the thumb, extending the wrist, and supinating the forearm, the palpation is performed transversely over the tendon.

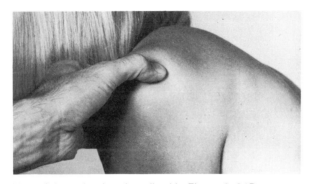

Figure 2–24E End position of the palpation described in Figure 2–24D.

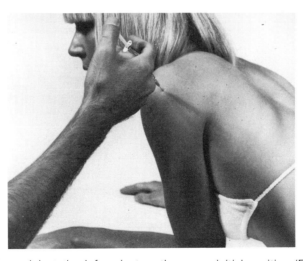

Figure 2–24F In order to inject the infraspinatus, the same initial position (Figures 2–24A–C) is recommended.

- Its *ventral wall* consists mainly of the lateral part of the pectoralis major, until its insertion at the crest of the greater tubercle. This muscle forms the easily palpable lateral part of the ventral axillary wall. Further medial, at the coracoid process, the pectoralis minor originates and runs in a mediocaudal direction. This muscle forms the medial part of the ventral axillary wall.
- The thorax forms the *medial wall* of the axilla covered by the serratus anterior. The individual muscle bellies of the serratus anterior are usually easy to palpate.
- The *dorsal wall* is formed mainly by the subscapularis, which covers the scapula. Note that this muscle inserts at the lesser tubercle. Thus, the dorsal wall of the axilla ends at the ventral aspect of the humerus, which means that the axillary fossa is situated relatively ventrally. The insertions of the teres major and latissimus dorsi together form the lateral part of the dorsal axillary wall. They also insert ventrally at the humerus (with the latissimus dorsi most ventrally located).
- The humerus forms the *lateral wall* of the axillary fossa. The tendon of the long head of the biceps runs the furthest laterally between the lesser tubercle (the insertion of the muscles of the dorsal wall) and the greater tubercle (on which the pectoralis major, the most important ventral wall muscle, inserts).

Upon abducting the arm, two longitudinal prominences appear within the axilla (between the axillary walls). The ventral prominence, directly behind the ventral wall, represents the course of the coracobrachialis and the short head of the biceps. Both muscles run from the coracoid process through the ventral axillary fossa to the arm. The dorsal longitudinal prominence consists of the neurovascular bundle. The subclavian artery becomes the axillary artery after it crosses the pectoralis minor, then runs through the axillary cavity, where it becomes the brachial artery. The subclavian artery is surrounded by the cords of the brachial plexus. In the axillary fossa, the cords give rise to the following main branches:

- axillary nerve
- radial nerve
- ulnar nerve
- median nerve

The subclavian artery and the cords of the brachial plexus are clearly palpable within the axilla.

With the arm in a relaxed hanging position, the glenohumeral joint can be palpated deeply within the axilla, with its firm labrum and sometimes palpable infraglenoid tubercle. Because the axillary nerve runs directly distal to the joint, palpation should be performed carefully in order not to irritate this nerve.

In the dorsal wall of the axilla, two openings can be found: the lateral opening is more clinically significant; the medial opening is not discussed further. The lateral opening, or quadrangular space, is located between the humerus, teres minor, long head of the triceps, and teres major. (The teres minor and the long head of the triceps lie behind the axilla; thus, the entrance to the quadrangular space, from the axilla, is located between the subscapularis and the dorsal axillary wall.) The posterior humeral circumflex artery and the axillary nerve run through the quadrangular space.

The posterior humeral circumflex artery is a branch of the axillary artery, which crosses the humerus posteriorly, then takes a more ventral course in order to form an anastomosis with the anterior humeral circumflex artery, which crosses the humerus ventrally. The axillary nerve is a branch of the posterior cord and innervates the deltoid and the teres minor.

In an inferior dislocation of the humerus, or in a poorly performed reduction after dislocation, the axillary nerve can become entrapped within the quadrangular space. Initially, weakness in abduction is found; later, atrophy of the deltoid is seen.

The floor of the axillary fossa consists of a collagenous layer of tissue upon which lymph nodes and sweat glands are located. The axillary lymph nodes, which are palpable with firm pressure, can be enlarged in many infectious and malignant processes. Increased size of the lymph nodes should be taken seriously, especially when they are not painful. Further examination by a physician is necessary. Swelling of the axillary sweat glands is also possible. Usually they are painfully inflamed, and thus easy to differentiate from malignant lymph nodes. Differentiation between swollen sweat glands and inflamed lymph nodes, however, is difficult.

Please see Appendix A, Schematic Topography of the Upper Extremity, for more information.

3

Examination of the Shoulder

Examinations of the shoulder are based on traditional positions that are used as the baselines from which measurements can be made. These positions are described briefly in this section, followed by a progressive procedure for conducting an examination.

GLENOHUMERAL JOINT

Zero Position

With the subject standing, if the relaxed arm is flexed to 90° in the elbow, the forearm does not lie in the sagittal plane; this indicates an apparent internal rotation of approximately 20° in the glenohumeral joint. This position is used as a reference for measurements and as a starting point for resisted tests.

Maximal Loose-Packed Position

Without internal or external rotation, there is 55° of abduction in the plane of the scapula (seen in relation to the anatomical planes, the shoulder is in 55° abduction and approximately 30° horizontal adduction, and the humerus is not internally or externally rotated).

Maximal Close-Packed Position

There is maximal glenohumeral abduction with maximal external rotation.

Capsular Pattern

External rotation is more limited and internal rotation less limited than glenohumeral

abduction. The ratio of limitations for external rotation, abduction, and internal rotation is 3:2:1, respectively (Figure 3–1).

ACROMIOCLAVICULAR AND STERNOCLAVICULAR JOINTS

Zero Position

This is the physiological position of the shoulder girdle. In other words, this is the position of the shoulder girdle during normal relaxed standing or sitting (different among individuals).

Maximal Loose-Packed Position

This is the same as the zero position.

Maximal Close-Packed Position

Acromioclavicular joint: there is 90° arm elevation through abduction.
Sternoclavicular joint: there is maximal arm elevation.

Capsular Pattern

Acromioclavicular joint: there is minimal to no limitation of motion, with pain at the end-range of each motion in which the shoulder girdle is involved.
Sternoclavicular joint: same as for the acromioclavicular joint, except that arm elevation can demonstrate a greater limitation of motion.

42

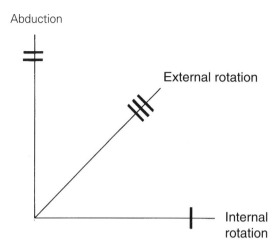

Figure 3–1 Capsular pattern of the glenohumeral joint.

OVERVIEW OF THE FUNCTIONAL EXAMINATION

General Inspection

When a patient enters the examination room, the practitioner immediately gathers information about the patient's condition by observing such things as general posture, facial expression, and the use of assistive devices. Attention is given to how the patient holds the affected arm and shakes hands. Whether the patient has a cast or a brace is also noted.

History

Age, Occupation, Hobbies, Sports

Some disorders occur only within a specific age group. (Refer to the section on arthritis in Chapter 4 for details.)

Insights concerning the problem and its possible cause can be gained by gathering information about the patient's occupation, hobbies, and sports activities. For instance, individuals who participate in throwing and racket sports often have problems related to stability of the shoulder.

The five most frequently seen disorders in the shoulder girdle and glenohumeral joint are as follows:

1. instability (particularly anterior or anteroinferior)
2. impingement (compression of the subacromial structures)
3. arthritis of the glenohumeral joint
4. pathology of the acromioclavicular joint
5. thoracic outlet (compression) syndrome

Chief Complaints

Depending on the type of shoulder pathology, complaints can consist of one or more of the following:

- pain
- limited motion
- locking
- weakness
- sensory disturbances
- paresthesia

Pain on top of the shoulder is likely caused by pathology of the acromioclavicular joint. Pain in the deltoid region can be caused by almost every other shoulder problem. In addition, there is often local tenderness in this area.

Usually, localization of pain and tenderness is misleading. The exact lesion can be determined (and then palpated) only after performing a thorough functional examination. Local treatment applied only to the areas of pain and local tenderness is usually ineffective. In some cases local surgery is even performed to determine the affected structure and relieve pain; results of such surgery are often unsatisfactory (Figure 3–2).

Limitations of motion can be caused by different shoulder disorders. The pathology most frequently causing limitations of motion is idiopathic arthritis.

Locking of the glenohumeral joint is seldom seen and is generally due to a dislocation or loose bodies.

Symptoms such as weakness, sensory disturbances, and paresthesia indicate a cervical problem, thoracic outlet syndrome, or a peripheral compression neuropathy, with or without accompanying shoulder (girdle) pathology.

Onset

In disorders of the shoulder girdle, it is important to distinguish whether the onset was sudden or gradual. For instance, if limited range of motion in a capsular pattern is found during the functional examination and the onset was gradual, the most probable diagnosis is an idiopathic arthritis. If the patient describes a trauma, after which first pain and then limited range of motion were experienced, there is likely to be a traumatic arthritis. If the patient is unable to raise the arm after a fall on the shoulder or outstretched hand, a rupture of the rotator cuff or a fracture (of the greater tubercle) should be suspected. Acromioclavicular joint pathology is considered if the patient complains of pain on top of the shoulder after a trauma.

Duration

Severe pain arising within a time span of a few hours or days may indicate an acute subacromial-subdeltoid bursitis. This acute bursitis has a rapid onset, but is limited to a period of only several days to a maximum of 2 weeks. On the other hand, a chronic subacromial-subdeltoid bursitis can cause a variety of changing symptoms lasting for years. The same is true for certain types of shoulder instability: Traumatic and idiopathic arthritis can last 1 to 2 years. Lesions of the rotator cuff tendons often exist for months.

Localization of the Complaints

Most glenohumeral problems cause radiating pain in the C5 dermatome. The more severe the pathology, the further, distally, the pain radiates.

Sternoclavicular and acromioclavicular pathology usually causes pain in the C4 dermatome. Because the sternoclavicular joint lies more proximal in the dermatome, there is

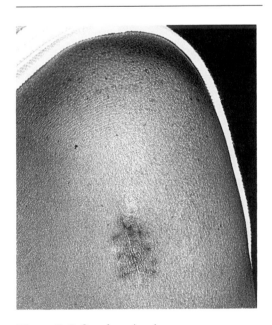

Figure 3–2 Scar from local surgery.

more referred pain. Pain from acromioclavicular lesions is generally local.

Ability To Lie on the Shoulder

Whether or not the patient can lie on the affected shoulder provides important indications of the severity of the lesion. In severe cases of arthritis, bursitis, and tendopathies, the patient complains of the inability to lie on the affected shoulder. Also, this is often true when there are acromioclavicular lesions.

Factors That Influence the Symptoms

Determining whether there is pain only during activity or also pain at rest provides significant information as to the stages of an arthritis or tendopathy. (Refer to Chapter 4 for a more detailed discussion.)

Pain during throwing or serving (such as in tennis) can indicate either an instability or an impingement. Pain in a position of maximal abduction-extension-external rotation (throwing, serving, or smashing), the so-called late cocking position, usually indicates an anterior or anteroinferior instability. If the pain is experienced particularly in the posterior aspect of the shoulder, a lesion of the posterior capsule or posterior part of the glenoid labrum usually is involved.

If pain is experienced during the acceleration phase of throwing, serving, or smashing, an impingement syndrome should be considered. Of course, combinations of instability and impingement also can be present.

To be certain that the symptoms are not caused by dysfunctions of the cervical spine, the examiner specifically asks the patient whether arm or neck movements provoke the complaints. Generally, if movements of the head and/or neck cause the symptoms, the cervical spine should be examined thoroughly. Pain provoked by arm movements is usually an indication of a shoulder problem. One area of difficulty is the thoracic outlet: in a thoracic outlet syndrome, both neck and arm movements induce the symptoms. In this instance, the specific tests for thoracic outlet syndrome are almost always positive.

Involvement of Other Joints

If the patient also has problems in other joints, the possibility of a systemic disease should be considered (eg, rheumatoid arthritis, psoriasis, or lupus erythematosus).

Previous Surgery

A patient's history of surgery is of particular importance if the operation concerned a malignant tumor. In this instance, the presence of metastases should always be ruled out.

Medication

Administration of mechanical therapy such as mobilization, manipulation, or transverse friction is contraindicated if the patient is taking anticoagulants. Exercise programs should be closely monitored (to ensure that the patient maintains proper breathing) in instances when the patient is on antihypertensive medication.

Antidepressant medication could indicate that the problem is multifactorial. It is also significant to note whether the patient is on nonsteroidal anti-inflammatory medication, and whether this has provided any relief of the symptoms.

For additional factors to consider, please refer to the section on history in *Diagnosis and Treatment of the Spine*, Chapter 6, Cervical Spine.

Specific Inspection

During the specific inspection, the examiner starts by making general observations of the patient. The positions of the patient's head, shoulders, and scapulae as well as overall posture are observed.

Specific attention is paid to the presence of local swelling or discoloration. In addition, the examiner looks for atrophy of the deltoid, supraspinatus, and infraspinatus muscles. The examiner also notices the position of the acromioclavicular and sternoclavicular joints, looking for signs of a subluxation or a dislocation.

Palpation

Before performing the functional examination, the examiner should feel for an increase in local skin temperature and the presence of swelling around the glenohumeral, acromioclavicular, and sternoclavicular joints. If swelling is noted, palpation is performed to test consistency (soft versus firm).

Functional Examination

Before the functional examination, the examiner determines whether the patient is experiencing symptoms at that specific moment. With each test, the examiner then notes whether the symptoms change.

The affected side is always compared with the nonaffected side. Thus, both sides are tested—first the nonaffected side (to have an idea of what is "normal") and then the affected side.

In the following description of the functional examination, the essential tests are indicated in ***boldface italic and underlined:*** these comprise the *basic functional examination.* The other tests are performed depending on the findings from the basic functional examination.

Even though it may be obvious from the history that the patient has a shoulder problem, *six quick tests to rule out involvement of the cervical spine are always performed first before proceeding further:*

1. cervical spine flexion
2. cervical spine extension (with the mouth open in order to relax the platysma muscle)
3. right rotation
4. left rotation
5. right sidebend
6. left sidebend

If one of these tests provokes the patient's chief complaint, the examiner should then conduct an appropriate functional examination of the cervical spine.

It is often necessary to differentiate between a shoulder problem and a possible thoracic outlet syndrome. Results of the Roos test are used to diagnose a thoracic outlet syndrome (refer to Chapter 8).

To obtain information about scapulothoracic mobility, as well as the sternoclavicular and acromioclavicular joints, the patient is instructed to perform four movements:

1. *bilateral shoulder girdle elevation*
2. *bilateral shoulder girdle protraction*
3. *bilateral shoulder girdle retraction*
4. *bilateral shoulder girdle depression*

The following tests are also performed in the functional examination of the shoulder.

Tests—Active Motions

3.1. ***Active bilateral arm elevation***
3.2.   Active unilateral arm elevation
3.3. ***Painful arc test***

Tests—Passive Motions (Alternating with Active Motions)

3.4. ***Passive arm elevation with overpressure in a medial direction***
3.5. ***Passive arm elevation with overpressure in a posterior direction***
3.6.   Active internal rotation in combination with extension
3.7. ***Passive internal rotation***
3.8. ***Passive glenohumeral abduction: mobility***
3.9.   Passive glenohumeral abduction: end-feel
3.10. Passive adduction from a position of internal rotation and extension
3.11. Passive horizontal adduction
3.12. Active external rotation

3.13. Passive external rotation
3.14. Biceps stretch test

Tests—Resisted Motions
3.15. Resisted adduction
3.16. Resisted abduction
3.17. Resisted external rotation
3.18. Resisted internal rotation
3.19. Resisted elbow flexion
3.20. Resisted elbow extension

Tests—Stability

3.21. Throwing test
3.22. External rotation test
3.23. Anterior subluxation test (apprehension test)
3.24. Anterior drawer test
3.25. Posterior drawer test

Tests—Differentiating between Bursitis and Rotator Cuff Tendinitis

3.26. Pull test with resisted abduction
3.27. Pull test with resisted internal and/or external rotation

Palpation

After the functional examination, the shoulder girdle region is again palpated for warmth and swelling. Based on the findings from the functional examination, the suspected affected structure is localized and palpated for tenderness.

Accessory Examinations in Limitations of Motion

If a limitation of motion in a noncapsular pattern has been found, the appropriate joint-specific, translatory tests should be performed to determine whether the limitation is in fact caused by the capsule.

Supplementary joint-specific testing should always be performed when a capsular pattern (pain with or without limitation) is noted in the acromioclavicular or sternocla-vicular joints. In this instance, the joint could be either hypermobile or hypomobile.

Other Examinations

If necessary, other examinations can also be performed, either to confirm a diagnosis or to gain further information when a diagnosis cannot be reached based on the functional examination:

- imaging techniques (such as conventional radiographs, computed tomography (CT) scan, arthrography, arthro-CT, magnetic resonance imaging (MRI), and ultrasonography)
- laboratory tests
- arthroscopy
- electromyography (EMG)

DESCRIPTION OF THE FUNCTIONAL EXAMINATION

Active Motions

The examination of active motions is performed to assess the amount of motion and the course of the movement. After the patient performs the active motion, the examiner immediately tests the passive performance of that motion.

3.1. Active Bilateral Arm Elevation

The patient is asked to elevate both arms actively. The examiner gives no further instructions, allowing the patient to raise the arms through abduction, flexion, or a combination of both.

A number of lesions of the shoulder girdle and the periarticular structures can cause pain and an active limitation of motion during arm elevation.

When arm elevation appears to be limited, the patient is asked to elevate both shoulders actively. If full range of motion is demonstrated in shoulder girdle elevation,

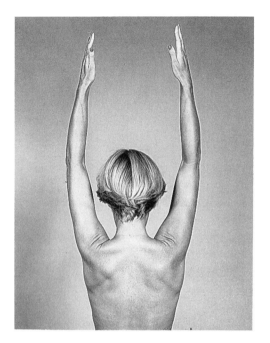

Test 3.1

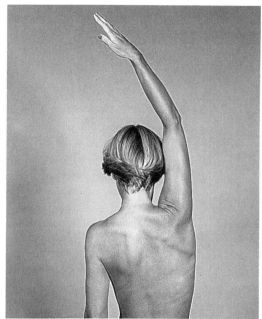

Test 3.2

scapulothoracic movements are normal. Even if there is a complete fusion of the glenohumeral joint, when scapulothoracic movement is normal, the patient should be able to elevate the arm to 60°.

3.2. Active Unilateral Arm Elevation

With both arms still elevated, the patient is asked to drop one arm and to move the still elevated arm as far as possible in a medial direction.

Generally the patient is able to bring the arm further into elevation. This occurs because the cervicothoracic junction rotates toward the elevated arm, allowing for more motion of the arm.

3.3. Painful Arc Test (A, B, C, D)

Starting with the shoulder in the zero position, the patient is instructed to elevate the affected arm actively, but *slowly*. The presence of a painful trajectory, preceded and followed by a trajectory without pain, has diagnostic significance (Figure 3–3).

A subacromial painful arc usually occurs between 60° and 120° of elevation. It results only when the affected structures lie between the head of the humerus and the roof of the shoulder (Figures 3–3, 3–4, 3–5, and 3–6). These structures are as follows:

- supraspinatus insertion (the lateral, or superficial, part of the insertion)
- infraspinatus insertion (the lateral, or superficial, part of the insertion)
- subscapularis insertion (the proximal part of the insertion)
- tendon or tendon sheath of the long head of the biceps
- subacromial-subdeltoid bursa
- acromion

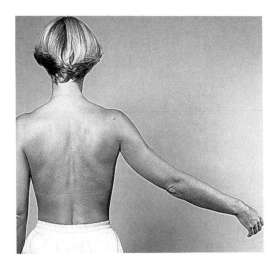

Test 3.3A The elevation starts without pain.

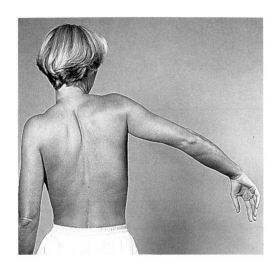

Test 3.3B The painful arc can begin at 60° elevation.

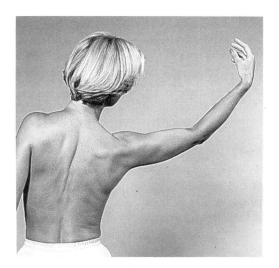

Test 3.3C The painful arc can continue at 130° elevation.

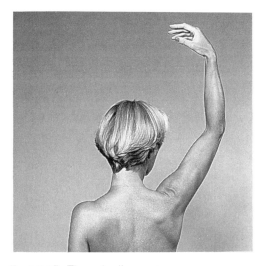

Test 3.3D The pain disappears.

- coracoacromial ligament
- lesser tubercle
- greater tubercle

In some cases, a painful arc is demonstrated near the end of elevation, between 160° and 180°. This can indicate a lesion of the acromioclavicular joint. However, acromioclavicular pathology generally causes pain at the end-range of both active and passive elevation. Sometimes there is also a small limitation of motion.

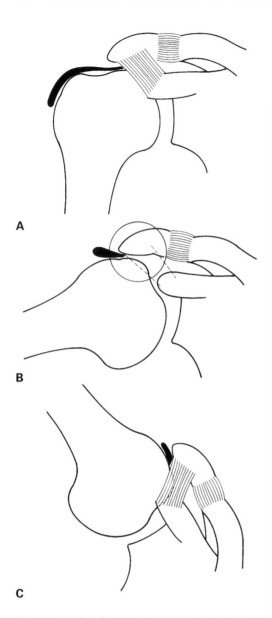

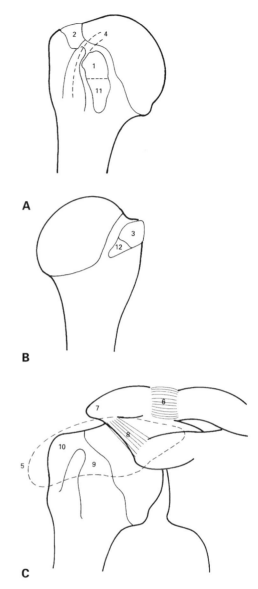

Figure 3–3 Painful arc, in this case caused by a subacromial-subdeltoid bursitis. **A**, No pain; **B**, pain; **C**, no pain.

Figure 3–4 Structures that can cause a painful arc. **A**, Right humeral head, anterior view; **B**, right humeral head, posterior view; **C**, right shoulder, anterior view. **1**, Subscapular muscle insertion, proximal part; **2**, supraspinatus muscle insertion; **3**, infraspinatus muscle insertion; **4**, tendon of the long head of the biceps muscle; **5**, subacromial-subdeltoid bursa; **6**, acromioclavicular joint; **7**, acromion; **8**, coracoacromial ligament; **9**, lesser tubercle; **10**, greater tubercle; **11**, subscapularis insertion, distal part (cannot cause a painful arc); **12**, teres minor insertion (cannot cause a painful arc).

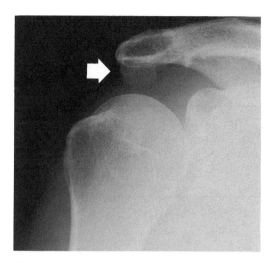

Figure 3–5 Exostosis underneath the acromion, causing a painful arc.

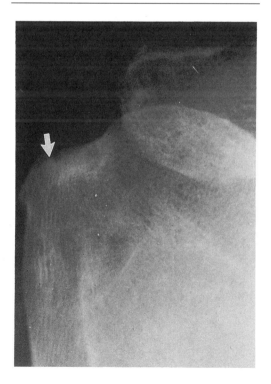

Figure 3–6 Irregular contour of the greater tubercle due to chronic supraspinatus muscle insertion tendopathy. The functional examination demonstrates a painful arc, but there are no signs of supraspinatus muscle pathology (resisted tests are not painful).

Passive Motions (Alternating with Active Motions)

The amount of motion found during the passive evaluation is compared with the active motion. In limitations of motion, differentiation is made between "capsular" and "noncapsular" patterns. Limitations of motion in a capsular pattern indicate arthritis or arthrosis (osteoarthrosis). Important information is also obtained by determining the end-feel. As with the active motions, provocation of the patient's symptoms is also noted.

3.4. Passive Arm Elevation with Overpressure in a Medial Direction

With the ipsilateral hand, the examiner grasps the patient's elbow and elevates the patient's arm through abduction, exerting slight overpressure in a medial direction at the end of the range of motion.

With the other hand, the examiner stabilizes the patient's upper body at the opposite shoulder (not illustrated). This test evaluates the range of motion (and end-feel) of the entire shoulder girdle. Thus, a limitation of motion could result from pathology of any of the

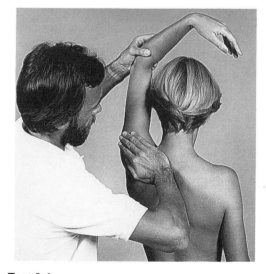

Test 3.4

shoulder girdle joints and junctions. Pain could be provoked as a result of pathology of one of these joints, or it could be caused by compression of the infraspinatus muscle insertion, supraspinatus muscle insertion, and subacromial-subdeltoid bursa against the glenoid labrum.

To compress specifically the structures lying between the greater tubercle and the acromion against the glenoid labrum, the examiner places the fixing hand on the superior angle of the scapula on the affected side (rather than on the opposite shoulder). When there is a lesion of the medial part of the supraspinatus or infraspinatus insertions, or in instances of a bursitis, testing passive arm elevation is much more painful on overpressure with the scapula fixed than with stabilization at the opposite shoulder.

3.5. Passive Arm Elevation with Overpressure in a Posterior Direction

The examiner stands next to the patient at the side to be tested. With the ipsilateral hand, the examiner grasps the patient's elbow, elevating the patient's arm through flexion. The other hand fixes the scapula on the same side. At the end of the range of motion, slight overpressure is exerted in a posterior direction.

Overpressure in a posterior direction compresses particularly the tendon (and tendon sheath) of the long head of the biceps against the acromion. In instances of pain provocation, this test can help to confirm a lesion of the tendon or tendon sheath of the long head of the biceps.

3.6. Active Internal Rotation in Combination with Extension (A, B)

The patient is instructed to bring the hand around the back and try to reach the opposite scapula.

In general, this test helps the examiner evaluate the available range of motion in the glenohumeral joint and the scapulothoracic junction during active internal rotation and extension. The sternoclavicular and acromioclavicular joints are also involved in this movement.

There is always a difference in the amount of motion between the right and left sides.

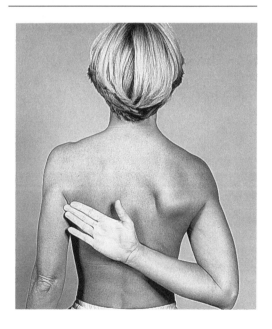

Test 3.5

Test 3.6A Right.

Usually, there is less range of motion on the dominant side. In the illustrations it is obvious that the model is right-handed; the movement on the right side is less than that on the left side.

3.7. Passive Internal Rotation

The examiner stands behind the patient, opposite the side to be tested, and places the lateral aspect of his shoulder against the posterior aspect of the patient's shoulder on that side. With the ipsilateral hand, the examiner grasps the patient's forearm (of the side being tested) just proximal to the wrist. The other hand stabilizes the patient's elbow against her body. Without extending the patient's arm, the examiner performs an internal rotation, exerting slight overpressure at the end of the range of motion.

The range of motion depends on the patient's general mobility, age, and gender. In some patients, this test cannot be performed as described here because of a severe limitation of motion. Usually the end-feel is firm.

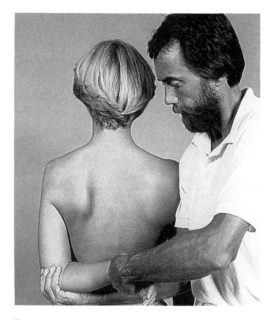

Test 3.7

Internal rotation is limited in the presence of a capsular pattern.

If the motion is only painful, and not limited, it is usually due to the stretch of an external rotator. Further diagnosis is required using resisted tests.

Passive internal rotation can also be performed in 90° of elevation through flexion (Kennedy test). If pain is provoked in this instance, there is probably an impingement syndrome.

3.8. Passive Glenohumeral Abduction: Mobility

With the contralateral thumb, the examiner fixes the lateral border of the patient's scapula, directly above the inferior angle. The other hand grasps the patient's forearm, just distal to the elbow. Starting from the zero position, and ensuring that no internal or external rotation occurs, the examiner brings the patient's shoulder into abduction until the lateral edge of the scapula pushes against the examiner's thumb.

The amount of motion generally varies between 70° and 120°, depending on the general

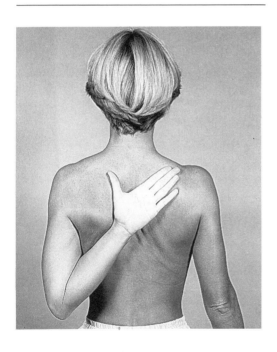

Test 3.6B Left.

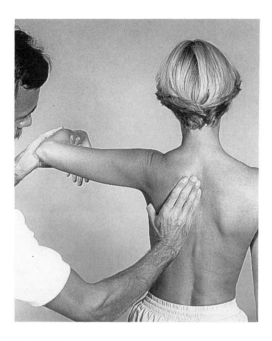

Test 3.8

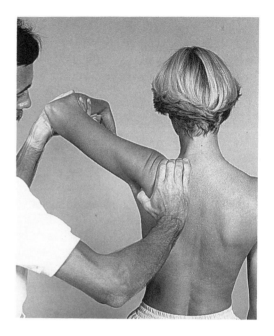

Test 3.9

mobility, age, and gender of the patient. If the motion is limited compared with the other side, there is usually a capsular disorder, and this limitation is part of a capsular pattern. The capsular pattern for the glenohumeral joint is such that the external rotation limitation is greater than the abduction limitation and the abduction limitation is greater than the limitation found in internal rotation, in a ratio of 3:2:1, respectively.

3.9. Passive Glenohumeral Abduction: End-Feel

To determine the end-feel in glenohumeral abduction, the examiner places the fingers of the contralateral hand on the patient's shoulder, palpating the lateral border of the scapula. The thumb and fingers fix the scapula while the other hand brings the patient's arm into abduction. Slight overpressure is exerted at the end of the motion.

The end-feel is usually hard, due to compression of the humerus (and subacromial structures) against the acromion.

3.10. Passive Adduction from a Position of Internal Rotation and Extension

The examiner stands behind the patient, opposite the side to be tested. The examiner brings the patient's hand of the side being tested behind the patient's back, and grasps the elbow of that side with the ipsilateral hand. Starting from this position of internal rotation in extension, the examiner brings the patient's shoulder into horizontal adduction. At the same time, the examiner stabilizes the patient's upper body by applying counter-pressure with the other hand against the anterior aspect of the patient's opposite shoulder. Slight overpressure is exerted at the end of the motion.

The end-feel is usually firm. If pathology of the acromioclavicular joint is suspected, this test can provoke the most pain. In these instances, the patient complains of pain at the top of the shoulder, sometimes radiating a very short distance ventrally to the clavicle or

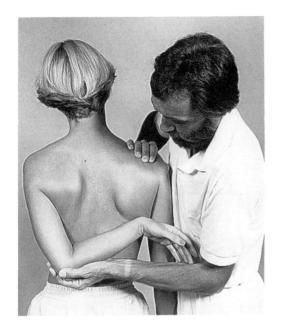

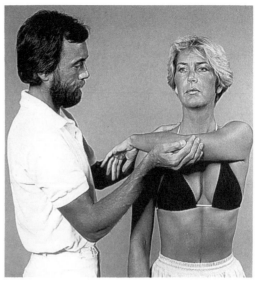

Test 3.11

Test 3.10

dorsally to the scapular spine (C4 dermatome).

3.11. Passive Horizontal Adduction

The examiner stands next to the patient, opposite the side to be tested. With the contralateral hand, the examiner grasps the patient's elbow of the arm being tested. After first elevating the shoulder to 90°, the examiner brings the arm into horizontal adduction. At the same time, the examiner stabilizes the patient's upper body by applying counterpressure with the other hand against the opposite scapula. Slight overpressure is exerted at the end of the motion.

The end-feel is usually soft. This test is very sensitive in the presence of acromioclavicular pathology. In these instances, the patient complains of pain in the C4 dermatome, and passive horizontal adduction is the most painful and limited motion in the functional examination. Unfortunately, this test is not specific. During horizontal adduction, the

shoulder abductors and external rotators are stretched, along with the suprascapular nerve. In addition, the distal insertion of the subscapularis muscle as well as various bursae are compressed. A lesion of any of these structures, however, usually provokes pain in the C5 dermatome.

3.12. Active External Rotation

The patient is instructed to flex both elbows to 90°, holding them close to the body. From this starting position, the patient is asked to rotate externally both shoulders.

The ranges of motion on both sides are compared.

3.13. Passive External Rotation

The examiner stands obliquely behind the patient, next to the side being tested. With the ipsilateral hand, the examiner grasps the patient's forearm just above the wrist. The examiner flexes the patient's elbow and stabilizes it next to the body by exerting slight axial pressure through the forearm. While bringing the patient's shoulder into external rotation, the examiner stabilizes the patient's

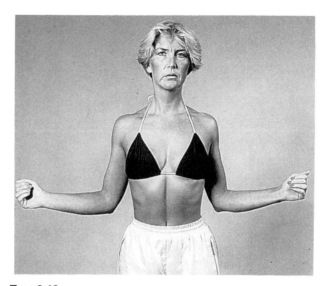

Test 3.12

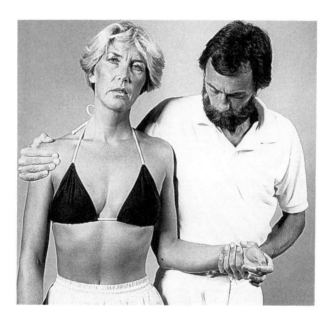

Test 3.13

upper body with the other hand, which has been placed on the patient's opposite shoulder. Slight overpressure is exerted at the end of the motion.

Depending on the patient's general mobility, age, and gender, range of motion varies between 60° and 110°. The end-feel is usually firm.

External rotation is the most limited motion in a capsular pattern of the glenohumeral joint. After a period of time, a rupture of the infraspinatus muscle leads to an external rotation limitation of motion.

In many cases, after an anterior dislocation of the glenohumeral joint, the external rotation is limited.

If the range of motion is not limited but only painful, this is likely due to a stretch of the anterior shoulder structures, such as the anterior aspect of the capsule and the insertion of the subscapularis.

3.14. Biceps Stretch Test

The examiner stands behind the patient and fixes the scapula on the side being tested with the contralateral hand. With the other hand, the examiner grasps the patient's forearm just above the wrist. While maintaining flexion in the patient's elbow, the examiner brings the patient's shoulder into extension in a plane that is perpendicular to the plane of the scapula. The forearm is then pronated, ensuring that the glenohumeral joint does not move into internal rotation. From this position of maximal glenohumeral joint extension

and forearm pronation, the examiner extends the patient's elbow.

This test is the most painful test when there is tenosynovitis of the long head of the biceps. When there is tendinitis, resisted elbow flexion will also be painful.

Resisted Motions

By performing isometric resisted motions, contractile structures are evaluated. In the shoulder examination, painful resisted tests usually indicate an insertion tendopathy. However, during isometric contraction, compression in parts of the shoulder joint and acromioclavicular joint also occurs. In addition, the subacromial-subdeltoid bursa is compressed. Differentiation can be made between these various structures by repeating the pain-provoking resisted tests while applying a pull on the arm (see Tests 3.26 and 3.27).

3.15. Resisted Adduction

The examiner stands next to the patient, at the side to be tested. The patient flexes the elbow to 90° and holds the upper arm against the body. With one hand, the examiner grasps

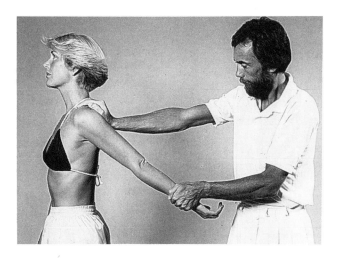

Test 3.14

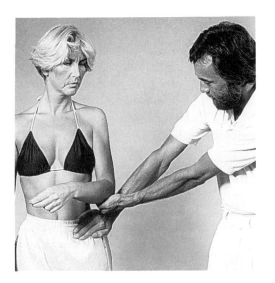

Test 3.15

the patient's elbow at its medial aspect. The other hand is placed on the patient's hip. The patient is instructed to bring the elbow in toward the body, while the examiner exerts maximal isometric resistance by pulling outward on the elbow and stabilizing the patient at the hip.

This is a test for the shoulder adductor muscles: latissimus dorsi, pectoralis major, teres major, and teres minor (the first three muscles are also internal rotators).

Resisted adduction is tested in 0° abduction so that the subscapularis is not facilitated. If resisted adduction is negative (as is usually the case) and resisted internal rotation is positive, there is likely to be a lesion of the subscapularis. If resisted adduction is negative and resisted external rotation is positive, pathology of the infraspinatus is suspected. An injury of the teres minor causes pain with resisted adduction and resisted external rotation.

Acromioclavicular problems, particularly arthritis, often cause pain during resisted adduction. In these instances the patient complains of pain in the C4 dermatome.

3.16. Resisted Abduction

The examiner stands next to the patient, at the side to be tested. The patient flexes the elbow to 90° and holds the upper arm against the body. The examiner places one hand at the lateral aspect of the patient's elbow. The other hand stabilizes the patient's opposite shoulder. The patient is asked to push the elbow away from the body, without rotating the arm. The examiner exerts maximal isometric resistance.

Resisted abduction is usually performed in 0° of abduction, but in order to assess strength or in instances of doubt, the test can be repeated at 30° and 60° of abduction.

This is a test for the shoulder abductors. Lesions of the deltoid muscle due to direct trauma or overuse are rare. Sometimes weakness of the deltoid occurs after a shoulder dislocation in which the axillary nerve has been injured.

The muscle most frequently causing pain during resisted abduction is the supraspinatus. Because the humeral head moves upward during resisted abduction, pain provoked during this test can also come from compres-

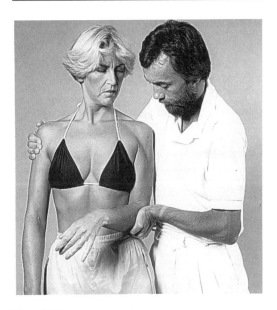

Test 3.16

sion of the inflamed subacromial-subdeltoid bursa between the humeral head and the roof of the shoulder. Bursitis can be differentiated from a supraspinatus tendopathy by performing resisted abduction while pulling on the arm (see Test 3.26).

3.17. Resisted External Rotation

The examiner stands next to the patient, at the side to be tested. With the ipsilateral hand the examiner grasps the patient's forearm just proximal to the wrist and brings the patient's elbow into 90° flexion. The other hand is placed on the patient's opposite shoulder to stabilize the upper body.

The patient is instructed to perform an external rotation (push the hand away from the body) while the examiner exerts maximal isometric resistance.

This is a test for the external rotators of the shoulder. The most frequently affected external rotator is the infraspinatus. The teres minor is rarely affected; if it is, the patient also has pain with resisted shoulder adduction. When resistance is applied to external rota-

tion, the supraspinatus contracts as well; however, if the supraspinatus is affected, resisted abduction will also be painful.

3.18. Resisted Internal Rotation

The examiner stands next to the patient, at the side to be tested. With the ipsilateral hand, the examiner grasps the volar aspect of the patient's forearm just proximal to the wrist, bringing the patient's elbow into 90° flexion. The other hand is placed on the patient's opposite shoulder in order to stabilize the upper body.

The patient is instructed to perform an internal rotation (bring the hand toward the body) while the examiner exerts maximal isometric resistance.

This is a test for the internal rotators of the shoulder. The most frequently affected internal rotator is the subscapularis (see Test 3.15 for further interpretation).

3.19. Resisted Elbow Flexion

The examiner stands next to the patient, at the side to be tested. With the ipsilateral

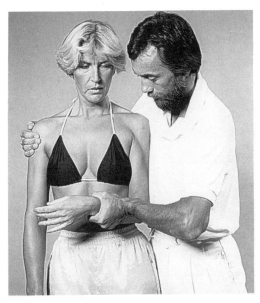

Test 3.17

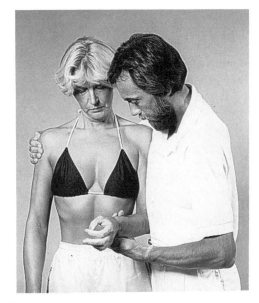

Test 3.18

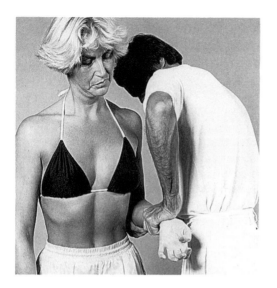

Test 3.19

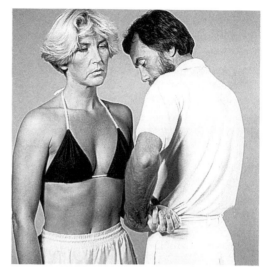

Test 3.20A Resisted elbow extension.

hand, the examiner grasps the volar aspect of the patient's forearm just above the wrist, positioning the patient's elbow in 90° flexion. The other hand supports the patient's elbow from posterior. The patient is instructed to flex the elbow, keeping the hand relaxed, while the examiner exerts maximal isometric resistance.

This is a test for the elbow flexors. However, in regard to shoulder problems, only the biceps is relevant. The biceps is the only muscle that could cause shoulder pain during resisted elbow flexion, because this is the only flexor which has function at each joint. If resisted elbow flexion provokes pain at the shoulder, the examiner can perform an extra test of resisted forearm supination. If this test also provokes the patient's shoulder pain, there is very likely to be a tendopathy of the long head of the biceps.

3.20. Resisted Elbow Extension (A, B)

The examiner stands next to the patient, at the side to be tested. With the ipsilateral hand, the examiner grasps the dorsal aspect of the patient's forearm just above the wrist, positioning the patient's elbow in 90° flexion.

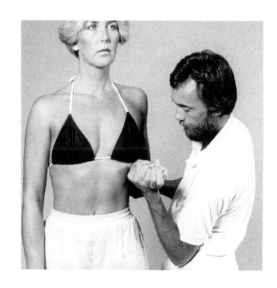

Test 3.20B Alternative performance.

The other hand supports the patient's elbow from a posterior position. The patient is instructed to extend the elbow, keeping the hand relaxed, while the examiner exerts maximal isometric resistance.

If the examiner is shorter than the patient, the test can be performed as illustrated in Test 3.20B.

This is a test for the elbow extensors. However, in regard to shoulder problems, only the triceps is relevant. Although triceps lesions in the shoulder region are rare, resisted elbow extension is often painful. This is due to the upward movement of the humeral head, leading to compression of the subacromial structures.

Stability Tests

Stability tests are performed to evaluate more specifically conditions in the glenohumeral joint. The most frequently seen instabilities in the glenohumeral joint are in an anterior direction and an anteroinferior direction. In these cases, lesions of the anterior capsuloligamentous structures are involved.

3.21. Throwing Test

The patient is instructed to position the arm in the throwing or "late cocking" position (90° to 120° abduction, maximal extension and external rotation). With the ipsilateral hand, the examiner grasps the volar aspect of the patient's distal forearm just proximal to

the wrist. The other hand is placed on the posterior aspect of the shoulder on that side in order to stabilize the trunk. The patient is instructed to perform an "explosive" throwing movement, while the examiner provides maximal isometric resistance.

The throwing test is most often positive (provoking the patient's symptoms) in instances of anterior and anteroinferior subluxations of the shoulder. Sometimes lesions of the long head of the biceps also cause pain during this test.

3.22. External Rotation Test (A, B, C)

The examiner starts testing with the patient's shoulder in the zero position. With the ipsilateral hand, the examiner grasps the volar aspect of the patient's forearm, just proximal to the wrist. The other hand is placed against the posterior aspect of the patient's elbow, which is flexed to 90°. The examiner performs a passive external rotation with the patient's arm, exerting a short, manipulative overpressure at the end of the motion. The movement is then performed in a position of slight abduction. By repeating the external rotation with overpressure in in-

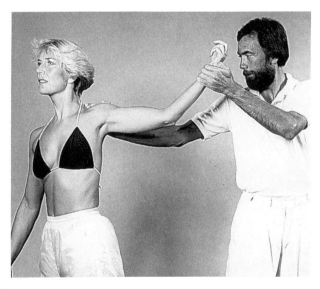

Test 3.21

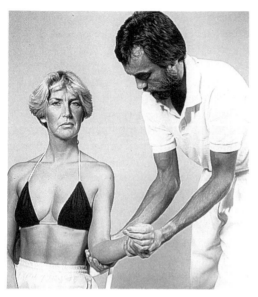

Test 3.22A External rotation test.

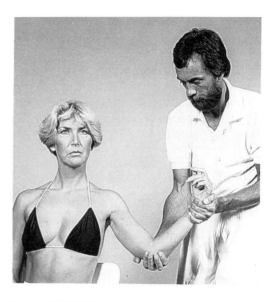

Test 3.22B With abduction.

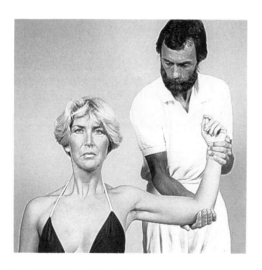

Test 3.22C In 90° abduction.

creasing amounts of abduction, tension is placed on different parts of the anterior joint capsule.

In instances of anterior and anteroinferior subluxations, this test is generally painful. The earlier the pain occurs, the more severe the instability.

3.23. Anterior Subluxation Test (Apprehension Test) (A, B, C)

After performing the external rotation test, and particularly in instances of a suspected slight instability, the apprehension test is performed. The test is performed with the patient in sitting position. The examiner stands behind the patient and grasps the volar aspect of the patient's forearm with the ipsilateral hand. The fingers of the other hand are placed at the front of the shoulder (the thumb at the back), in such a way that the tip of the index finger rests on the lesser tubercle and the tips of the other fingers on the coracoid process. The thumb rests on the humeral head, just lateral and inferior to the posterior angle of the acromion.

The patient is instructed to relax while the examiner brings the patient's arm into the position that caused pain during the external rotation test (Test 3.22). From this position, the examiner pushes the patient's humeral head anteriorly with the thumb in a manipulative way, by abruptly extending the wrist.

If this manipulative movement does not provoke the patient's pain, the test is re-

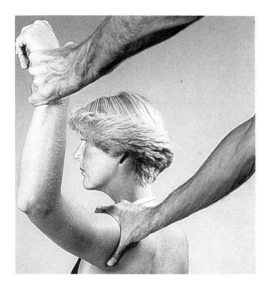

Test 3.23A Initial position.

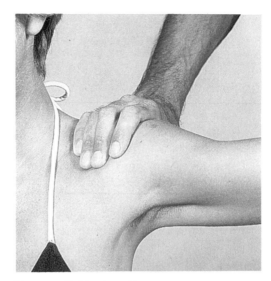

Test 3.23B Hand position.

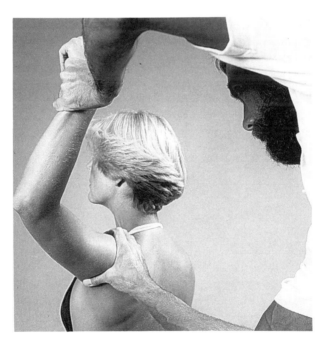

Test 3.23C End position.

peated with a manipulative push of the thumb against the posterior humeral head in an anteroinferior direction.

Sometimes an anterior subluxation is felt: the tip of the index finger (on the lesser tu-

bercle) "passes" the tips of the other fingers on the coracoid process. Occasionally a click is heard or felt. A *painful* click generally indicates a lesion of the glenoid labrum, also called a Bankart lesion. The test is considered positive when the patient's pain is provoked, with or without noting a subluxation or click. Frequently, patients with an anterior or anteroinferior instability react with a strong protective contraction of the muscles: apprehension.

3.24. Anterior Drawer Test (A, B, C)

The patient lies in a supine position on the examination table. The table is brought to a level of midthigh to the examiner. The examiner stands next to the patient, at the side to be tested, and places the patient's hand in his axilla, fixing it between his trunk and upper arm. The patient's shoulder is positioned in approximately 80° abduction, 20° horizontal adduction, and 30° external rotation.

With the ipsilateral hand, the examiner fixes the patient's scapula against the plinth in such a way that the fingers grasp the scapular spine and the thumb exerts pressure on the anterior aspect of the coracoid process. The other hand grasps the patient's humerus

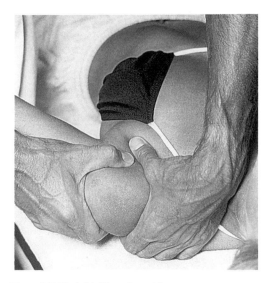

Test 3.24B Initial hand position.

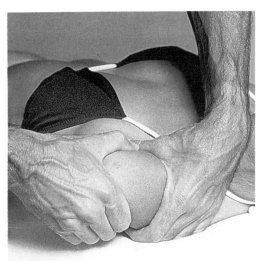

Test 3.24C Ending hand position.

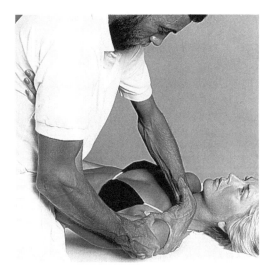

Test 3.24A Initial position.

as close as possible to the joint, with the thumb anterior and the fingers posterior.

The examiner brings the patient's humerus in an anterior direction as far as possible. The humerus is then returned to its initial position, and the test is repeated several times in order to assess the amount of movement properly. At the end of the last anterior movement, the examiner exerts overpressure to determine the end-feel.

During the anterior movements, instability can be clearly felt when the thumb on the humerus passes the thumb on the coracoid process. Sometimes a click is heard or felt. A *painful* click indicates a lesion of the glenoid labrum, the so-called Bankart lesion. If necessary, the lesion can be confirmed by an arthroscopic or arthrographic examination. If anterior laxity is not found in this position, the test can be repeated with the patient's arm in the "late cocking" position (maximal glenohumeral abduction, external rotation, and horizontal abduction).

3.25. Posterior Drawer Test (A, B)

The patient lies in a supine position on the examination table. The table is brought to a level of midthigh to the examiner. The examiner stands next to the patient, at the side to be tested. With the ipsilateral hand, the examiner grasps the patient's forearm just proximal to the wrist. The thumb of the other hand is placed on the anterior aspect of the humeral head as close as possible to the joint (just lateral to the coracoid process). The index and middle fingers of this hand rest against the scapular spine.

After flexing the patient's elbow to 90°, the examiner brings the patient's arm into approximately 80° abduction and 20° horizontal adduction. From this position, the examiner performs a combined movement of internal rotation while moving toward approximately 45° flexion. At the same time, the examiner pushes the humeral head posteriorly with the thumb.

Laxity is evident when the thumb on the humerus glides past the coracoid process in a posterior direction. Although the test rarely is

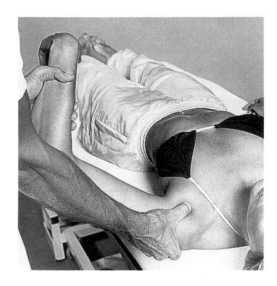

Test 3.25A Initial position.

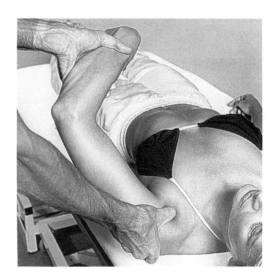

Test 3.25B End position.

painful, minimal to moderate muscle splinting often occurs. Only in the last instance is the test considered clinically positive. Many people demonstrate hypermobility in a posterior direction without corresponding symptoms. In this instance, the hypermobility is normal.

Tests Differentiating between Bursitis and Rotator Cuff Tendinitis

When one or more of the resisted tests are painful and there are also signs of an impingement (for instance, a positive painful arc test), the examiner should have the patient repeat the painful resisted motion while the examiner exerts pull on the humerus. During this pull on the humerus, space between the humeral head and the roof of the shoulder increases. If the resisted test is negative (not painful) with a pull on the arm, but positive (painful) without the pull, the bursa is affected.

3.26. Pull Test with Resisted Abduction (A, B)

The test is performed with the patient either sitting or standing. The examiner stands next to the patient's affected side, and grasps the patient's elbow, exerting a slight inferior pull on the arm. The fingers of the other hand palpate the increase in space between the acromion and the humeral head. The patient is then instructed to abduct the arm slowly and with increasing force, while the examiner exerts maximal isometric resistance. Because the deltoid also contracts, the space between the head of the humerus and the roof of the shoulder can no longer be palpated. The more force the patient exerts, the more inferior pull the examiner performs.

If resisted abduction without inferior pull is painful and the pain disappears during resisted abduction with a pull on the arm, there is a subacromial-subdeltoid bursitis. How-

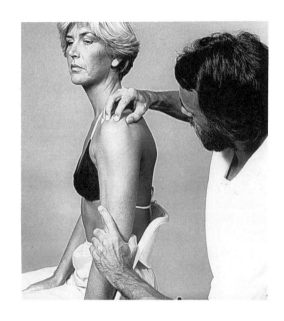

Test 3.26A Initial position, lateral view.

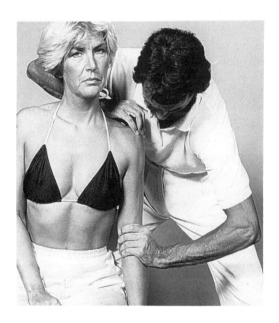

Test 3.26B Anterior view.

ever, if the pain increases during resisted abduction with a pull on the arm, the supraspinatus is affected. Sometimes there is no change in the pain during resisted abduction, with or without a pull. In this instance, the supraspinatus is likely affected, either alone or in conjunction with a bursitis.

3.27. Pull Test with Resisted Internal and/or External Rotation (A, B)

It is also possible to test resisted rotations while applying an inferior pull on the arm. The patient lies in a supine position with the elbow flexed 90°. With one hand the examiner grasps the patient's elbow and exerts an inferior pull on the arm. Depending on the motion to be tested, the other hand is placed either against the dorsal or the volar aspect of the patient's forearm, just proximal to the wrist. The patient is instructed to push into the examiner's hand, in either an external rotation (dorsal pressure) or an internal rotation (volar pressure), while the examiner exerts maximal isometric resistance. The more force the patient exerts, the more inferior pull the examiner performs.

In this test, differentiation can be made between a subacromial-subdeltoid bursitis and a tendinitis of either the infraspinatus or subscapularis. If a resisted rotation without inferior pull is painful and the pain disappears during the resisted rotation with a pull on the arm, there is a subacromial-subdeltoid bursitis. If the pain increases during the resisted rotation with a pull on the arm, however, the tendon is affected. Sometimes there is no change in the pain during resisted rotation, with or without a pull. In this instance, the tendon is likely affected, either alone or in conjunction with a bursitis.

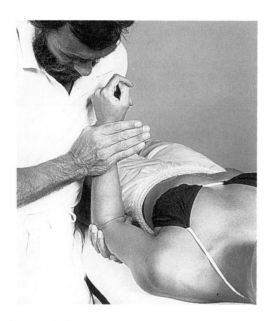

Test 3.27A External rotation.

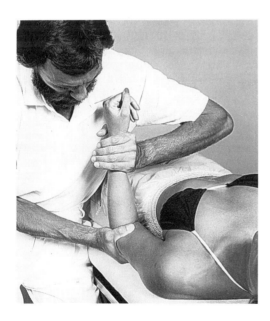

Test 3.27B Internal rotation.

4

Pathology of the Shoulder

4.1 GLENOHUMERAL JOINT PATHOLOGY

PATHOLOGY WITH LIMITED MOTIONS IN A CAPSULAR PATTERN

Arthritis

In every form of glenohumeral arthritis, the so-called frozen shoulder occurs, which is a limitation of passive motions in the capsular pattern. The capsular pattern for the glenohumeral joint is a greater limitation of external rotation than abduction and a greater limitation of abduction than internal rotation, in a ratio of 3:2:1, respectively.

"Frozen shoulder" is not really a diagnosis. Arthritides have many causes, including trauma, immobilization, and idiopathic, as well as systemic diseases such as rheumatoid arthritis, ankylosing spondylitis, gout, and Reiter's disease. Based on the patient history and laboratory tests, the cause of an arthritis can be determined. The most frequently occurring arthritides are discussed in the following section. Although there are many other types of arthritis (McCarty[8] describes over 200 possible causes of arthritis), they are seldom encountered.

Traumatic Arthritis

Traumatic arthritis is rarely seen in individuals who are younger than 45 years. Generally the patient experiences a relatively insignificant trauma, and several days later, pain in the deltoid region develops. Unfortunately, traumatic arthritis is also frequently seen after a shoulder arthroscopy or arthrographic procedure. At first, pain is experienced only during specific movements. The pain gradually increases, however, so that after 3 to 5 weeks, pain is present even at rest.

The pathogenesis of this disorder is unknown. Schwartzman and McLellan[9] mention the possible involvement of a sympathetic dystrophy.

Sometimes after a shoulder trauma, motions appear to be restricted in a capsular pattern, but the pain radiates diffusely over the entire (particularly posterior) shoulder region. In the functional examination, passive horizontal adduction is the most limited and painful test. In this instance, a traumatic compression neuropathy of the suprascapular nerve may be responsible for the symptoms.[10] However, one way to differentiate between an arthritis and a suprascapular neuropathy is that in the suprascapular neuropathy the limited motion is active, due to muscle splinting; passively, the range of motion is full. In an arthritis of the shoulder, both the active *and* passive motions are limited.

Clinical Findings

Glenohumeral joint arthritis can be organized into three clinical stages:
Stage 1
- Pain occurs only in the shoulder or upper arm, or both.
- Pain occurs only during movement.
- Lying on the shoulder is not painful.

Stage 2

- Stage 2 is an intermediate form of stages 1 and 3.

Stage 3

- Pain radiates distal to the elbow.
- There is constant pain.
- Lying on the affected shoulder is painful.

In every stage, the functional examination reveals a capsular pattern of limitations. In stage 1, during the passive motion tests, the examiner first feels resistance to the motion, and then the patient experiences the resulting pain.

In stage 2, pain and resistance to further movement occur at the same time.

In stage 3, the patient first experiences pain, and then the examiner feels resistance to the motion.

Treatment

Treatment depends on the stage. In medical literature, many forms of therapy are described. Following are recommended treatment methods with which we have had the most success. For the most part, these methods agree with treatments described by Murnaghan.[11]

For stage 1, joint-specific mobilization, with respect for the patient's pain, is the treatment of choice.

For stage 2, if the end-feel is firm, good results can be expected from gentle, joint-specific mobilization, with respect for the patient's pain. If the end-feel is hard, the patient can best be treated with just manual traction. With the glenohumeral joint in its maximal loose-packed position, the humerus is moved perpendicularly away from the glenoid cavity.

If improvement is not achieved with mobilization, an intra-articular injection of corticosteroid and local anesthetic is indicated.

For stage 3, the treatment of choice is an intra-articular injection of corticosteroid and local anesthetic. If an injection is contraindicated, pain-relieving treatment consisting of gentle glenohumeral traction can be tried.

If a traumatic arthritis is not treated, the pain and limitations of motion continue to increase for approximately 4 months. Later, the pain gradually decreases. After about 1 year, the shoulder functions normally again. Thus, traumatic arthritis is a self-limited disorder.

Immobilization Arthritis

Immobilization arthritis can occur at any age. However, it is seen most often in elderly patients, usually after the arm (for whatever reason) has been placed in a sling or a cast for a considerable period of time. A patient with hemiplegia or other neurological lesions in which the arm is paralyzed can also develop an immobilization arthritis, particularly if the patient has received inadequate advice on exercise therapy. As a matter of fact, if proper advice and guidance were given after immobilization or in instances of arm paralysis, this disorder would not occur.

Clinical Findings

Immobilization arthritis is divided into three stages similar to those described under traumatic arthritis. In the functional examination, a capsular pattern is demonstrated.

Treatment

Prophylactic: passive range of motion exercises are given during the immobilization period. Therapeutic: treatment for immobilization arthritis is the same as that described for traumatic arthritis—it depends on the stage of the disorder.

Idiopathic Arthritis

In people between 45 and 60 years of age, a limitation of motion in a capsular pattern can occur without any previous trauma or immobilization of the shoulder. In medical literature, it is this disorder in particular that is referred to as the frozen shoulder.

One possible cause of an idiopathic arthritis is the spreading of an inflammatory reaction from the supraspinatus tendon to the joint capsule. The actual etiology is unknown, however. Some authors describe adhesions between the capsule and humeral head, particularly at the anterior aspect of the joint.[12]

In approximately 25% of all idiopathic arthritis cases, the patients have diabetes mellitus. These patients either tend to have the arthritis bilaterally, or it appears first on one side and later on the other side.[13]

Differential Diagnosis

Differential diagnosis includes other arthritides, such as rheumatoid arthritis, bacterial arthritis, ankylosing spondylitis, gout, or Reiter's disease.

Clinical Findings

The same stages described for the traumatic and immobilization arthritides are used in classifying idiopathic arthritis.

Initially, there is pain only during arm movement. The pain progresses rapidly over the next 2 months, radiating down the upper arm to the elbow and later into the forearm. At approximately 3 to 4 months, the pain is at its worst.

Patients complain of pain particularly at night, making it difficult to fall asleep, or causing them to wake up repeatedly during the night. Often, relief can be obtained by taking a few minutes to perform gentle swinging and rotational motions of the shoulder, within the limits of pain.

In the functional examination, glenohumeral motions are significantly limited in the capsular pattern.

Resisted tests are often painful, particularly abduction and internal and external rotation. Because the rotator cuff insertions and the joint capsule actually form one structure, tension in (part of) the rotator cuff provokes pain due to a pull on the affected capsule. As the pain gradually decreases, and the motion subsequently increases, pain elicited during resisted tests also diminishes.

Treatment

Without treatment, the symptoms gradually begin to decrease after about 6 months. In mild cases of idiopathic arthritis, the patient recovers completely within 1 year. In more severe cases, it can take up to 2 years to fully recover. It is very important to explain the self-limited nature of this disorder to the patient. The patient is then reassured and can decide to go on with treatment or wait for the self-healing process. In the latter case, it is recommended that the patient be seen monthly for follow-up.

Treatment consists of a series of intra-articular injections with a weak solution of corticosteroid. With this form of arthritis, it is important to keep the joint under the influence of medication so that the pain can be well tolerated. Thus, the second injection (2 mL of triamcinolone acetonide and 3 mL of 1% lidocaine) is administered 1 week after the first. If necessary, third and fourth injections can be administered to control the pain.

It is essential that the dosage of corticosteroid be kept to a minimum, otherwise the rotator cuff can become weakened. In patients with well-controlled diabetes mellitus, a corticosteroid injection can temporarily disturb the balance.

The patient is instructed to perform gentle range of motion exercises, remaining within the limits of pain, every hour during the waking day. The limitation of motion responds to this treatment much more slowly than the pain.

An alternative to the intra-articular injection series is the so-called distention therapy in which local anesthetic (in the lowest concentration possible) is injected intra-articularly in a larger amount than the joint cavity can actually contain. The goal of this technique is to break adhesions between the capsule and the humeral head. This results in an immediate increase in motion and often a significant decrease in the pain. Sometimes the same phenomenon happens during an arthrography.[14,15]

The patient must maintain the regained mobility through a daily intensive (although still remaining within the limits of pain) exercise program.

Manipulation under general anesthesia is the final choice when intra-articular injections and distention therapy do not provide satisfactory results. If performed according to the rules of arthrokinematics, the results generally are favorable.

In medical literature, opinions regarding manipulation under general anesthesia are divided.[16,17] Although mobility generally improves, according to Lundberg[18] the duration of the self-healing process is not influenced. After the manipulation under general anesthesia, a corticosteroid intra-articular injection should be given.

The remaining (painless) limitation of motion should be treated with joint-specific mobilization techniques.

Shoulder-Hand Syndrome

This relatively rare disorder is the most frequent manifestation of sympathetic dystrophy without a traumatic cause. The disorder can occur unilaterally or bilaterally, usually between the ages of 50 and 70 years.

Clinical Findings

Shoulder-hand syndrome usually begins with burning pain in the shoulder region, which increases with activity. Almost simultaneously, diffuse swelling develops, particularly at the dorsal aspect of the hand and fingers. The volar aspect of the hand is markedly hyperhidrotic.

The fingers cannot be fully extended and are held in a flexed position (capsular pattern). Even lightly touching the skin is extremely painful (hyperesthesia).

Two stages are differentiated.

Hypertrophic Stage

The hypertrophic stage is characterized by diffuse swelling of the hand, combined with hyperemia, hyperhidrosis, and severe pain in the shoulder, upper arm, and hand. A signifi-cant capsular pattern of limitations occurs in the shoulder. This stage lasts from 6 months to 1 year.

Atrophic Stage

In the atrophic stage, swelling of the hand disappears and the skin becomes taut, pale, and often cold. The pain diminishes significantly, and there is a gradual increase in the range of motion. This stage can last for years, and often there is a remaining limitation (particularly true of finger motions).

Radiographs of the hand, after approximately 3 months, show spotty atrophy of the bones in the hand (Sudeck's bone atrophy).

Treatment

- The patient should perform gentle range of motion exercises regularly.
- Every form of physical therapy by which the microcirculation is stimulated can have a positive effect, such as lymph drainage massage.
- Oral or intra-articular corticosteroids often provide some relief.
- A stellate ganglion block often results in significant improvement.

Rheumatic Polymyalgia

This rare disorder is seen primarily in patients over the age of 60. The etiology is unknown. Actually, the term "polymyalgia" is not correct, because the pathology lies in the joints, not in the muscles.

Clinical Findings

- Initially, shoulder symptoms are the patient's chief complaint. The patient complains of constant pain and stiffness in the shoulders and hips, bilaterally. The onset is usually acute.
- In the functional examination, limitations in a capsular pattern are found in the shoulders and hips, bilaterally.
- In 30% of the cases, temporal arteritis is also present. This disorder must be identified quickly; otherwise circulation to

the eye can be affected, leading to irreversible sight impairment.

- When suspecting this disorder, the examiner should always specifically question whether the patient is experiencing headaches or disturbed vision.
- General symptoms such as loss of appetite, weight loss, and general malaise also accompany rheumatic polymyalgia.

Treatment

Treatment should be administered by a physician. Usually administration of oral corticosteroids is begun immediately.

Arthrosis (Osteoarthrosis)

Arthrosis is seen less often in the glenohumeral joint than in the knee or hip joints. Usually, it develops after a trauma or some other disorder (particularly septic arthritis). In other words, glenohumeral arthrosis is generally a secondary disorder.

In arthrosis, a mild trauma, (relative) overuse, or immobilization can lead quickly to a traumatic (in the first two instances) or immobilization arthritis.

Clinical Findings

- Most of the time, patients with glenohumeral arthrosis experience minimal or no pain.
- Crepitation is often clearly audible or palpable.
- The functional examinations reveal slight limitations of motion in a capsular pattern.

Treatment

- If the shoulder arthrosis does not provoke symptoms, treatment is not indicated.
- If a traumatic or immobilization arthritis occurs based on the arthrosis, treatment depends on the stage of the arthritis. (Refer to Traumatic Arthritis for suggested treatment.)

Milwaukee Shoulder (Rotator Cuff Tear Arthropathy)

In 1981 Garancis et al.[19] described a type of shoulder pathology, which they termed *Milwaukee shoulder*. This disorder is observed mostly in elderly people, usually women, who have glenohumeral arthritis in conjunction with a complete (full thickness) tear of the rotator cuff. Neer et al.[20] described the same lesion, but they called it "rotator cuff tear arthropathy." Approximately 4% of all total (full thickness) ruptures of the rotator cuff develop a rotator cuff tear arthropathy.

Neer et al. performed total shoulder replacement surgery on 26 shoulders with this disorder. Women were involved in 75% of the cases. The average age was 69 years, and 20% of the patients had the problem bilaterally. Because trauma was involved in only 25% of the cases, a degenerative etiology was suspected.

Clinical Findings

- The patient complains of pain and limited motion.
- On inspection, marked swelling of the shoulder is noted, along with atrophy of the musculature. There is almost always a rupture of the tendon of the long head of the biceps.
- Active and passive arm elevation is possible to only approximately 90°. Passive external rotation is limited by approximately 60°, glenohumeral abduction is limited by approximately 40°, and internal rotation is limited by approximately 20°. Thus, there is a capsular pattern of limited motions. Resisted abduction and external rotation are very weak.
- Usually, radiographs demonstrate collapse of the proximal part of the humeral head (Figure 4–1). Erosion of the glenoid cavity, greater tubercle, and both acromioclavicular joint surfaces also often is visible.

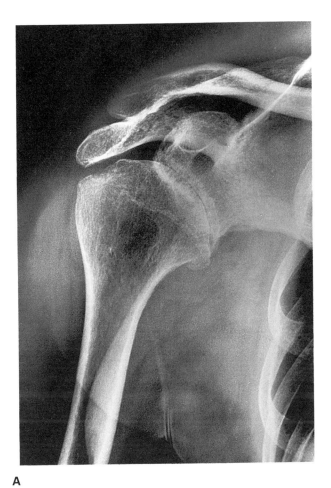

A

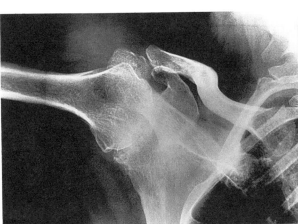

B

Figure 4–1 Conventional radiograph showing severe arthrotic changes in the glenohumeral joint. **A**, Relaxed position; **B**, maximal elevation.

Treatment

Treatment in these rare cases is not simple, and it is still in an experimental phase.[21] Various operative procedures for total shoulder replacement are being tried.

PATHOLOGY WITH LIMITED MOTIONS IN A NONCAPSULAR PATTERN

Pain and limited range of motion in a noncapsular pattern can be caused by a number of shoulder disorders. One frequent cause for a solitary limitation in external rotation, internal rotation, or arm elevation is glenohumeral instability. In this instance, increased motion is usually noted in another motion. This phenomenon occurs as a result of a malalignment of the joint surfaces. (Refer to the sections on instability for more detailed information.)

Although tightness of the posterior capsule may not cause pain in itself, it often leads to a subacromial-subdeltoid bursitis. In this instance, the functional examination indicates the bursitis, but a slight limitation of motion in internal rotation is also found. (Refer to the section on subacromial-subdeltoid bursitis for more detailed information.)

Another cause of a noncapsular limitation of glenohumeral motions is a loose body (Figures 4–2 to 4–4).

In rare cases, an incomprehensible limitation of motion is caused by a tumor in or around the joint (Figure 4–5).

Severe limitations of motion in a noncapsular pattern are also seen in instances of acute dislocation of the glenohumeral, sternoclavicular, or acromioclavicular joints; in fractures; and in acute subacromial-subdeltoid bursitis.

Loose Bodies

Loose bodies can result from trauma, osteochondrosis dissecans, synovial osteochondromatosis, or unknown causes.

Clinical Findings

- Usually, symptoms include sudden locking of the joint and limitation of one or more motions.
- In weight lifters, sometimes a loose body is found in the subscapular bursa (between the tendon of the subscapularis and the joint). In this case, horizontal adduction is the most painful and limited motion.
- Since the development of shoulder arthroscopy, the diagnosis of loose bodies occurs much more frequently than before.

Treatment

Treatment is almost always by means of arthroscopy.

PATHOLOGY OF THE CAPSULOLIGAMENTOUS COMPLEX

Anterior and Anteroinferior Instability

Anterior and anteroinferior instabilities can be traumatically induced or become habitual. Differentiation is made between subluxation and dislocation.

Subluxation

Most of the time, subluxation is a typical sports injury, related to throwing (Figure 4–6), using a racket, or swimming.

During movements such as throwing, serving, smashing, and backstroke, particularly when the arm is in maximal glenohumeral abduction, extension, and external rotation (the so-called late cocking phase), the anterior and anteroinferior aspects of the joint capsule endure an enormous amount of tension. The same holds true for the tendon of the subscapularis. In addition, several structures at the posterior aspect of the joint are compressed, particularly the posterior capsule, the glenoid labrum, and the infraspinatus insertion. (If one of the latter three structures is injured, this compression provokes

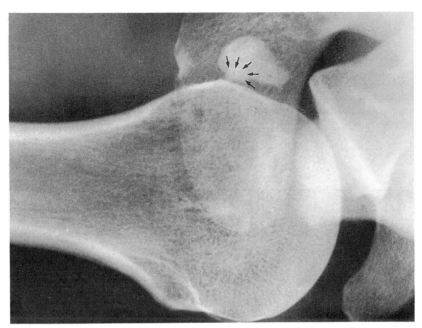

Figure 4–2 Conventional radiograph, view from above. There is a large loose body in the abducted glenohumeral joint. In this view, the loose body (**arrows**) is partially covered by a calcification in the tendon of the supraspinatus muscle. In this case, the etiology is unknown. The diagnosis was arthroscopically confirmed.

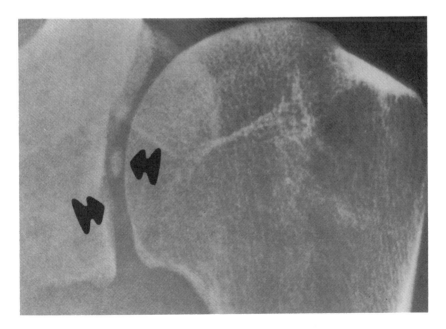

Figure 4–3 Conventional radiograph: osteochondrosis dissecans of the glenoid cavity. A loose body is visible between the glenoid cavity and the humeral head. In addition, there is a defect in the glenoid cavity.

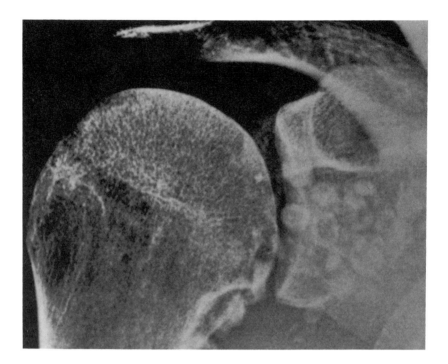

Figure 4–4 Multiple loose bodies in the glenohumeral joint. In this case, the loose bodies are the result of synovial osteochondromatosis.

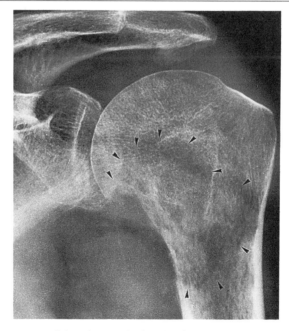

Figure 4–5 Malignant tumor medial to the surgical neck of the humerus. There is irregular decalcification in the spongiosa of the humeral head and neck with erosion of the edge of the medial aspect of the surgical neck. This radiograph was made after finding a severe noncapsular pattern of limited shoulder motions.

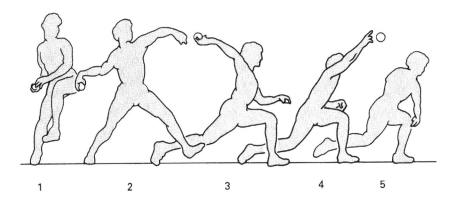

1   2   3   4   5

Figure 4–6 The five phases of throwing. Analysis of the throwing movement in baseball: With minor differences, this analysis can be adapted to the various phases in all throwing, smashing, and serving movements. **1**, *Wind up*, or preparation phase—preparatory activity in which the shoulder muscles demonstrate minimal activity (the emphasis lies in trunk rotation while the ball is held with both hands); **2**, *early cocking*—abduction and external rotation of the shoulder, which begins the instant the nonthrowing hand lets go of the ball; **3**, *late cocking*—this phase begins when the forward foot contacts the ground (the phase ends the instant the shoulder is maximally externally rotated); **4**, *acceleration*—the phase in which the shoulder is moved forward (this phase ends the instant the ball leaves the hand); **5**, *follow-through*—the end of the throwing motion, in which the arm is decelerated in front of the body. *Source:* Glousman R, et al. Dynamic electromyographic analysis of the throwing shoulder with glenohumeral instability. *Journal of Bone and Joint Surgery.* 1988; Vol. 70A, 2:220–226.[3]

the typical posterior shoulder pain about which throwing athletes, tennis players, and swimmers so often complain.)

Normally the humeral head shifts slightly posterior during early cocking. This posterior shift results because the posterior rolling component of the movement is larger than the simultaneous "compensatory" anterior gliding. During late cocking, the shift increases because of stretch on the intact anterior structures.[22,23]

Instability caused by excessive or repeated throwing-like motions has two possible mechanisms of injury: the anterior structures remain strong while the posterior structures fail, or the anterior structures weaken with a resultant change in the arthrokinematic behavior of the humeral head. If the anterior and anteroinferior capsule as well as the subscapularis tendon stretch out, the humeral head shifts anteriorly instead of posteriorly during early and late cocking motions. The anterior glide component of the motion becomes larger than the posterior rolling (Figure 4–7).

During late cocking, overstretch of the subscapularis and anterior capsule causes pain. Immediately after the "late cocking" motion, during the acceleration phase, the subscapularis and other internal rotators and adductors (particularly the latissimus dorsi) should normally contract forcefully. However, when there is pain present, the contraction is inadequate or absent. Dynamic electromyographic (EMG) research by Glousman et al.[3] clearly demonstrates this phenomenon (Figures 4–8 and 4–9).

The serratus anterior, which moves the scapula forward during the acceleration phase, also shows decreased EMG activity (Figure 4–10). Thus, it is important to incorporate serratus anterior exercises in the rehabilitation program of an anterior or anteroinferior instability.

In an attempt to stabilize the humeral head, the supraspinatus, infraspinatus, and biceps

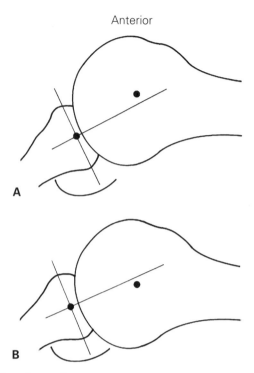

Figure 4–7 Representation of an axillary radiograph of a patient with an anterior shoulder instability (**A**) and of a normal shoulder (**B**). **A**, Abnormal anterior translation of the humeral head (3 mm) when the shoulder is in the late cocking position; **B**, diagram of a normal shoulder: a posterior translation occurs.

muscles perform extra work. The deltoid muscle demonstrates no changes during throwing in athletes with unstable shoulders.

Anterior subluxations occur most often in persons whose glenohumeral ligaments (particularly the medial and inferior glenohumeral ligaments) (Figure 4–11) are either poorly developed or absent. Of course, this form of instability can also occur in nonathletes as a result of a trauma in which the arm is forced into abduction (extension) and external rotation.

Anterior or anteroinferior instabilities are often seen in combination with an impingement syndrome. In athletes participating in throwing sports, lesions of supraspinatus insertion and (less often) the tendon of the long head of the biceps frequently occur because of instability. The latter case is often observed during arthroscopy and has little clinical significance. Eventually, the subacromial-sub-

deltoid bursa and the acromioclavicular joint also undergo pathological changes.

An instability can be anticipated from the patient's history: an instability causes pain particularly during the late cocking phase, while impingement problems cause pain particularly during the acceleration phase. As the problem becomes more chronic, the patient also complains of pain on top of the shoulder caused by secondary acromioclavicular problems.

Clinical Findings

The patient complains of an inability to throw, serve, smash, or perform the backstroke forcefully. Sharp shooting pain is experienced when attempting one of these movements. Depending on the severity of the problem, pain can radiate down into the fingertips. Symptoms can also include a "para-

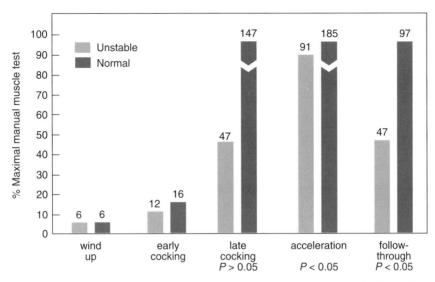

Figure 4–8 Activity of the subscapularis muscle in a shoulder with an anterior instability compared with a normal shoulder.[24] There is a statistically significant difference between the groups ($P < 0.05$).

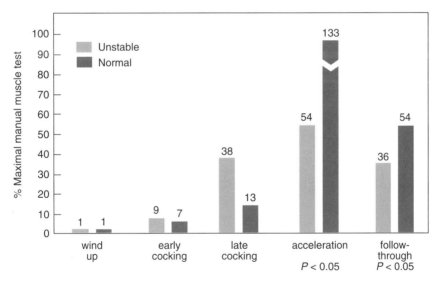

Figure 4–9 Activity of the latissimus dorsi muscle in a shoulder with an anterior instability compared with a normal shoulder.[3] There is a statistically significant difference between the groups ($P < 0.05$).

lyzed" or "dead" feeling in the arm, the so-called dead arm syndrome. This acute pain disappears rather quickly, but the arm sometimes feels weak and sore for several hours afterward.

Approximately 50% of all patients actually feel the subluxation ("it's as if the arm goes out of joint"). Sometimes they also describe feeling a click.

Functional Examination

Passive external rotation can be painful due to a stretch of the anterior structures. Because the rotator cuff muscles have to

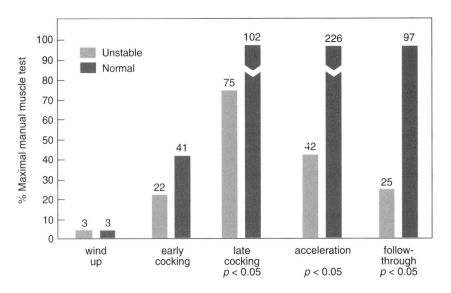

Figure 4–10 Activity of the serratus anterior muscle in a shoulder with an anterior instability compared with a normal shoulder.[3] There is a statistically significant difference between the groups ($P < 0.05$).

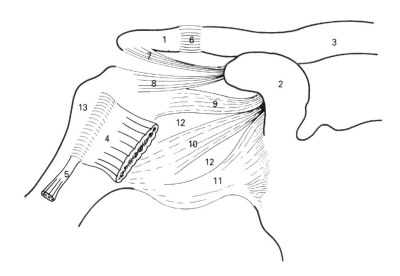

Figure 4–11 The glenohumeral joint capsule, anterior view. **1**, Acromion; **2**, coracoid process; **3**, clavicle; **4**, subscapularis muscle; **5**, long head of the biceps muscle; **6**, acromioclavicular joint; **7**, coracoacromial ligament; **8**, coracohumeral ligament; **9**, superior glenohumeral ligament; **10**, middle glenohumeral ligament; **11**, inferior glenohumeral ligament; **12**, articular capsule; **13**, transverse ligament.

compensate for the lack of intrinsic stability, insertion tendopathies can result from overuse. Thus, frequently, one or more resisted tests (particularly abduction or external rotation) will cause pain. Passive internal rotation can also cause pain due to a stretch on the supraspinatus or infraspinatus tendons.

Significant stability tests include the throwing, external rotation, anterior subluxation (should be performed only in instances of doubtful instability), and anterior drawer tests. While undergoing these tests, the patient may react with sudden forceful muscle splinting. This reaction is commonly termed *apprehension*.

If a patient experiences a painful click during the stability tests, a lesion of the glenoid labrum (the so-called Bankart lesion) should be suspected (Figure 4–12). A Bankart lesion is often seen in conjunction with a Hill-Sachs lesion, which is an impression of the humeral head caused by pressure of the labrum against the head in the subluxated position (Figures 4–13 and 4–14).

Treatment

Treatment is primarily focused on the cause of the problem. Athletes participating in throwing and racket sports should have their techniques evaluated.

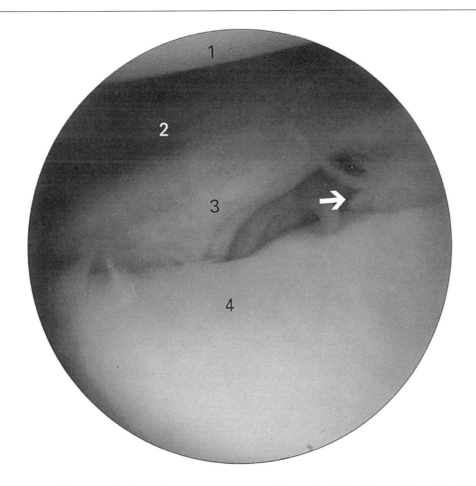

Figure 4–12 Arthroscopic view demonstrates a tear *(arrow)* of the labrum from the glenoid. **1**, Humeral head; **2**, capsule; **3**, labrum; **4**, anterior edge of the glenoid.

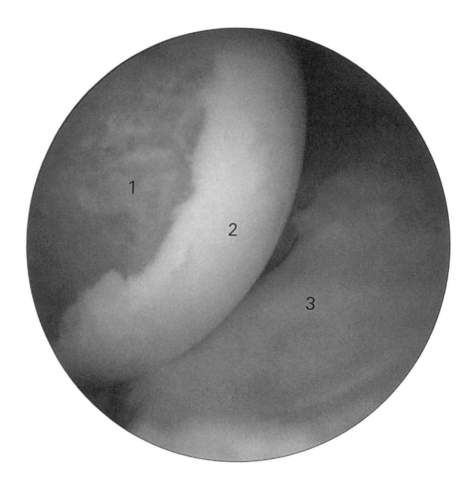

Figure 4–13 Arthroscopic view in the same patient as in Figure 4–12, but now from more posterior in the joint. **1**, Hill-Sachs lesion: the cartilage is completely gone from the humeral head; **2**, cartilage of the intact part of the humeral head; **3**, glenoid.

During throwing or serving motions, the hand should be brought over the shoulder through the sagittal plane. The further the hand is from the sagittal plane in which the shoulder lies, the more force is applied against the inferior capsuloligamentous structures. For an athlete with poor technique, this often means significantly changing "bad" habits. However, if the technique cannot be remedied, the patient's only options are to undergo corrective surgery or quit the sports activity entirely. Surgery may repair the damage, but the technique must still be changed.

Occasionally, the athlete is unable to acquire the proper technique due to lack of motion in a neighboring joint, or junction. For example, the pectoral muscles may be tight (possibly due to a protracted position of the shoulders) or there may be hypomobility of the thoracic spine. If this is the case, the causal treatment is first aimed at increasing muscle length through stretching or increasing thoracic range of motion through mobili-

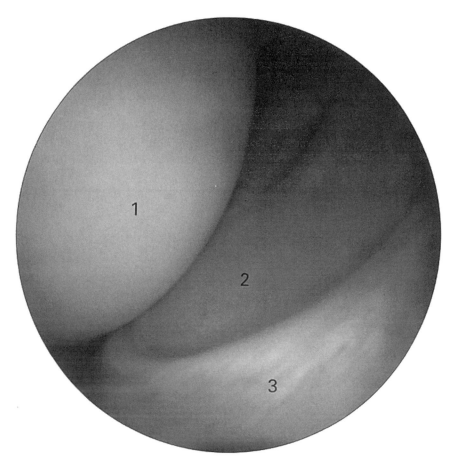

Figure 4–14 Arthroscopic view in the same position as in Figure 4–13, but now in a normal shoulder. **1**, Humeral head; **2**, glenoid; **3**, posterior capsule.

zation, and then improving the throwing technique.

Accompanying insertion tendopathies are treated with local transverse friction and cautious stretching.

As soon as the resisted tests are negative, isometric and isokinetic muscle strengthening should be initiated. Emphasis is placed on strengthening the shoulder adductors and internal rotators, as well as the serratus anterior.[24]

In therapy-resistant cases (minimal to no improvement after 6 months of treatment), arthroscopic evaluation and treatment may be indicated. In these instances, there is often a labrum lesion at the level of the insertion of the long head of the biceps (Figure 4–15).

Dislocation (Luxation)

Traumatic dislocations are usually caused by a force applied against the abducted, externally rotated arm. Once the capsule is torn, recurrent dislocations happen easily. Repeated dislocations can ultimately lead to habitual dislocation. In other words, the glenohumeral joint dislocates (almost) every time the shoulder is brought into a certain position. In the case of anterior dislocation (Figures 4–16 and 4–17). This happens especially in abduction and external rotation.

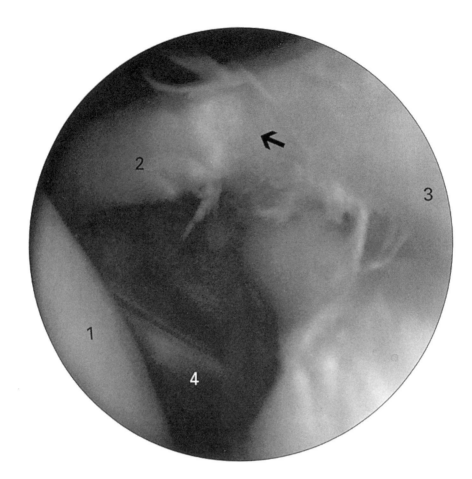

Figure 4–15 Arthroscopic view demonstrating a so-called SLAP (superior labrum, anterior to posterior) lesion, a lesion of the glenoid labrum at the level of the insertion of the tendon of the long head of the biceps. In this case there is an obvious tear *(arrow)*. **1**, Humeral head; **2**, tendon of the long head of the biceps; **3**, glenoid labrum; **4**, subscapularis tendon.

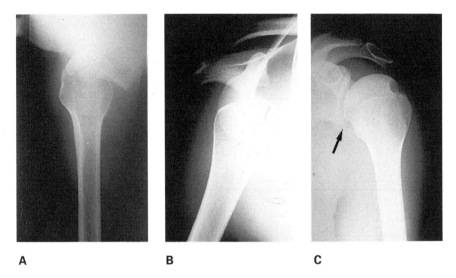

A   B   C

Figure 4–16 Conventional radiograph of an anteroinferiorly dislocated shoulder. **A**, Axial view: the humeral head is located anterior (right) to the glenoid; **B**, anteroposterior view: in this view, the anteroinferior dislocation is best visualized; **C**, in internal rotation, the Hill-Sachs lesion is visible *(arrow)*.

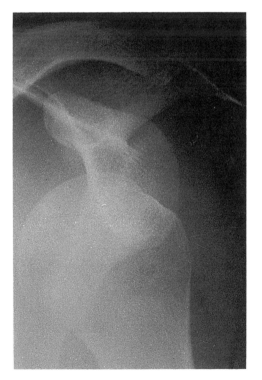

Figure 4–17 Conventional radiograph: Anterior dislocation of the shoulder.

Clinical Findings

In a traumatic anterior dislocation, the patient experiences severe pain. The contour of the shoulder changes: the normal curve of the deltoid is flattened or there may be an obvious lateral indentation. The patient supports the arm in an adducted position in front of the body. In instances of traumatic dislocation, radiology should be used to rule out the possibility of a fracture.

In cases of habitual dislocation, the patient experiences much less pain in comparison to traumatic cases. The anterior instability tests will produce pain or discomfort.

Treatment

Traumatic dislocations should be repositioned by an orthopaedic surgeon.

Habitual dislocation is treated in the same way as habitual subluxation. Unfortunately, results are often poor in conservative treatment with athletes participating in throwing and racket sports. In these instances, surgical treatment is indicated (Figure 4–18). Cur-

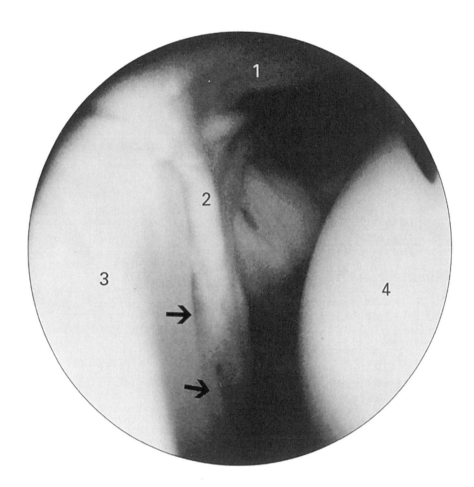

Figure 4–18 Arthroscopic view of a shoulder with recurrent anterior dislocations. On this view, significant posttraumatic and degenerative lesions of the glenoid labrum can be seen. The lesions *(arrow)* are the result of recurrent anterior shoulder dislocations. At the top of the view, the insertion of the long head of the biceps is visible. **1**, Tendon of the long head of the biceps brachii muscle; **2**, glenoid labrum; **3**, glenoid cavity; **4**, humeral head.

rently, functional stabilization through reconstruction of the capsuloligamentous complex is replacing the extraarticular stabilization as the operation of choice. The advantage to the former procedure is that the postsurgical function is much better. For instance, the external rotation usually has full range of motion. This full range of motion is very important for any athlete participating in throwing or racket sports, and for swimmers as well.

Posterior Instability

Using clinical and radiological techniques, diagnosis of posterior instability is often missed.

As with anterior instability, in a posterior instability both subluxations as well as complete dislocations can occur. Posterior subluxations and dislocations usually result from falling on the abducted arm or from a forced internal rotation of the glenohumeral joint.

Posterior instability often occurs in combination with anterior and inferior instability.

Clinical Findings

Sometimes patients complain only of pain, weakness, or an unstable feeling when load is placed on the flexed and internally rotated shoulder (such as when performing push-ups). Occasionally patients are able to subluxate actively (or even dislocate) their shoulder(s) by performing a flexion and internal rotation movement.

A traumatic posterior shoulder dislocation is extremely painful and the patient holds the arm in adduction and internal rotation. On the radiograph, the dislocation is difficult to identify; in the most obvious cases, the edge of the glenoid cavity is projected too far laterally (Figure 4–19).

Functional Examination

In posterior instabilities, the posterior drawer test demonstrates increased motion, often with a click, in comparison to the other side.

Treatment

Because posterior instability often occurs as part of a complex instability, all of the muscles around the shoulder require strengthening, both isometrically and isokinetically. If there is an isolated lesion, the shoulder extensors and external rotators are emphasized in the rehabilitative exercise program.

Conservative rehabilitation treatments should be performed for at least 6 months in order to prevent reoccurrence.

If therapeutic results are unsatisfactory, surgical treatment is indicated.

In traumatic posterior shoulder dislocations, the humerus is repositioned by performing a very slow external rotation while pulling on the arm.

Inferior Instability

An inferior instability is almost always one component of a complex instability.

Clinical Findings

This form of instability is usually part of a complex instability, and all of the clinical findings from the anterior and posterior instabilities may apply. Often the patient is able actively to dislocate the shoulder inferiorly.

Functional Examination

Refer to the sections on anterior and posterior instability.

When exerting an inferior pull on the arm, a significant amount of space is visible (and palpable) between the acromion and humeral head.

Treatment

If the inferior instability is an isolated problem, isometric and isokinetic muscle strengthening can be tried in order to stabilize the shoulder. Emphasis is placed on the supraspinatus and deltoid muscles.

If the inferior instability is part of a complex shoulder instability, all of the shoulder muscles should undergo rehabilitative treatment for at least 6 months.

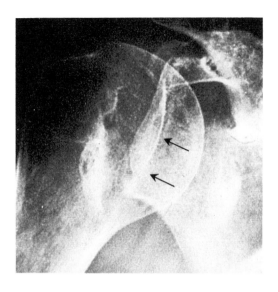

Figure 4–19 Conventional anteroposterior radiograph of the right shoulder: posterior dislocation. The edge of the glenoid cavity is projected too far laterally *(arrows)*.

As with other instabilities, if results are unsatisfactory after at least 6 months of treatment, surgery is indicated.

Complex Instability

This form of shoulder instability occurs relatively often. It involves instabilities in two or more directions and may be a combination of anterior, posterior, and inferior.

Clinical Findings

Refer to the clinical findings and functional examinations described under the sections on anterior, posterior, and inferior instabilities.

Treatment

Refer to treatment as described under the sections on anterior, posterior, and inferior instabilities.

4.2   ACROMIOCLAVICULAR JOINT PATHOLOGY

Pathology of the acromioclavicular (AC) joint can be primary or secondary. Primary disorders are almost always the result of direct or indirect trauma. Secondary acromioclavicular joint pathology is often seen in patients with chronic shoulder problems, regardless of the type of problem.

Almost every shoulder (girdle) dysfunction eventually leads to overuse of the AC joint, which in turn causes degenerative changes in the joint. Because of disturbances in joint function, the clavicle reaches its end position too early during arm elevation. Ultimately, this can lead to compression of the brachial plexus in the thoracic outlet.

After a trauma of the AC joint, secondary changes often occur. These changes can include degenerative changes of the joint, osteolysis, and periarticular calcifications.

Differentiation is made between traumatic and nontraumatic lesions.

TRAUMATIC LESIONS

Traumatic lesions of the AC joint are classified according to the severity of the lesion (in other words, the number of structures that have been injured). The classification was first established by Tossy et al.[25] in 1963. Allman[26] modified the classification in 1967, and more recently, further modifications were made by Post[27] and Rockwood and Young.[28] The following classification is described according to Allman, and supplemented by Rockwood and Young.[28]

Mechanism of Injury

The most frequent AC joint trauma is a direct trauma, such as falling on top of the shoulder (acromion) with the arm adducted and slightly internally rotated. In this instance, the scapula is forcefully moved in a caudal direction. This results in a lesion of the AC ligaments, the coracoclavicular ligaments, and possibly including a clavicle fracture, sometimes combined with a fracture of the coracoid process. If the clavicle does not fracture, a sequence of injuries occurs depending on the force of the trauma: first the AC ligaments are sprained, then they rupture, next the acromioclavicular ligaments are sprained, followed by a rupture, and finally the deltoid and trapezius insertions tear away from the clavicle. At that point, the ligamentous connection between the upper extremity and lateral end of the clavicle is severed. A sagging of the entire upper extremity occurs in relation to the clavicle (which remains relatively in place).

In medical literature regarding dislocations of the AC joint, focus is almost always placed on the "elevated" position of the clavicle. In reality, there is minimal upward displacement of the clavicle due to pull from the trapezius.

Another form of direct trauma is a severe blow against the cranial aspect of the lateral end of the clavicle, in which the arm is positioned in abduction and the scapula in retraction. According to Rockwood and Young,[28] this results in a type VI lesion.

In rare cases, an indirect trauma causes an AC lesion. For instance, a fall on the outstretched hand in which the humeral head is pushed against the acromion can result in a solitary lesion of the AC ligament. In severe cases, a fracture of the acromion occurs.

Classification According to Allman[26] and Rockwood and Young[28]

Type I.
- Acromioclavicular ligaments are sprained.
- AC joint is intact.
- Coracoclavicular ligaments are intact.
- Deltoid and trapezius are intact.

Type II.
- AC capsuloligamentous complex ruptures.

- AC joint space widens: the acromion is slightly lower in comparison to the nonaffected side.
- Coracoclavicular ligaments are sprained.
- Sometimes the coracoclavicular space slightly increases (visible on a radiograph).
- Deltoid and trapezius muscles are intact.

Type III.
- AC capsuloligamentous complex ruptures.
- AC joint dislocates; the upper extremity (plus scapula) is displaced distally in relation to the clavicle.
- Coracoclavicular ligaments rupture.
- Coracoclavicular distance increases 25% to 100% in relation to the nonaffected side.
- Deltoid and trapezius muscles are usually torn from the lateral end of the clavicle.
- In children under 13 years of age, a clavicle fracture usually occurs. Sometimes a pseudodislocation occurs: the scapula dislocates caudally and the intact coracoclavicular ligaments pull the periosteum from the clavicle.
- In rare cases, the coracoid process fractures.

Type IV.
- AC capsuloligamentous complex ruptures.
- AC joint dislocates; the clavicle is displaced dorsally in or through the trapezius muscle.
- Coracoclavicular ligaments rupture.
- Due to posterior displacement, the coracoclavicular distance appears normal on the anteroposterior radiographs.
- Deltoid and trapezius muscles tear away from the lateral end of the clavicle.

Type V.

- AC capsuloligamentous complex ruptures.
- AC joint severely dislocates. Due to spasm of the trapezius, the clavicle is sometimes pulled upward as far as the base of the neck.
- Coracoclavicular ligaments rupture.
- Coracoclavicular distance can be up to 300% greater than on the nonaffected side.
- Deltoid and trapezius muscles tear away from the lateral end of the clavicle.

Type VI.

- AC capsuloligamentous complex ruptures.
- AC joint dislocates; the clavicle is displaced caudally in relation to the acromion and coracoid process.
- Coracoclavicular ligaments rupture.
- Coracoclavicular distance diminishes.
- Deltoid and trapezius muscles tear away from the lateral end of the clavicle.

Dislocations are seen four times more often in the AC joint than in the sternoclavicular joint. The lesion is seen more frequently in men than in women; in medical literature the numbers vary from 5:1 to 10:1.[28]

Clinical Findings

Type I.

- There is tenderness and mild pain at the AC joint.
- Sometimes there is a high, painful arc (160°–180°) during active arm elevation.
- Passive horizontal adduction is painful; usually passive adduction with the arm behind the back is also painful.
- Passive arm elevation, external rotation, and internal rotation can be painful at the end-range of motion.

- Resisted adduction is often painful; occasionally resisted abduction is painful.

Type II.

- There is moderate to severe local pain.
- There is tenderness in the region of the coracoclavicular space.
- The clavicle may appear to be slightly higher than the acromion (actually, the acromion is positioned lower than the clavicle) (Figure 4–20).
- All passive motions are painful at the end-range of motion; horizontal adduction is the most painful motion.
- Usually both resisted adduction and resisted abduction are painful.
- Passive posteroanterior translation of the clavicle in relation to the acromion is abnormally large.
- Sometimes there is a slight "piano key" phenomenon: after pushing the clavicle caudally, it springs back to its original position.

Type III.

- The patient with a complete dislocation of the AC joint usually holds the arm in a slightly adducted position against the body, exerting upward axial pressure through the humerus in order to decrease the pain.
- Usually an obvious gap is visible between the acromion and the clavicle (Figure 4–21).
- Usually the pain is moderate, although at first it is quite severe.
- All active motions are painful, especially abduction.
- Passive motions usually have full range of motion if performed very cautiously.
- Palpation of the AC joint, the coracoacromial space, and the cranial lateral one fourth of the clavicle is painful.
- The piano key phenomenon is evident.
- Most of the resisted tests are painful.

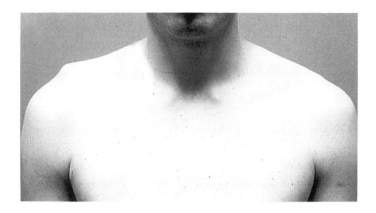

Figure 4–20 Clinical view of an acromioclavicular subluxation, type II. The lateral aspect of the clavicle can be clearly seen.

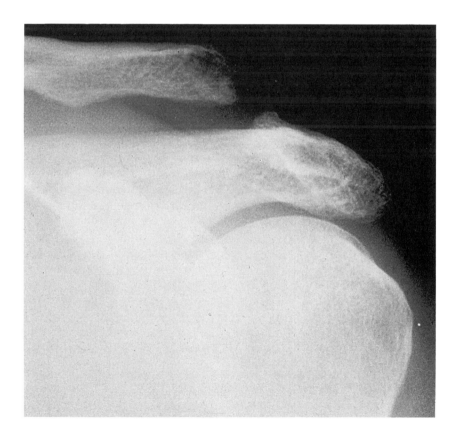

Figure 4–21 Acromioclavicular dislocation, type III. The scapula is dislocated caudally in relation to the clavicle.

Type IV.

- More or less the same clinical findings are found as in type III, except that here the patient has severe pain, and the clavicle is displaced posteriorly. This is particularly obvious when inspecting the AC joint from above. Sometimes the clavicle pushes the skin further posteriorly.
- Passive and resisted motions are much more painful than in type III.

Type V.

- This is the worst form of type III; the distance between the clavicle and coracoid process is extremely large, and is sometimes accentuated because of a spasm of the trapezius, which pulls the clavicle upward.
- Pain is more severe than in type III.
- There is tenderness to palpation over the entire lateral half of the clavicle, due to tearing of the soft tissue structures.

Type VI.

- The cranial aspect of the affected shoulder is flatter than the nonaffected side.
- The acromion appears to be higher (on palpation) than the clavicle (although it is the clavicle that is actually lower).
- Often there are fractures of the clavicle and upper ribs, as well as injury to the brachial plexus. Because of the severe amount of swelling, this lesion is not always recognized.

Supplementary Examination

Radiological examination is necessary for every lesion except type I. In order to visualize the AC joint, a special view is made. One technique, the so-called Zanka technique, visualizes the AC joint in an anteroposterior direction from an angle of 10° to 15° below the horizontal.

Stress views should also be taken. A 5- to 8-kg weight is attached to the arm,which allows for better evaluation of the coracoclavicular distance. When examined in this manner, a le-sion that appears to be type II can actually turn out to be type III (due to the weight, the coracoclavicular distance increases).

Treatment

Type I. Local treatments, such as transverse friction massage and application of ice, are administered to relieve pain. Active range of motion exercises should be performed within the limits of pain. Full recovery should be attained in 1 to 2 weeks.

Type II. Although medical literature is in agreement that treatment should be conservative, the suggested treatment programs differ greatly. Usually a bandage, a brace, or a cast is applied with the clavicle in depression in order to bring the ruptured structures closer to each other. Unfortunately, stabilizing the clavicle in depression often leads to compression of the brachial plexus in the costoclavicular space.

In actuality, however, the scapula and arm have dislocated distally; the clavicle has not dislocated superiorly. Thus, it would be more logical to devise a brace in which the entire arm is brought up toward the clavicle. In such a brace, compression of the brachial plexus could be prevented.

Our best results have been obtained with immediate range of motion exercises, both actively and passively, within the limits of pain. This is initiated on the day of the trauma, along with ice applications.

From the fourth day postinjury, transverse friction massage is used to relieve pain.

In rare instances, when improvement is not noted with this treatment program, there may be interposition of soft tissue or an internal derangement due to a detached disc or meniscus in the joint. In such cases, surgical treatment is indicated.

Type III. Medical literature differs greatly regarding the appropriate treatment of type III lesions. There are strong advocates of conservative as well as operative treatment.

In 1989, Bannister et al.[29] published research involving 60 patients. Thirty-three patients were conservatively treated, and 27 were surgically treated. The follow-up averaged 4 years (in 54 patients). The patients who were treated conservatively recovered motion significantly faster and returned to work and sports-related activities earlier than the patients who underwent surgery. Only when the coracoacromial distance was greater than 2 cm did the surgical patients have a better score. Bannister et al. conclude that conservative treatment is the treatment of choice for the majority of acute dislocations. Younger patients with severe dislocation, however, benefit from early operative reduction and stabilization.

Dias et al.[30] published their own research concerning 44 patients who were conservatively treated for AC joint dislocations (and had long-term follow-up of an average of 5 years), along with a comparative literature review on operative versus conservative treatment. Dias et al. conclude that subjective and objective results were satisfactory in every case, except in one with a painful dislocation. From the literature review, results were poor in only 7 of the 185 conservatively treated patients. Of the 181 surgically treated patients, the results were poor in 16 cases; this is over 100% more than in the conservatively treated group.

Wojtys and Nelson[31] evaluated strength and endurance in 22 patients with a type III dislocation. Strength and endurance of the affected shoulder were compared with that of the nonaffected shoulder. Along with a low discomfort level, the long-term follow-up (average 2.6 years) indicated only slight tenderness in the AC joint area after performing vigorous activities with the shoulder.

Regarding the type of conservative treatment, there is also little agreement. Almost all of the authors immobilize the joint for a period of 3 to 6 weeks. Afterward, an exercise program is initiated, either with or without guidance. None of the authors described their precise rehabilitation program.

Our rehabilitation begins the day after the trauma with range of motion exercises, staying within the limits of pain. The patient is instructed to grasp the affected arm at the elbow and push axially upward through the humerus. From this position, shoulder girdle elevation, protraction, and retraction are performed. During these exercises, the patient ipsilaterally sidebends the head in order to take tension off the injured trapezius muscle. As soon as possible, usually after a few days, the other arm motions are performed in the same manner as the initial exercises (in other words, assisted by the other hand). Most patients are able to resume training for sports within 2 to 3 weeks.

When a springy, rubberlike end-feel is found during passive upward movement of the scapula (achieved by exerting axial pressure upward through the humerus) with simultaneous fixation of the clavicle (opposite performance of the piano key test), there is probably soft tissue or articular disc or meniscus interposition in the joint. In these cases, conservative therapy is usually unsuccessful, particularly when this phenomenon is still present 2 weeks after the trauma. Surgery is indicated.

Types IV, V, and VI. Because the dislocation is so severe and disfigurement remains after conservative treatment, surgery is indicated.

Complications

In both the conservatively treated and surgically treated patients, symptoms occasionally arise again, months to years later. This is usually due to degenerative changes in the joint, which are generally not significant enough to warrant treatment.

If the patient requires treatment for degenerative changes in the AC joint, therapy should first consist of joint-specific mobilization. If adequate improvement is not achieved, an intra-articular injection of corticosteroid is indicated. If an injection does not provide acceptable results, resection of the lateral 2 cm of the clavicle may be necessary.[28]

Follow-up studies of patients who have experienced AC dislocations indicate that calcification of the coracoclavicular ligaments occurs frequently. Less often there is an osteolysis of the clavicle. Neither of these complications necessarily causes symptoms.

If dislocation recurs, operative stabilization is indicated. Recurrence is also seen in surgically treated patients, moreover, at a slightly higher rate than in patients conservatively treated.

Clavicle fractures can be treated either conservatively or surgically. The rare, coracoid fracture should be surgically treated.

NONTRAUMATIC LESIONS

Arthritis

As in every joint, arthritis can also occur in the AC joint. Rheumatoid arthritis is the most frequently seen nontraumatic arthritis in this joint.

Clinical Findings

The patient complains of local pain in the C4 dermatome. In the functional examination all passive shoulder movements are painful at the end-range of motion, and may be very slightly limited. Horizontal adduction is generally the most painful and limited motion.

Treatment

In both acute and chronic cases, the pain is treated by administering one or more intra-articular injections of corticosteroid.

Arthrosis (Osteoarthrosis)

Arthrosis of the AC joint is usually a secondary disorder (Figures 4–22 and 4–23). Treatment should consist first of joint-specific mobilization. If adequate improvement is not noted, an intra-articular injection of corticosteroid is indicated. If an injection does not provide sufficient results, resection of the lateral 2 cm of the clavicle may be indicated.[28]

Primary arthrosis often occurs but rarely causes problems. If treatment is necessary, it is the same as described for secondary arthrosis: joint-specific mobilization and, if needed, an intra-articular injection.

Osteolysis

In most cases, osteolysis is the result of a past trauma, usually a dislocation or, less often, a fracture (Figure 4–24). Occasionally this secondary osteolysis leads to subsequent

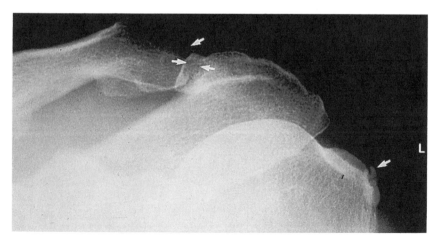

Figure 4–22 Conventional radiograph. Past patient history of an AC dislocation. Arthrotic changes are visible (**arrows**).

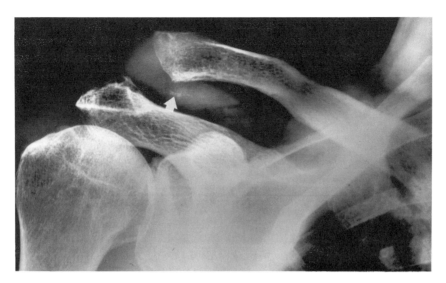

Figure 4–23 Conventional radiograph. Chronic, complete dislocation of the AC joint. An avulsion fracture exists at the caudal aspect of the clavicle.

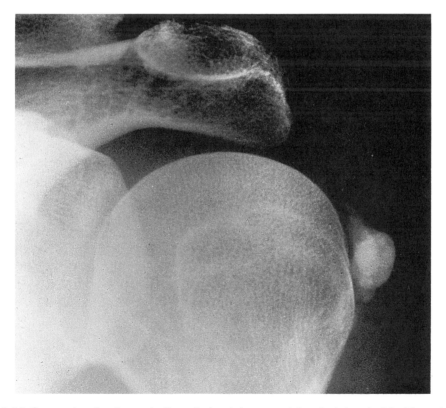

Figure 4–24 Conventional radiograph. Osteolysis of the acromial end of the clavicle. There is significant calcification at the level of the teres minor insertion. This calcification had no clinical significance.

complaints. In these cases, conservative therapy is worthless. Excision of the lateral 2 cm of the clavicle is the only effective measure.

Primary osteolysis is rare. Some authors propose that the disorder has a microtrau-matic etiology.[32] Others, however, report cases of the lesion without a history of over-use, particularly in women.[33] As in posttrau-matic osteolysis, treatment consists of exci-sion of the lateral 2 cm of the clavicle.

4.3   STERNOCLAVICULAR JOINT PATHOLOGY

As in pathology of the AC joint, pathology of the sternoclavicular (SC) joint is also clas-sified into traumatic and nontraumatic le-sions. Traumatic lesions are seen less often in the SC joint than in the AC joint.

TRAUMATIC LESIONS

Type I: sprain of the sternoclavicular liga-ments, where the joint is completely stable

Type II: subluxation; partial tear of the capsular ligaments, the intra-articular disc, or the costoclavicular ligaments

Type IIA: ventral subluxation: most fre-quently seen

Type IIB: dorsal subluxation

Type IIIA: ventral dislocation

Type IIIB: dorsal dislocation

Type IV: habitual dislocation (rare)

Mechanism of Injury

As the result of a direct blow (car accident, sports trauma) against the medial aspect of the clavicle, a dorsal subluxation (or disloca-tion) can occur. Biomechanically considered, a direct blow could also easily cause a ventral subluxation or dislocation. The latter lesion, however, is usually the result of an indirect trauma. Generally this involves a blow against the anterolateral aspect of the shoulder or a fall on this part of the shoulder.

Clinical Findings

Type I.
- On inspection, sometimes slight local swelling is visible.
- The patient complains usually of local pain.
- All passive movements of the shoulder are painful at end-range. Passive hori-zontal adduction is the most painful mo-tion.

Type II.
- The findings are similar to those in type I, but here the pain can radiate into the C4 dermatome.
- All the shoulder motions are very painful at end-range.
- The subluxation is usually visible, whether a type IIA (ventral subluxation) or a type IIB (dorsal subluxation) is con-cerned.

Type III.
- Pain is severe in the acute stage.
- The dislocation is visible (type IIIA or IIIB).
- The patient usually holds the shoulder in protraction, supporting the arm in front of the body.

Type IIIA.

- Ventral dislocation: the medial aspect of the clavicle may still be fixed or just very easily movable.

Type IIIB.

- Dorsal dislocation is more painful than ventral dislocation.
- The sternal part of the SC joint is palpable.

Complications

Complications caused by pressure on the structures lying directly dorsal to the medial end of the clavicle (such as the common carotid artery, subclavian vein, trachea, or esophagus) may include venous congestion in the arm or neck, breathing problems, choked feeling, or swallowing problems.

In every type II lesion, a computed tomography (CT) scan is indicated, because local swelling sometimes gives the appearance of a ventral subluxation or dislocation although a dorsal subluxation or dislocation is actually present. Correct diagnosis is extremely important in order to select an effective treatment program.

Treatment

Type I. Cryotherapy is indicated in the acute phase. Encourage movement within the limits of pain. Full recovery is usually attained in 5 to 10 days.

Type II. Cryotherapy is indicated in the acute phase. Encourage movement within the limits of pain, although most practitioners apply a sling or figure-eight bandage such as used in clavicle fractures. Full recovery is usually attained in 2 to 4 weeks. Surgery is rarely indicated (only when severe complications arise).

Type IIIA. In medical literature, treatment of this lesion is still a topic of discussion. In the first instance, conservative reduction should be tried (either with or without general anesthesia).

The patient lies in a supine position with an 8- to 10-cm thick sandbag between the scapulae. With the arm in 90° abduction, a gentle pull is exerted on the arm. Manual reduction is performed in a dorsal direction.

If the joint remains in position while the shoulders are held in retraction, a figure-eight brace (as used in clavicle fractures) is applied.

If the joint re-dislocates, the figure-eight bandage is *still* applied; however, the joint usually remains unstable. The bandage is worn until the patient no longer has symptoms.

Operative fixation is sometimes performed; however, the chance of complication is great.

Type IIIB. If the CT scan demonstrates a dorsal dislocation, and if both the CT scan *and* the clinical examination indicate that structures lying dorsal to the medial end of the clavicle are affected, a closed reduction is performed.

The technique is similar to that used for ventral dislocations; only in this instance a spontaneous reduction usually occurs when the arm is slowly abducted and a gentle pull is exerted on the arm (in line with the clavicle). One person pulls on the arm and another fixes the patient's thorax. If necessary, the clavicle is grasped between thumb and fingers in order to pull the clavicle ventrally. As soon as the reduction takes place, a firm figure-eight brace is applied while the shoulders are held in retraction. The brace is worn 3 to 4 weeks, after which activities involving the joint can be increased gradually and progressively.

Recent medical literature advises against operative treatment.

Type IV. Habitual dislocation after a traumatic ventral or dorsal dislocation is extremely rare; either the joint remains stable after the reduction or it remains permanently dislocated. In people younger than 25 years, the CT scan may show that the "dislocation" is in fact a slipping of the epiphysis from the medial end of the clavicle. Before the age of

18 years, the epiphysis is not visible on conventional radiographs. It is the last epiphysis to close in the human body (about the age of 25).[24] A ventrally slipped epiphysis is left untreated; a dorsally slipped epiphysis should be treated with closed reduction.

NONTRAUMATIC LESIONS

Spontaneous Subluxation or Dislocation

Nontraumatic subluxations or dislocations are seen particularly in young people under age 20 and more often in women than in men. The lesion can occur unilaterally or bilaterally.

Clinical Findings

- Usually there is only local pain.
- During active arm elevation, the SC joint subluxates or dislocates, and reduction occurs as the arm is slowly lowered again.

Treatment

In regard to pain, the condition is self-limited. Thus, patients should be reassured by explaining that every form of "treatment" is unsuccessful, and operative "treatment" would likely increase the symptoms. With time, usually within a few months to years, the pain gradually resolves on its own.

Arthritis

As in other synovial joints, nontraumatic arthritis can also occur in the SC joint. Usually it occurs as a result of systemic disease; sometimes it involves septic arthritis.

Clinical Findings

- The patient complains of local pain, sometimes radiating into the C4 dermatome.

- All shoulder motions are painful at end-range. Horizontal adduction is the most painful motion.

Treatment

Treatment depends on the cause. Except for cases of septic arthritis, an intra-articular injection of corticosteroid usually provides excellent results. The use of a 1-cm long needle is recommended because of the blood vessels running directly behind the joint.

Subacute Degeneration of the Sternoclavicular Joint

The cause of subacute degeneration of the SC joint, also called postmenopausal arthrosis, is unknown. It is seen most often in women who have gone through menopause. In the patient history, there is no indication of a previous trauma or arthritis. Usually the dominant side is affected.

Clinical Findings

- Sudden swelling is visible, particularly at the medial end of the clavicle. Sometimes there are mild signs of inflammation. The pain is usually moderate.
- All passive shoulder motions are painful at the end-range of motion; passive horizontal adduction is the most painful motion. Scapula retraction is also painful.
- The radiograph indicates obvious sclerosis along with ventral subluxation of the joint.

Treatment

Because the symptoms are generally mild, treatment is rarely necessary. Usually the symptoms gradually disappear on their own. Stubborn cases can be treated with an intra-articular injection of corticosteroid.

Condensing Osteitis (Sclerosing Osteitis)

This disorder is rare and is seen mostly in women over the age of 40 years. The cause is unknown—possibly chronic microtrauma plays a role.

Clinical Findings

- The patient complains of local pain. Swelling of the SC joint is visible.
- During the functional examination the patient experiences slight pain and slight limitation of every shoulder motion. Horizontal adduction is the most painful and most limited motion.
- The aberration is best visualized on a CT scan; the bone marrow is replaced by bone tissue.

Treatment

Because the symptoms are mild, treatment is generally conservative. In severe cases, nonsteroidal anti-inflammatory medications or an intra-articular injection of corticosteroid is administered.

Sternocostoclavicular Hyperostosis

This rare disorder is seen equally in men and women between the ages of 30 and 50 years. Initially, the costoclavicular ligaments ossify. Afterward, the calcification process spreads to the sternum. Ultimately a large block of bone results, which is several centimeters thick and extends over the sternum, clavicle, and first rib. In this instance, the SC joint has disappeared.

Clinical Findings

Pain is minimal, but there is a severe limitation of shoulder girdle and shoulder range of motion.

Treatment

In medical literature, opinions vary in regard to the appropriate treatment. Although treatment aimed at pain relief is often beneficial, the pain usually resolves itself.

4.4 PATHOLOGY OF THE BURSAE

ACUTE SUBACROMIAL-SUBDELTOID BURSITIS

The subacromial-subdeltoid bursa can be seen as the joint cavity of the "subacromial joint". The capsule of the bursa is firmly connected to the greater tubercle as well as to the supraspinatus and infraspinatus insertions. At its superior aspect, the bursa merges with the acromion and coracoacromial ligament. The lateral part of the bursa moves freely.

Etiology

An acute subacromial-subdeltoid bursitis is thought to be an inflammatory reaction to calcium breaching into the bursa from a calcium deposit in the rotator cuff (usually the supraspinatus tendon) (Figure 4–25).

Acute bursitis can also be pyogenic, or the first sign of rheumatoid arthritis, gout, or primary villonodular synovitis.

Clinical Findings

- After a few hours or days, pain in the shoulder region, upper arm, and forearm becomes unbearable.
- There is a limitation of motion in a noncapsular pattern; the abduction is severely limited and the rotations are less limited.

Treatment

- This disorder is self-limited, and within 4 to 6 weeks the patient has recovered fully.
- In the acute stage, the bursa can be injected with a solution of corticosteroid and local anesthetic.

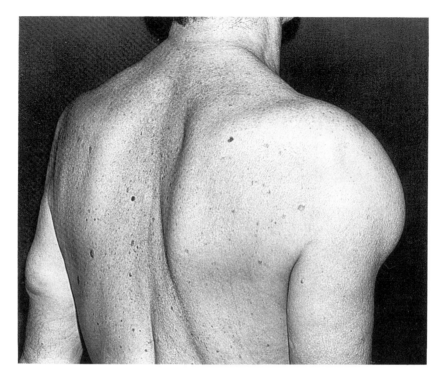

Figure 4–25 Acute subacromial-subdeltoid bursitis.

CHRONIC SUBACROMIAL-SUBDELTOID BURSITIS

Primary Chronic Bursitis

Neither the primary nor secondary chronic bursitis develops from the above-described acute subacromial-subdeltoid bursitis.

Two kinds of primary chronic bursitis are defined: in both cases, the complaints are *not* preceded by other shoulder problems. In the first case, the term *primary* actually is incorrect: there are symptomless degenerative changes, especially of the supraspinatus and AC joint, that cause the bursitis. Because of the increased volume of the degeneratively changed structures, the subacromial space decreases, resulting in diminished room for the bursa. This leads to an inflammatory reaction of the bursa. Thus, this form of bursitis is

actually secondary and is often responsible for the pain manifested in the impingement syndrome.

The second case is the only really primary bursitis. Inflammation of the bursa is based on a systemic disease. Like the joint capsule and tendon sheath, the bursa is partly a synovial structure and can therefore become inflamed as the result of a systemic disease. Sometimes a bursitis is the only clinical sign in a patient with rheumatoid arthritis.

Clinical Findings

Pain develops gradually in the shoulder and lateral deltoid region. Often the pain radiates into the upper arm, in the C5 dermatome.

The functional examination reveals a positive painful arc test. Sometimes one or more passive motions are painful at end-range. Passive internal rotation with the shoulder in maximal glenohumeral abduction is painful (due to compression of the bursa against the roof of the shoulder). Often one or more resisted tests are painful. If this is the case, when the resisted tests are repeated with an inferior pull on the arm, no pain is incurred.

Occasionally during shoulder movements, subacromial crepitation is palpable.

Treatment

The treatment of choice is an injection of 5 mL of local anesthetic. If the situation has improved after 1 week, the injection is repeated. If improvement was only temporary, the injection is repeated, but this time with a mixture of 3 mL of local anesthetic and 2 mL of corticosteroid. Usually two to four injections are necessary to achieve complete relief.

Arthroscopic treatment is seldom indicated in this form of bursitis.

Secondary Chronic Bursitis

Secondary chronic bursitis occurs more frequently than primary chronic bursitis. It is the result of other shoulder pathologies, such as those pertaining to the supraspinatus and infraspinatus muscles; the tendon of the long head of the biceps muscle; lesions of the AC joint; or irregularities of the acromion, greater tubercle, or lesser tubercle.

Clinical Findings

Pain develops gradually in the shoulder and lateral deltoid region. Often the pain radiates into the upper arm, in the C5 dermatome.

The patient experiences pain during the painful arc test, performed as part of the functional examination. Sometimes one or more passive motions are painful at end-range, but there is no limitation of motion. Passive internal rotation with the shoulder in maximal glenohumeral abduction is painful (due to compression of the subacromial structures against the roof of the shoulder).

Often one or more resisted tests (particularly abduction and internal or external rota-

tion) are painful. In this instance, the resisted tests are repeated while an inferior pull is exerted on the arm. If the bursa, and not the muscles, is responsible for the symptoms, the pain disappears. If one or more contractile structures are affected in conjunction with the bursa, the pain usually decreases, but does not completely disappear.

Occasionally, during shoulder movements, subacromial crepitation is palpable.

Sometimes there is a varying pattern of symptoms; during the functional examination certain resisted tests are painful, but a few days later when the functional examination is repeated, the patient experiences pain during *other* resisted tests.

Treatment

Generally, the bursa is treated in the same way as for a primary chronic bursitis. The treatment of choice is an injection of 5 mL of local anesthetic. If the situation has improved after 1 week, the injection is repeated. If improvement was only temporary, the injection is repeated, but this time with a mixture of 3 mL of local anesthetic and 2 mL of corticosteroid. Usually two to four injections are necessary to achieve complete relief.

For secondary bursitis, the primary lesion should also be treated (causal treatment) in order to prevent recurrence of the bursitis. Refer to Subacromial Impingement Syndrome, section 4.5, for more detailed description of the appropriate therapy.

CALCIFIC BURSITIS

Primary calcifications of the bursa itself are very rare. When the radiographic demonstrates a cloudy calcium shadow, this calcification is usually localized in the rotator cuff tendon and is not actually a bursitis.

Clinical Findings

Although the calcification usually does not cause symptoms, there are cases where problems do arise. Refer to Tendopathy with Calcification in section 4.6 for more detailed information on this topic.

Treatment

If the bursa is inflamed because of a calcium deposit, the treatment of choice is an injection of 5 mL of local anesthetic. If the situation has improved after 1 week, the injection is repeated. If improvement was only temporary, the injection is repeated, but this time with a mixture of 3 mL of local anesthetic and 2 mL of corticosteroid. Usually two to four injections are necessary to achieve complete relief.

SUBCORACOID BURSITIS

Subcoracoid bursitis is a rare lesion of the bursa located between the tendon of the subscapularis and the coracoid process. Sometimes the subcoracoid bursa is connected to the subacromial-subdeltoid bursa. The etiology of the bursitis is similar to that described for the subacromial-subdeltoid bursitis.

Clinical Findings

- Usually the patient complains of local pain.
- In the functional examination, passive external rotation is particularly painful. This pain disappears, however, when passive external rotation is performed in 90° shoulder abduction.
- Occasionally, calcification of this bursa is observed (Figure 4–26).

Treatment

Initially, treatment consists of administering an injection of a local anesthetic. If the results are only temporary, the injection is repeated, but with a corticosteroid added to the solution.

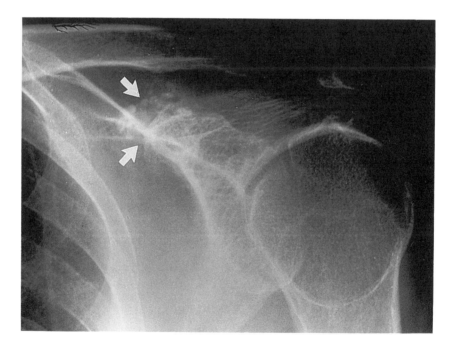

Figure 4–26 Calcific subcoracoid bursitis.

4.5 SUBACROMIAL IMPINGEMENT SYNDROME

The subacromial impingement syndrome involves painful compression of one of the soft tissue structures located between the head of the humerus and the roof of the shoulder (acromion, coracoacromial ligament, coracoid process, or AC joint) during arm elevation and rotations of the arm. The only soft tissue structures that can be affected in a subacromial impingement syndrome are the rotator cuff, subacromial-subdeltoid bursa, joint capsule, and the tendon of the long head of the biceps.

Although in this book bursitis, tendinitis, and AC joint pathology are discussed separately, there is often an interrelation among the various lesions.

The diagnosis of impingement syndrome is frequently used. It is easy to assume a single cause for this syndrome. In reality, it is a composite of several separate lesions. For the specific clinical findings and treatment of the separate lesions, refer back to the descriptions of pathology of the subacromial-subdeltoid bursa, supraspinatus, infraspinatus, subscapularis, biceps, and AC joint in previous sections.

The term *impingement syndrome* was introduced by Neer in 1972.[34] He describes three stages:

stage 1: reversible small bleeding and edema in the rotator cuff, in patients younger than 25 years

stage 2: fibrosis and tendinitis of the rotator cuff in patients between 25 and 40 years

stage 3: osteophytes of the acromion and the AC joint and (partial) tear of the rotator cuff in patients over the age of 40 years

Various factors play a role in the development of an impingement syndrome, including the following

- form of the acromion

- vascularization of the rotator cuff
- function of the rotator cuff and biceps muscles
- glenohumeral joint stability
- condition of the AC joint
- occupation and hobbies of the patient

Form of the Acromion. Regarding its relevance in the impingement syndrome, the form of the acromion is best evaluated by a lateral-view radiograph, the so-called supraspinatus outlet view. Three forms of the acromion can be differentiated (Figure 4–27):

1. type I: flat
2. type II: concave
3. type III: hooked

Most patients (70% to 80%) with a local rupture (full-thickness tear) appear to have a type III acromion.[35]

Vascularization of the Rotator Cuff. As described in Chapter 1, vascularization of the rotator cuff is not always fully developed, particularly of the supraspinatus muscle and part of the tendon of the long head of the biceps muscle. Certain positions of the shoulder interfere with the vascularization even more, such as during throwing activities. A direct result of this lack of blood supply is edema, later fibrosis, and finally a rupture of the tendon fibers.

Function of the Rotator Cuff and Biceps Muscles. The rotator cuff and the tendon of the long head of the biceps are primary stabilizers and depressors of the humeral head. In glenohumeral joint instability, lesions of the rotator cuff and biceps (long head) occur more easily due to overuse. In the presence of inflammation, the affected structure increases in size, leading to impingement.

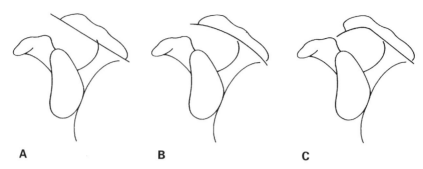

A   **B**   **C**

Figure 4–27 The acromion is differentiated into three types according to Beglianni, Morrison, & April. **A**, Flat type; **B**, concave type; **C**, hooked type. *Source:* Reprinted with permission from C.A. Rockwood and F.A. Matsen, III, *The Shoulder,* © 1989, W.B. Saunders.

Glenohumeral Joint Stability. If the glenohumeral joint is stable, other factors such as the type of acromion, vascularization of the rotator cuff, or daily activities of the patient can lead to degenerative changes of the rotator cuff. If rotator cuff function diminishes, the humeral head migrates upward. This leads to a narrowing of the space between humeral head and roof of the shoulder, again resulting in impingement.

Condition of the AC Joint. Osteophytes at the caudal aspect of the AC joint also decease the subacromial space. During arm elevation, impingement of the bursa and rotator cuff occurs.

Occupation or Hobbies of the Patient. If the patient's occupation or sports activities involve frequent elevation with internal rotation of the shoulder, repetitive diminishing of the subacromial space occurs. Furthermore, in this position the "critical zone" (area of decreased vascularization) of the supraspinatus lies underneath the acromial arch, which results in an even further decrease in the local blood supply.

Clinical Findings

The most significant symptom is pain, particularly manifested during abduction or flexion with internal rotation movements. Often in this position crepitation and loss of strength are noted. The pain is usually experienced in the lateral deltoid region, often just at the insertion.

Findings from the functional examination depend on the number of affected structures. The most definitive symptom is the painful arc during arm elevation in the plane of the scapula, whereby the arm is simultaneously positioned in internal rotation.

For more detailed information, refer to the separate sections discussing clinical findings for the various structures that are involved in the impingement syndrome.

Treatment

Considering the moderate results in operative treatment of athletes, the importance of nonsurgical treatment should be emphasized. The same is true for patients whose occupation is responsible for the onset of symptoms. Matsen and Arntz state emphatically, "Exercises and job modification before acromion modification."[35] In general the conservative treatment program should consist of the following:

- preventing the painful movements as much as possible
- if necessary, improving limitations of motion by means of stretching exercises,

particularly for the supraspinatus and infraspinatus (Often the posterior capsule needs to be stretched by means of joint-specific mobilization techniques.)

- muscle strengthening, particularly of the scapula stabilizing and rotator cuff muscles: internal rotators and adductors more than external rotators and abductors (The rotator cuff muscles are very important for holding the humeral head down.)
- maintaining or improving general physical condition
- modification of work or sports activities as necessary to avoid trauma

Matsen and Arntz[35] list several conditions that, if met, can lead to good results from a subacromial decompression, but only after conservative treatment (of at least 6 months) has had unsatisfactory results:

- motivated patient over 40 years of age
- no limitation of motion, particularly of the posterior structures (capsule, supraspinatus, and/or infraspinatus)
- presence of subacromial crepitation
- disappearance of pain after a subacromial infiltration with local anesthetic
- pathology not related to the patient's occupation

4.6 PATHOLOGY OF THE MUSCLE-TENDON UNIT— ROTATOR CUFF PATHOLOGY

SUPRASPINATUS LESIONS

Tendopathy

Lesions of the supraspinatus muscle are seen frequently. They can be classified according to cause and according to age.

Classification According to Cause

There are several factors that lead to a tendopathy, either by themselves or in combination.

Instability. One of the most frequent causes for a tendopathy in athletes is the anterior or anteroinferior instability of the glenohumeral joint. Because stability of the capsuloligamentous complex is insufficient, the rotator cuff muscles are overloaded. This is especially true for athletes participating in

throwing and racket sports, during which the shoulder is brought into maximal glenohumeral abduction, external rotation, and extension.

Poor Vascularization. The supraspinatus teno-osseous insertion or part of the tendon (total length approximately 1 cm) is moderately to poorly vascularized. This poorly vascularized area is called the "critical zone." In activities generating greater than normal pressure, such as those involving objects heavier than usual, local inflammatory reactions can occur in the tendon's critical zone.

"Wringing Out" Phenomenon. When the arm hangs alongside the body (an adducted position), the already minimal amount of blood in the vessels of the tendon and teno-osseous insertion is pushed away by the round surface of the humeral head. This is called the "wringing out" phenomenon, and leads to problems especially in swimmers (due to the adduction phase in almost all the strokes) and long-distance runners.

Narrow Space between Humeral Head and Roof of the Shoulder. There is only a small amount of room between the humeral head and the roof of the shoulder. This space decreases even more during sideways arm elevation, in which the space is narrowest between 60° and 120°. This is also the range where the painful arc occurs.

Differential Diagnosis

Subacromial-Subdeltoid Bursitis. In an impingement syndrome as well as subacromial-subdeltoid bursitis, resisted abduction is often painful. In the instance of a bursitis, resisted abduction performed while exerting an inferior pull on the arm is not painful. Tendopathies of the supraspinatus often lead to a subacromial-subdeltoid bursitis.

Classification According to Age. In young people, particularly athletes participating in throwing sports, racket sports, or swimming, a supraspinatus insertion tendopathy often arises as a result of overuse. The lesion is usually localized directly at the insertion on the greater tubercle (Figure 4–28). This can be seen by use of magnetic resonance imaging (MRI).

In the age group of 30 to 40 years, degenerative supraspinatus lesions can occur. Because of poor vascularization of the tendon or insertion, degeneration caused by overuse occurs, causing pain. The location of this lesion is medial to the insertion, at the level of the critical zone (Figure 4–28). Sometimes calcium deposits are found in the degenerated tissue. Usually the calcium is gradually reabsorbed.

Clinical Findings

In a tendinitis, five clinical stages are identified:

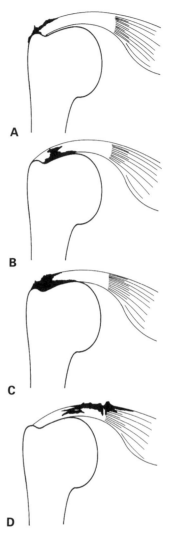

Figure 4–28 Tendopathy of the supraspinatus. It should be understood that combinations of the following can also occur.
A, *Location:* Lateral part of the insertion (particularly in young athletes). *Clinical findings:* Pain with resisted abduction; painful arc. **B**, *Location:* Medial part of the insertion (particularly in 30- to 45-year-olds). *Clinical findings:* Pain with resisted abduction; pain at end-range passive arm elevation with overpressure in a medial direction. **C**, *Location:* Entire insertion (particularly in 30- to 45-year-olds). *Clinical findings:* Pain with resisted abduction; pain at end-range passive arm elevation with overpressure in a medial direction; painful arc. **D**, *Location:* Musculotendinous junction (rare) (2 to 3 cm medial to the insertion). *Clinical findings:* Pain only on resisted abduction.

Stage 1.
- The pain is usually felt in the lateral deltoid region.
- Pain is experienced after activity and is of short duration.
- Resisted testing (of abduction) is painful only on release of the resistance.

Stage 2.
- The pain sometimes radiates down the arm to the elbow.
- Pain is experienced at the beginning of the activity and for a short while (a few hours) afterward.
- Resisted testing (of abduction) is painful.
- The painful arc test is usually positive.
- Sometimes there is also pain at end-range of passive arm elevation.

Stage 3.
- The pain can radiate distal to the elbow.
- Pain is experienced during and after the activity; however, the activity (whether work or sports related) is not significantly influenced. Pain after the activity sometimes lasts 1 day or longer.
- Resisted testing (of abduction) is very painful.
- Often the patient experiences a painful arc during active elevation or has pain at the end-range of passive arm elevation.

Stage 4.
- Pain is experienced during and after the activity, with the activity being clearly affected. Pain at rest can last several days after the activity.
- Severe pain is experienced on resisted testing (of abduction).
- The patient generally experiences a painful arc during active elevation. Passive arm elevation is usually painful at end-range.

Stage 5.
- Performance of the activity is impossible because of pain. There is also pain at rest.

- Severe pain is experienced on resisted testing (of abduction).
- The patient generally experiences a painful arc during active elevation. Passive arm elevation is usually painful at end-range.

A painful arc during elevation indicates that the lesion is localized in the lateral part of the supraspinatus tendon. This affected part of the insertion "bumps" against the acromion or coracoacromial ligament during arm elevation, causing the so-called painful arc.

Pain at the end-range of passive elevation with overpressure in a medial direction indicates that the more medial aspect of the tendon is affected. In this position, this affected part of the insertion is pressed against the glenoid labrum.

If only the resisted abduction is painful, there is likely to be a lesion of the supraspinatus musculotendinous junction. This lesion is rare, however.

In the resisted tests, external rotation sometimes also is painful, because the supraspinatus also contracts when resistance is applied to external rotation. A lesion of both the supraspinatus and infraspinatus can be ruled out by injecting a local anesthetic or performing transverse friction massage (analgesic effect) to the supraspinatus insertion. If the patient no longer has pain during resisted external rotation (as well as abduction), the supraspinatus lesion is confirmed, and a lesion of the infraspinatus is unlikely.

When abduction and external rotation are painful against resistance, the tests should always be repeated while exerting a pull on the arm in order to rule out a bursitis. In instances of a tendinitis, the tests are usually just as, or even more, painful with a pull on the arm. Combined lesions are often seen.

Treatment

Treatment of a supraspinatus tendinitis is primarily cause oriented. It also depends on the stage of tendinitis. For instance, if the lesion is a consequence of glenohumeral instability, muscle strengthening must be achieved to stabilize the joint functionally. Efforts are also made to correct the throwing, smashing, or swimming techniques.

In addition to treating causes, the following therapeutic procedures can be used.

Stage 1. Transverse friction massage and stretching exercises (performed also as a home exercise program) are begun. Muscle-strengthening procedures are initiated after the functional examination produces no pain. Usually four to eight transverse friction massage treatments are necessary before muscle-strengthening procedures can be initiated.

Stage 2. Transverse friction massage and stretching exercises are begun. If necessary, the sports or work activity is decreased to the point where the patient feels no pain. Usually 6 to 12 treatments of transverse friction and stretching are necessary before muscle strengthening procedures can be initiated.

Stage 3. Daily transverse friction massage is initiated. Activities involving the affected extremity are restricted. If there is no obvious improvement after six treatments, a local anesthetic can be injected into the affected site. This injection is repeated two more times at the most (one time per week). Usually, muscle-strengthening treatments can be initiated after 4 to 8 weeks.

Stage 4. Treatment is the same as for stage 3; however, if improvement is not achieved, one or two injections of a mild solution of corticosteroid can be administered. After each injection, the arm is kept in a sling for 3 days.

Stage 5. Treatment is the same as for stage 4. Often prolonged treatment is necessary (from 3 to 9 months). Sometimes surgery is indicated, such as an acromioplasty proposed by Neer et al.[20] This arthroscopic procedure entails resection of the coracoacromial ligament and shaving underneath the ventrolateral aspect of the acromion. Often, resection of the lateral part (approximately 1 cm) of the clavicle is indicated. This is because in chronic cases, acromioclavicular problems also occur.

Tendopathy with Calcification

Frequently, a calcium deposit in the supraspinatus tendon is visible on a radiograph (Figure 4–29). This finding is of clinical relevance, however, only when there are accompanying clinical signs and symptoms.

Clinical Findings

- The pain can radiate distal to the elbow.
- Pain is experienced during and after the activity. Often the activity (whether work or sports related) is significantly influenced. Pain after the activity sometimes lasts 1 day or longer.
- Resisted testing (of abduction) is very painful.
- The patient almost always experiences a severely painful arc during active elevation and has pain at the end-range of passive arm elevation.

Treatment

Usually one to three injections of a local anesthetic are sufficient for treating the symptoms. Transverse friction massage is not indicated; it can make the pain even worse.

For large calcium deposits, a thick needle can be used to "needle" the deposit. This breaks up the calcium deposit, after which the pieces are gradually reabsorbed. In therapy-resistant cases, arthroscopic treatment is indicated (excision of the calcium deposit and Neer[36] acromioplasty).

Partial or Complete Tear of the Tendon

In a *complete* tear of the tendon, there is a tear through the entire thickness of the tendon, from the articular surface to the bursa.

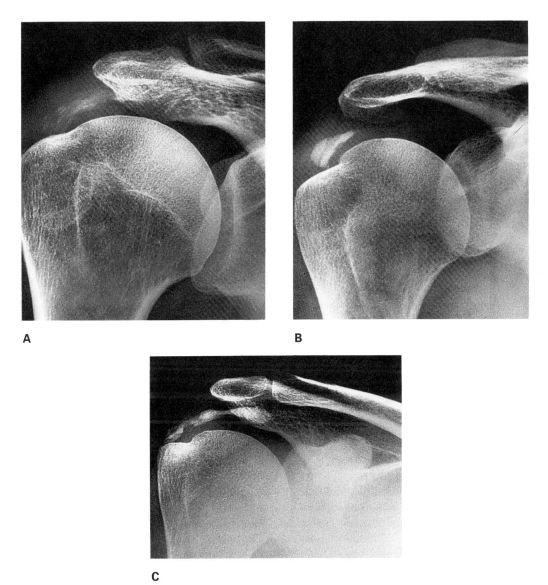

A

B

C

Figure 4–29 Conventional radiographs demonstrate calcification in a rotator cuff tendon. Three different forms of calcification are visible in **A**, **B**, and **C**.

Complete tears are more frequent than once presumed. Based on cadaver studies, researchers report findings varying from less than 5% to 26.5%.[20,37]

A *partial* tear can be superficial (in the middle of the tendon) or deep (lying at the articular surface). Partial tears are seen twice as often as complete tears.

An *acute* partial tear occurs as the result of a trauma. A *chronic* partial tear occurs gradually as degenerative changes occur in the tendon (critical zone) (Figure 4–30). After an apparently insignificant trauma, or without an obvious cause, the still-intact fibers can rupture, causing a sudden increase in the symptoms.

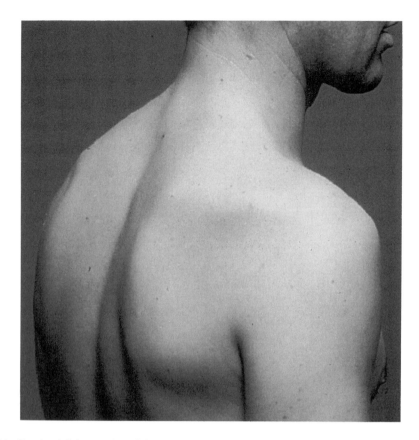

Figure 4–30 Clearly visible atrophy of the supraspinatus and infraspinatus muscles in a patient with a chronic rotator cuff tear.

Most partial tears are found at the level of the articular surface and are thus visible during intra-articular arthroscopy. Tears on the bursa side (superficial) are less frequent, but usually cause the most symptoms because the bursa also becomes inflamed. These tears are almost always located in the critical zone of the tendon. In severe cases, a gap is often palpable.

Partial tears in athletes occur particularly at the level of insertion. Usually the deep fibers are involved. Complete tears in athletes under the age of 40 years always have a traumatic cause, but are very rare; traumatic fractures or tears in the capsule are more common.

Rotator cuff tears are often seen in conjunction with dislocations. Petersson[38] found a partial rotator cuff tear in 30% of patients over 40 years who had experienced anteroinferior shoulder dislocations. In patients over 60, the amount increased to 60%.

Often, in complete tears of the supraspinatus tendon, the tendon of the long head of the biceps also ruptures.

Supplementary Examination

Arthrography, arthro-CT, and arthroscopy are invasive procedures that can be performed to visualize the lesions (Figure 4–31). Ultrasonography is becoming a more popular imaging technique because it is noninvasive

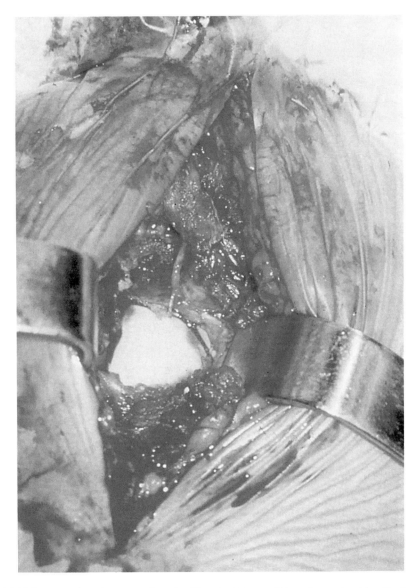

Figure 4–31 This operative view reveals a significant rotator cuff tear through which the humeral head is visible.

and is a relatively simple method of evaluating the extent of the lesion.

Clinical Findings

- In a partial tear there is usually severe pain with almost every shoulder motion, especially abduction.

- Resisted abduction not only is painful, but also weak. Many patients are unable to elevate the arm actively.

- In a complete tear, usually there is pain only in the acute phase. The pain disappears within a few days.

- Resisted abduction is weak, but not painful.
- In the chronic phase, crepitation and clicking in the shoulder often can be felt, particularly when performing internal rotation from a position of maximal glenohumeral abduction.

Complications

In rare instances, a cuff tear arthropathy occurs in elderly patients.

Treatment

In many elderly patients, a partial tear occurs without the development of symptoms. In such cases, treatment is not indicated. If the shoulder does become a source of symptoms, treatment is aimed at relieving pain, improving function, and preventing recurrence or progression.

Injections of corticosteroid, once into the subacromial space and once into the joint, can help to decrease symptoms. Repeated injections weaken the tendon fibers, however, increasing the chance of residual problems or progression of the problem.[39] In such cases, later surgical treatment has a poorer prognosis because of the weak tendon tissue.

Partial Tear. Transverse friction and cautious stretching can be effective for a partial tear. The patient should perform mobility exercises within the limits of pain. Therapy can be supplemented with nonsteroidal anti-inflammatory medication.

A one-time injection of corticosteroid can be administered, but only in therapy-resistant cases (minimal to no improvement within 2 months). The patient receives the injection in the subacromial space for superficial tears and intra-articularly for deep tears (as indicated by ultrasonography).

If recovery is smooth, muscle-strengthening exercises (without weight) should be prescribed.

Complete Tear. In principle, all young patients (under the age of 40) and older athletes with complete supraspinatus tendon tears should be treated surgically. In the other cases, treatment is administered as described for the partial tear. Sometimes the patient is unable to lift the arm actively, because the deltoid pulls the greater tubercle cranially due to deficiency of the supraspinatus. In this instance, the patient can learn to lever the arm into elevation through depression and external rotation of the humeral head.

INFRASPINATUS LESIONS

Infraspinatus pathology is seen less often than supraspinatus pathology (Figure 4–32). One reason there are fewer degenerative changes in the tendon and the teno-osseous insertion of the infraspinatus is that vascularization is better.

There are three locations for an infraspinatus tendopathy: (1) the lateral aspect of the insertion, (2) the medial aspect of the insertion, and (3) the body of the tendon. A tear of the infraspinatus is usually located at the tendon. Refer to the discussion on partial and complete tears of the supraspinatus for more detailed information.

Clinical Findings

- The patient complains of pain in the shoulder, of radiating pain in the C5 dermatome (lateral deltoid region to the dorsolateral aspect of the forearm), or both.
- The clinical stages of tendinitis, as described for supraspinatus, apply to the infraspinatus also. In this case, external rotation is the painful resisted motion.
- In a complete tear, after a period of time, a limitation of both active and passive external rotation occurs. This happens because full external rotation can no longer be performed by the teres minor alone.

Insertion Tendinitis, Lateral Aspect.

- A painful arc is experienced during active elevation.

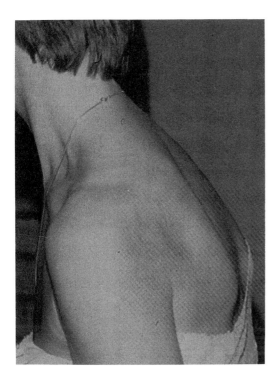

Figure 4–32 Severe atrophy of particularly the infraspinatus. The patient has the clinical findings of a complete tear of the infraspinatus.

- Resisted external rotation is painful.
- Passive horizontal adduction and passive internal rotation are sometimes painful because of stretch.

Insertion Tendinitis, Medial Aspect.
- Pain is encountered during the functional examination at end-range passive elevation (because of compression of the affected medial part against the glenoid labrum).
- Resisted external rotation is painful.
- Passive horizontal adduction and passive internal rotation are sometimes painful because of stretch.

Tendinitis, Body of the Tendon.
- In the functional examination, only resisted external rotation is painful.

- Passive horizontal adduction and passive internal rotation can be painful because of stretch.

Treatment

Treatment is the same as described for lesions of the supraspinatus and also will depend on the cause and stage of the tendinitis.

SUBSCAPULARIS LESIONS

Of the muscles belonging to the rotator cuff, the subscapularis has the best vascularization at the level of the insertions.

Lesions of the subscapularis are often due to overuse. Problems with this muscle are seen particularly in athletes participating in throwing sports, because of the tremendous load placed on the muscle during throwing motions, including smashing and serving. In order to be able to suddenly and maximally contract the muscle, the athlete first brings the arm backward over the head, increasing tension and stretch of the muscle. In various forms of anterior instability, the subscapularis and other internal rotators lose substantial strength due to pain. (Refer to the section on anterior instability in section 4.1 for more thorough information.)

Without demonstrable cause, tendopathies are sometimes seen in women between the ages of 40 to 60 years.

Clinical Findings
- The patient complains of pain at the anterior aspect of the shoulder, sometimes with radiating pain in the arm (C5 dermatome).
- If the proximal part of the subscapularis insertion is affected, the patient will experience a painful arc during active elevation.
- Resisted internal rotation is always painful. Passive external rotation can be painful because of stretch. (If resisted adduction is tested from an abducted position, or resisted abduction is tested

from 90° of abduction, these tests will also be painful.)

- If the distal part of the subscapularis is also affected, passive horizontal adduction is painful. In this test, the distal part of the insertion is compressed against the coracoid process.

Treatment

As for the other rotator cuff lesions, treatment for a subscapularis tendinitis is primarily causal. Athletes participating in racket or throwing sports should have their techniques evaluated.

If there is no obvious demonstrable cause, subscapularis insertion tendopathy usually reacts very well to a one-time injection of corticosteroid. It is seldom necessary to administer a second injection. After the injection, the arm should be supported in a sling for 3 days.

Transverse friction massage and stretching exercises are also effective; however, it takes much longer to achieve full recovery. In instances of a sports injury, specific muscle strengthening is also indicated. Muscle strengthening is begun only after the functional examination produces no pain.

PATHOLOGY OF THE MUSCLE-TENDON UNIT—BICEPS LESIONS

Tenosynovitis and Tendinitis of the Long Head

Because many patients complain of shoulder pain and tenderness in the region of the biceps tendon, the biceps tendon is often incorrectly blamed for these symptoms. Basing the diagnosis solely on palpation usually provides misleading information. The functional examination is decisive.

The tendon of the long head of the biceps runs intra-articularly as well as extra-articularly. It is surrounded by synovial membrane. Intra-articularly, the tendon sometimes lies imbedded in a capsular fold. The tendon sheath extends approximately 4 to 5 cm distally from the point where the tendon pierces the joint capsule. During shoulder movements, the tendon hardly moves. The humeral head glides underneath the static tendon.

As is the case with the supraspinatus, the tendon of the long head of the biceps has a "critical zone" where vascularization is diminished. With the arm in a hanging position, the critical zone is 1 to 2 cm long and is located just distal to the acromion. Ruptures of the tendon almost always occur at this level.

The tenosynovitis, which usually contributes to an impingement syndrome, is seen particularly in young athletes participating in throwing and racket sports, or in swimmers. Lesions of the tendon or tendon sheath are often caused by poor throwing, serving, or swimming techniques. Overuse can also result from an anterior instability of the glenohumeral joint.

Clinical Findings

- The patient usually complains of pain at the anterior aspect of the shoulder, often radiating along the length of the biceps.
- In the functional examination, if resisted elbow flexion is painful at the shoulder, the diagnosis is obvious: tendinitis of the long head of the biceps. However, because the tendon sheath is not a contractile structure, if the tendon sheath alone is affected the functional examination will be negative. In this instance an extra test is performed: the biceps stretch test (Test 3.14 in Chapter 3). The stretch test entails fixing the patient's scapula, then performing passive glenohumeral extension, forearm pronation, and finally elbow extension. If the tendon sheath is affected, this test provokes the patient's shoulder pain.
- In addition, passive arm elevation with overpressure in a posterior direction at the end-range of motion is also painful

due to compression of the tendon and tendon sheath against the acromion.

- The throwing test (Test 3.21 in Chapter 3) may also be positive. Glenohumeral stability should always be checked in instances of tendinitis and tenosynovitis of the long head of the biceps.

Treatment

In addition to causal treatment, local transverse friction is applied. Depending on the severity of the problem, it may also be necessary to reduce the pain-provoking (sports) activities.

For a further discussion of the treatment, refer to section 4.5.

Dislocation of the Tendon of the Long Head

Sometimes the tendon of the long head of the biceps dislocates out of the intertubercular sulcus. In medical literature, reports have attributed this to an abnormal groove formation, whereby the repeated external rotation and abduction movements overstretch or tear the transverse humeral ligament.

Occasionally a dislocation occurs as a result of a trauma.

Clinical Findings

The patient rarely complains of severe pain. However, the click, felt particularly during external rotation and abduction motions, can be very annoying.

Treatment

Treatment consists of avoiding temporarily the pain- and click-provoking movements. To relieve pain, transverse friction massage can be very effective. In severe cases, surgical treatment may be indicated.

Total Rupture of the Tendon of the Long Head of the Biceps

The total rupture is seen especially in middle-aged patients and is often associated with a rotator cuff tear (Figure 4–33). The rupture almost always occurs in the critical zone of the tendon, which can tear under a relatively small amount of strain.

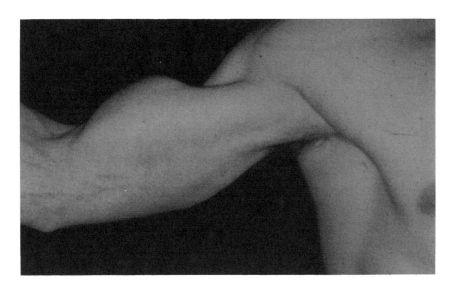

Figure 4–33 Total rupture of the tendon of the long head of the biceps.

Clinical Findings

- Most patients report hearing or feeling a "snap." Pain, when present, is rarely severe and is almost always temporary (lasting 3 to 7 days).
- During contraction of the biceps, swelling of the muscle belly occurs close to the elbow instead of in the middle of the upper arm.

Treatment

Usually the patient only requires reassurance, without further treatment. In some instances surgery is performed whereby the tendon is fixed in the intertubercular sulcus instead of its original insertion. The remaining part of the tendon is resected.

With or without surgery, rupture of the tendon of the long head of the biceps results in decreased stability of the glenohumeral joint. Another disadvantage to this lesion is that the chance for developing an impingement syndrome increases because the short head of the biceps pulls the humeral head upward. The opposite force from the long head (which used to push the head downward) is absent.

4.7   NEUROLOGICAL DISORDERS

ACCESSORY NERVE LESION

The accessory nerve (eleventh cranial nerve) innervates the trapezius and sternocleidomastoid muscles. The trapezius muscle is also innervated by the C3 and C4 nerve roots.

Clinically, differentiation is made between two types of accessory nerve paresis. In one case, the sternocleidomastoid, as well as the trapezius (pars descendens), is affected. In this instance, severe pathology should be suspected, such as a tumor at the base of the skull near the foramen magnum.

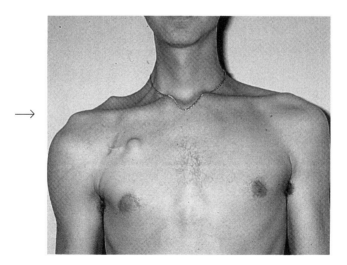

Figure 4–34 Iatrogenic (postoperative) lesion of the accessory nerve. The trapezius muscle has almost disappeared; the superior angle of the scapula is visible.

More often, there is only a paresis of the descending part of the trapezius. This type of accessory nerve lesion is seen after surgery (Figure 4–34), for instance after excision of a lymphoma at the posterior edge of the sterno-cleidomastoid.

Clinical Findings

- On inspection, there is an obvious, medially rotated position of the scapula: the inferior angle moves toward the spinal column, and the superior angle moves laterally. The entire scapula stands slightly further away from the spinal column.

- Weakness, without complete deficit, is noted in the trapezius muscle and pars descendens. During active arm elevation, there is sometimes a limitation of motion; passively, the range of motion is full.

- In many cases, the only complaints of the patient are neck and shoulder pain.

Treatment

Treatment has little influence on the pain and weakness. The prognosis is poor and recovery is rare.

For an overview of the common pathologies of the shoulder refer to Appendix B, Algorithms for the Diagnosis and Treatment of the Upper Extremity.

5

Treatment Techniques in Lesions of the Shoulder

GLENOHUMERAL JOINT ARTHRITIS

Functional Examination

- Capsular pattern of limitation:
  1. External rotation is more limited than abduction.
  2. Internal rotation is less limited than abduction.
  3. These three motions are limited in a ratio of external rotation: abduction:internal rotation = 3:2:1.
- One or more resisted tests can be painful (due to the tight connection between the joint capsule and the rotator cuff muscles).

Injection

An intra-articular injection is the treatment of choice for stage III traumatic, postimmobilization, and idiopathic arthritides. Other indications include arthritides of a rheumatoid nature, such as rheumatoid arthritis, gout, ankylosing spondylitis, and Reiter's disease.

Position of the Patient

The injection can be administered with the patient in one of two positions:

1. The patient lies prone on the table. The affected arm is positioned in internal rotation; the patient lies on the forearm, and the head is rotated away from that side (Figure 5–1).
2. The patient sits with the affected arm resting at the side (Figure 5–2A and B).

Position of the Physician

The physician stands at the affected side of the patient next to the treatment table.

Performance

The physician palpates the tip of the coracoid process with the index finger and the posterior angle of the acromion (junction between the scapular spine and the lateral edge of the acromion) with the thumb. Approximately 1 cm distal to the posterior angle, a 5-cm long needle is inserted and pushed in the direction of the coracoid process. After approximately 4 cm, the needle generally meets "tough" resistance (of the thickened joint capsule), which can be overcome by slightly increasing the push on the needle. After passing through the joint capsule, the resistance reduces significantly and the tip of the needle is now intra-articular.

At this point, 5 mL of solution (2 mL of triamcinolone acetonide, 10 mg/mL, and 3 mL of local anesthetic) is injected into the joint. By using a somewhat larger volume of solution, the procedure has a better influence on the joint capsule. If too much pressure is required to empty the syringe, the needle should be withdrawn approximately 3 cm and reinserted more specifically in the direction of the lower edge of the coracoid process.

Usually the patient will be able to lie on the affected shoulder that night. On the other hand, if the patient experiences severe pain after the injection (that night), it is likely that the solution was not deposited intra-articularly.

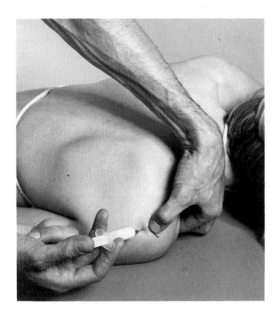

Figure 5–1 Intra-articular injection in the gleno-humeral joint, with patient prone.

When administering an intra-articular injection, a posterior approach offers the advantage that solution cannot be deposited into the subacromial-subdeltoid bursa, and large blood vessels are not in danger of being hit (which is possible when the needle is inserted from anterior).

Follow-Up

For the first 2 days following the injection, the patient should not force movements in the shoulder. Afterward, the patient is instructed to move the arm *within the limits of pain*.

The patient is seen again 2 weeks later, and the shoulder is reevaluated. If necessary, a second injection is given. Usually, a maximum of three injections are administered over a period of 3 months. More than three injections can cause a weakening of the rotator cuff tendons and lead to a rupture of the cuff years later.

Usually, after one to three injections, stage 1 is again attained and further treatment consists either of specific joint mobilization or waiting for the joint to recover by itself.

Note: Often in patients with diabetes mellitus, a stubborn arthritis of the shoulder occurs. *In these cases, joint-specific mobilization is contraindicated.* Sometimes an injection with triamcinolone acetonide can cause a minimal imbalance in metabolism. In the authors' experience, however, no significant side effects have ever been noted.

ANTERIOR DISLOCATION OF THE GLENOHUMERAL JOINT

Reduction Technique According to Hippocrates[40]

Position of the Patient

The patient lies in a supine position, with the affected side as close as possible to the edge of the table.

Position of the Physician

The physician stands on one leg at the patient's affected side. The leg closest to the table is extended and the physician places the foot in the patient's axilla. The physician grasps the patient's forearm using both hands (Figure 5–3).

Performance

The physician cautiously exerts an axial inferior pull on the patient's arm.

Note: In regard to the neurovascular bundle, this maneuver should not be performed on patients over age 60 years.

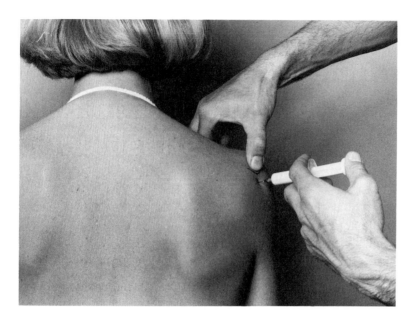

Figure 5–2A Intra-articular injection in the shoulder, with patient sitting.

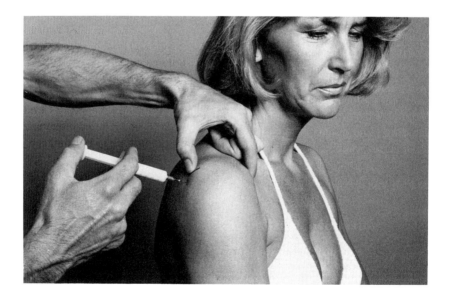

Figure 5–2B View from the side.

Reduction Technique According to Manes[41]

The Manes maneuver (Figure 5–4) is es-pecially appropriate for reducing anterior shoulder dislocations in patients over age 60 years.

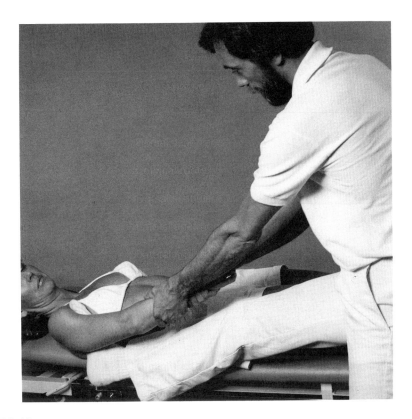

Figure 5–3A Hippocrates maneuver.

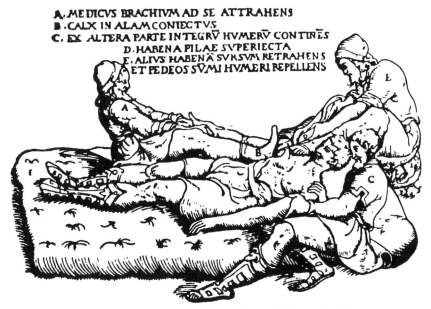

A. MEDICVS BRACHIVM AD SE ATTRAHENS
B. CALX IN ALAM CONIECTVS
C. EX ALTERA PARTE INTEGRV HVMERV CONTINES
D. HABENA PILAE SVPERIECTA
E. ALIVS HABENA SVRSVM RETRAHENS
ET PEDEOS SVMI HVMERI REPELLENS

Figure 5–3B Reduction of the dislocated shoulder according to Hippocrates.[40]

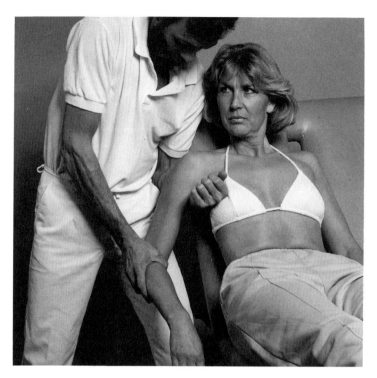

Figure 5–4 Manes maneuver.[41]

Position of the Patient

The patient sits on a chair or inclined against the raised end of the treatment table.

Position of the Physician

The physician stands next to the treatment table, diagonally behind the patient's affected side. If the right shoulder is affected, the physician places the left forearm (with elbow in 90° flexion) in the patient's axilla. The other hand grasps the patient's elbow.

Performance

With the right arm, the physician exerts a slight axial pull on the patient's humerus while the left forearm in the patient's axilla pulls the humerus in a proximolateral direction until the reduction occurs. Afterward, the pull is slowly released.

SPRAIN OF THE CRANIAL ACROMIOCLAVICULAR LIGAMENTS

Functional Examination

- Passive arm elevation, internal rotation, and external rotation of the shoulder are painful at end-range.
- Passive horizontal adduction is painful and limited.
- Often, resisted adduction is also painful.

Transverse Friction Massage

One seldom sees an isolated lesion of the cranial acromioclavicular ligaments. Usually a combination of treatments is used in dealing with acromioclavicular pathology, such as transverse friction massage and joint-specific mobilization, or injection and joint-specific mobilization.

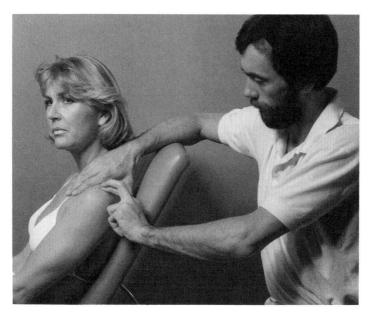

Figure 5–5 Transverse friction of the cranial acromioclavicular ligaments.

Position of the Patient

The patient sits on the treatment table with the affected side as close to the edge of the table as possible. The arm hangs in a relaxed position, with the forearm resting in the patient's lap.

Position of the Therapist

The therapist sits at the affected side of the patient, behind the treatment table. After localizing the joint, the therapist places—when the patient's left shoulder is affected—the left index finger on the anterior aspect of the joint. The other hand can rest on the patient's shoulder just medial to the acromioclavicular joint (Figure 5–5).

Performance

The transverse friction massage consists of a movement of the wrist from a neutral position, or slight palmar flexion, into dorsal extension. During this movement, pressure is exerted with the tip of the index finger, which is reinforced by the middle finger (Figure 5–6A). The wrist then moves into palmar flex-

ion, at which time the fingers relax. During the relaxation phase only enough pressure is exerted so that the therapist's finger and the patient's skin move as one unit (Figure 5–6B).

Duration of Treatment

Usually 2 to 4 weeks of treatment are required, whereby the patient is seen three to five times per week. The transverse friction massage should last approximately 10 minutes.

During the treatment period, vigorous activities should be avoided. When the functional examination is completely pain free, the patient can slowly increase daily activities and gradually return to participating in sports.

ACROMIOCLAVICULAR JOINT ARTHRITIS

Functional Examination

- Passive arm elevation, internal rotation, and external rotation of the shoulder are painful at end-range.

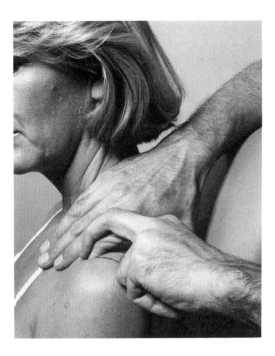

Figure 5–6A Starting position of transverse friction.

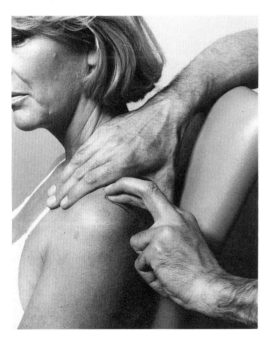

Figure 5–6B End position of transverse friction phase.

- Passive horizontal adduction is painful and limited.
- Often, resisted adduction is also painful.

Injection

Injection is indicated for subluxation, traumatic arthritis, and arthritides that are rheumatoid in nature, such as rheumatoid arthritis, Reiter's disease, ankylosing spondylitis, and gout.

Position of the Patient

The patient sits on the treatment table and leans back against the head of the table, which is inclined approximately 120°. The arm of the affected side hangs over the edge of the table; in this way gravity exerts a slight pull in the acromioclavicular joint, resulting in a widening of the joint line.

Position of the Physician

The physician stands at the affected side of the patient next to the treatment table.

Performance

After carefully localizing the acromioclavicular joint, a 3- to 4-cm needle (with 2 mL syringe) is inserted vertically into the ventral V-shaped indentation between the clavicle and acromion.

Upon passing through the cranial ligaments, the joint space is reached, followed by the caudal ligaments. At this point, the caudal ligaments are injected from ventral to dorsal (Figure 5–7) in a dropwise fashion, using approximately 0.5 mL of solution. Next, 0.5 mL is injected intra-articularly, and finally 0.5 mL is injected into the cranial ligaments (again in a dropwise fashion).

Follow-Up

Activities are limited for 1 week (no vigorous activities should be performed). The patient is rechecked in 1 week. Usually two or three injections, given over a time period of 4 to 6 weeks, are required for complete relief of pain.

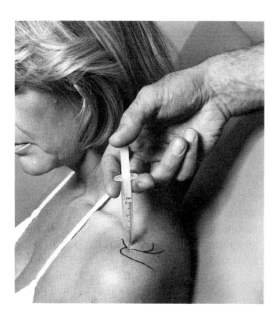

Figure 5–7A Injection of the caudal acromioclavicular ligaments, ventral part.

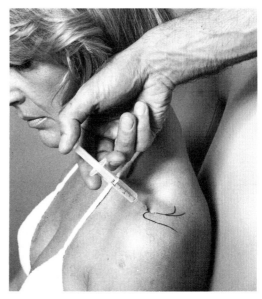

Figure 5–7B Injection of the caudal acromioclavicular ligaments, dorsal part.

When there is only minimal to no improvement, surgery may be indicated.

STERNOCLAVICULAR JOINT ARTHRITIS

Functional Examination

- End-range passive arm elevation, internal rotation, and external rotation of the shoulder are painful in the region of the sternoclavicular joint.
- All active motions of the shoulder girdle *can* be painful.
- Passive horizontal adduction is painful in the region of the sternoclavicular joint and limited.

Injection

An injection is particularly beneficial in relieving pain in patients suffering from a traumatic arthritis of the sternoclavicular joint (which is often seen in conjunction with a ventrocaudal subluxation of the clavicle).

This is also true in cases of rheumatoid arthritis and subacute joint degeneration.

Usually, residual limited motion can be restored by means of joint-specific mobilization.

Position of the Patient

The patient sits on the treatment table and leans back against the inclined head of the table.

Position of the Physician

The physician stands or sits at the affected side of the patient, next to the treatment table.

Performance

The physician carefully locates the sternoclavicular joint. Sometimes, slightly contracting both of the sternocleidomastoid muscles makes the palpation easier.

The injection is performed with a 2-cm long needle, which is inserted directly medial to the sternal end of the clavicle (Figure 5–8). The needle is then guided in a dorsal and

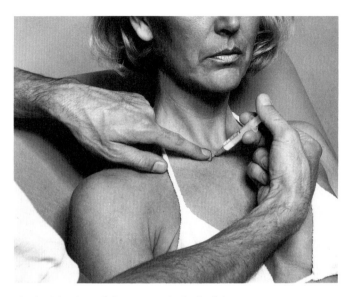

Figure 5–8 Intra-articular injection of the sternoclavicular joint.

slightly medial direction; after approximately 1 cm, the tip of the needle is intra-articular. At this point, 0.5 to 1 mL of solution is injected into the joint.

The needle should not be any longer than 2 cm; otherwise there is danger of puncturing the large blood vessels running directly behind the joint.

The patient should wear a sling for 3 days, followed by 1 week of minimal activity.

Follow-Up

After 2 weeks, the patient is seen for follow-up.

Usually, one or two injections over a period of 4 to 6 weeks are required for complete relief of pain.

Generally, the patient remains permanently free of pain after this treatment.

SUBACROMIAL-SUBDELTOID BURSITIS

Functional Examination for a Chronic Bursitis

- A painful arc is encountered during active arm elevation.

- The impingement test provokes pain (passive internal rotation performed with the shoulder in 90° flexion).
- One or more passive tests can be painful, usually at end-range.
- One or more resisted tests can be painful, particularly abduction. However, when the resisted tests are repeated with an inferior pull exerted on the arm, pain is no longer provoked.

Functional Examination for an Acute Bursitis

- There is severe limitation of arm elevation.
- Passive abduction is significantly more limited than the rotation motions.

An acute bursitis is often the result of a calcium deposit in the supraspinatus tendon that has protruded into the bursa.

A chronic bursitis is never the result of an acute bursitis. This lesion develops through mechanical irritation and almost always occurs in conjunction with other pathology of the shoulder, such as a rotator cuff lesion or an acromioclavicular joint problem.

Injection for Acute Bursitis

For an acute bursitis, the injected solution consists of 3 to 5 mL of triamcinolone acetonide, 10 mg/mL, and 2.5 mL of a strong local anesthetic (2% lidocaine) (Table 5–1).

After 2 days, the patient is again seen in the clinic. Generally, significant improvement already will have been achieved. Solution is again injected into the bursa, but this time using less solution. Rarely are more than two injections necessary for complete relief of pain.

Injection for Chronic Bursitis

The first time the patient receives an injection, the solution should consist only of 3 to 5 mL of a local anesthetic (for example, 1% lidocaine) (Table 5–1). Immediately after the injection, the functional examination is repeated and should now be painless.

Two possible situations exist when the patient is reevaluated 1 week later: (1) No improvement is noted: in this case, solution is again injected into the bursa but this time with an additional 1 to 2 mL of triamcinolone acetonide, 10 mg/mL. (2) Improvement is noted: injection of a local anesthetic is repeated.

Position of the Patient

The patient sits on the treatment table, with the affected side as close to the edge of the table as possible. The patient leans back against the head of the table, which is inclined approximately 120°. The arm of the affected side hangs over the edge of the table.

Position of the Physician

The physician stands or sits at the affected side of the patient, next to the treatment table.

Performance

The physician palpates the lateral border of the acromion and then—indirectly—the subdeltoid part of the bursa.

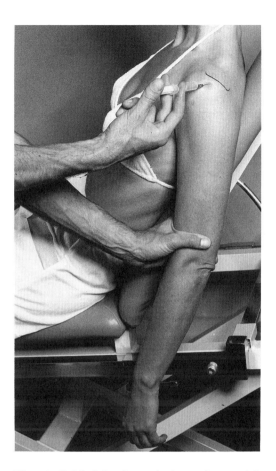

Figure 5–9A Injection of the subacromial-subdeltoid bursa, while pulling on the arm.

First the subdeltoid part of the bursa is injected with a 5-cm needle; this is followed by injection of the subacromial part. If the hanging arm does not afford enough room between the humerus and the acromion, the physician can exert a slight inferior pull on the patient's distal humerus in order to increase the subacromial space even more (Figure 5–9).

Injection Technique

In treatment of the subdeltoid part of the bursa, the needle is inserted 0.5 to 1 cm distal from the lateral edge of the acromion at an angle of 45° below the horizontal; if the subacromial part is to be injected, the needle is

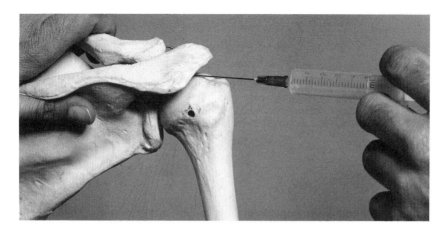

Figure 5–9B Skeletal model.

inserted horizontally. Should the needle contact bone, the needle is guided slightly more superior (in instances where the head of the humerus is reached) or slightly more inferior (in cases where it has hit the acromion).

The bursa receives the injection corresponding to the patient's pain. When the needle passes through the wall of the bursa, the patient typically experiences pain. At this point, the needle is inserted further until the pain is no longer felt. *The solution is then injected as the needle is withdrawn from this area.* This insertion, then withdraw, and inject method is repeated in all directions until the entire painful area of the bursa has been injected (Figure 5–10). If the needle enters a nonpainful area, no solution is injected.

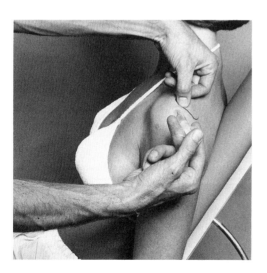

Figure 5–10A The subacromial-subdeltoid bursa is injected in all directions, the anterior part . . .

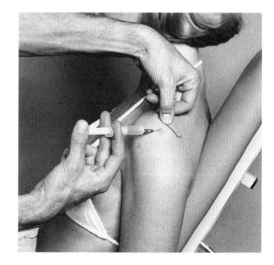

Figure 5–10B . . . and the posterior part.

Follow-Up

For a few days after the injection, patients should limit their activities as much as possible. The goal of the injection is to reduce the inflammatory reaction of the bursa as quickly as possible in order to begin the appropriate causal treatment.

An exercise program is initiated as soon as the functional examination provokes no pain (usually after 1 week, unless a second injection is necessary for complete relief) (Table 5–1). The exercise program is aimed at increasing the subacromial space. This can be achieved by strengthening muscles that insert on the humeral head and function to move the head distally. Emphasis is put on the adductors, internal rotators, and external rotators of the shoulder. The patient is encouraged to perform the home exercise program daily.

SUPRASPINATUS INSERTION TENDOPATHY

Functional Examination

- Active elevation of the arm can be painful.
- Passive elevation of the arm can be painful at end-range (when the medial part of the insertion is affected).

- A painful arc is encountered during active arm elevation (when the lateral part of the insertion is affected).
- Passive internal rotation can be painful (due to stretch).
- Passive horizontal adduction is sometimes painful (due to stretch).
- Resisted abduction is painful, and sometimes weak.
- Resisted external rotation is often painful (the supraspinatus is also active with external rotation against resistance).
- If the resisted tests are repeated with a pull on the arm (to rule out involvement of the bursa), the tests are just as painful if not more so.

Transverse Friction Massage

With these symptoms one must differentiate between an insertion tendopathy of the supraspinatus and a chronic subacromial-subdeltoid bursitis. Repeating the resisted test with a pull on the arm makes this possible. In cases of tendopathy, the resisted test with a pull on the arm is at least as painful as it is without the pull.

Position of the Patient

The patient sits on the treatment table with the affected side as close to the edge of the

---

Table 5–1 Regimen for Injection for Acute and Chronic Bursitis

Treatment	Acute Bursitis	Chronic Bursitis
Length of needle	5 cm	5 cm
Volume of solution	5–10 mL	4–7 mL
Solution	Triamcinolone acetonide, 10 mg/mL, + 2% lidocaine	1% lidocaine + possibly triamcinolone acetonide, 10 mg/mL
No. of injections required	Two	One to a maximum of three
Advice after injection	Limited activities	Limited activities for 1 week, then home exercise program

table as possible. The patient leans back against the head of the table, which is inclined approximately 120°. In this position, the part of the greater tubercle where the supraspinatus inserts lies in the horizontal plane.

The patient places the forearm of the affected side behind the back (with this, the shoulder is in internal rotation, extension) whereby the arm is in approximately 10° abduction. (This slight abduction of the humerus is necessary because circulation in the hypovascular zone of the supraspinatus is diminished even more if the arm is in 0° abduction.)

From this position, the supraspinatus insertion is brought in front of the acromion and is the most accessible for both palpation and injection.[42]

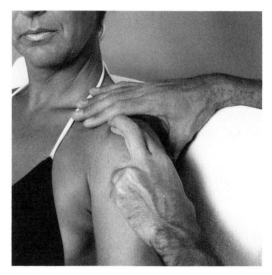

Figure 5–11A Transverse friction massage of the supraspinatus insertion.

Position of the Therapist

The therapist stands or sits at the affected side of the patient, next to the treatment table.

The ventral corner of the acromion is located (possibly with a slight pull on the arm), and from here, with the end phalanx of the index finger—now horizontal, the plateau of the greater tubercle is palpated in a medial direction. Usually, the medial border is clearly palpable. Due to the thick fibers of the deltoid, it is impossible to palpate the supraspinatus tendon itself.

If the right side is affected, the therapist places the tip of the right index finger directly medial to the plateau of the greater tubercle; the thumb rests vertically under the index finger (Figure 5–11A).

Performance

The middle finger reinforces the index finger (Figure 5–11B). Pressure is exerted while the wrist is brought into dorsal extension, which moves the index finger transversely over the supraspinatus insertion. Subsequent palmar flexion in the wrist occurs during the relaxation phase. In order to be able to perform the transverse friction massage over a longer period of time, the therapist slightly adducts the shoulder during the "friction" phase.

When the patient experiences a painful arc during active elevation, the lateral part of the insertion is affected. This is best treated by exerting pressure during the transverse friction in an inferior direction. In this instance, the thumb is placed on the humerus, in a position along a vertical line distal to the index finger (Figure 5–11A–C).

When the patient has pain at the end-range of elevation, the medial part of the insertion is affected. This is treated by exerting pressure in a posteroinferior direction. To accomplish this, the thumb is placed in a position dorsal and inferior to the index finger (Figure 5–12).

Unsatisfactory results from the transverse friction may be due to the following:

- When there is a calcium deposit in the tendon, there is usually minimal to no pain relief during the treatment; instead, the pain can even increase. In this case, an injection of a local anesthetic may be indicated.

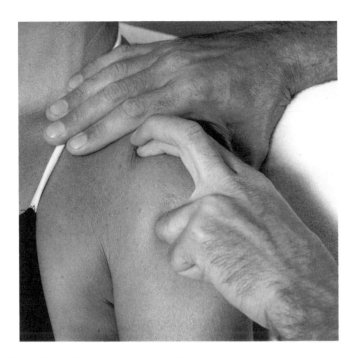

Figure 5–11B Initial position of the transverse friction massage.

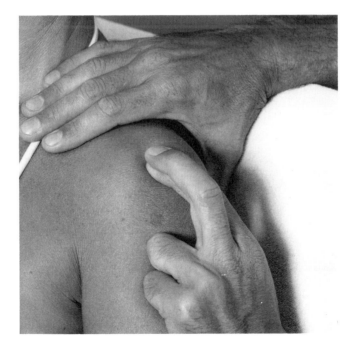

Figure 5–11C End position of the transverse friction massage.

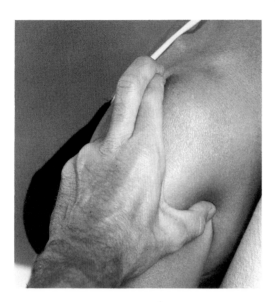

Figure 5–12 Hand position for transverse friction when the medial part of the supraspinatus insertion is affected.

- If a chronic subacromial-subdeltoid bursitis is present, there is unlikely to be improvement in the pain. Generally bursitis does not react well to mechanical local treatment, and the pain will increase significantly during the transverse friction. Normally, this lesion can be differentiated from the insertion tendopathy by the "pull" test. Again, in this instance, an injection is indicated (see Subacromial-Subdeltoid Bursitis).

Duration of Treatment

The frequency of treatment can range from two to five times per week. Athletes, however, should be seen daily for treatment. Each session of transverse friction should last approximately 15 minutes. Depending on the stage of the tendinitis, it may take 2 to 6 weeks for complete recovery.

The treatment of transverse friction should always be combined with stretching of the supraspinatus muscle. During the recovery

period, activities should be reduced: in stage 2 by 50%; in stage 3, sports activities should be stopped temporarily. In cases where the treatment is unsuccessful or the patient has recurrent problems, an injection may be indicated.

As soon as the functional examination provokes no pain, a muscle-strengthening exercise program should be initiated. If the lesion is the result of a shoulder instability, emphasis is placed on strengthening the appropriate muscles for that particular type of instability.

Stretching for Supraspinatus and Infraspinatus Tendopathies

Stretching for a supraspinatus insertion tendopathy is always combined with transverse friction massage. The patient is also instructed to perform a self-stretching exercise several times daily at home.

Position of the Patient

The patient lies supine with the unaffected side as close as possible to the edge of the table.

Position of the Therapist

The therapist stands at the unaffected side of the patient next to the treatment table. If the right side is to be treated, the therapist brings the patient's right shoulder into depression and retraction and then fixes the scapula with the left hand by pushing the lateral border of the scapula into the table (Figures 5–13A and B).

The therapist grasps the patient's elbow with the right hand, bringing the patient's shoulder into approximately 90° flexion (the patient's forearm is held between the therapist's right upper arm and body).

Performance

Slight axial pressure is exerted proximally through the patient's humerus, and the therapist brings the patient's arm slowly into horizontal adduction (Figure 5–13C). If necessary, slight internal rotation can be added to

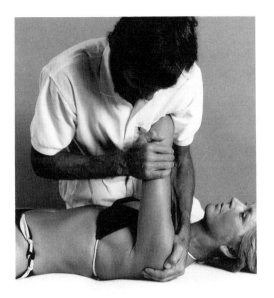

A

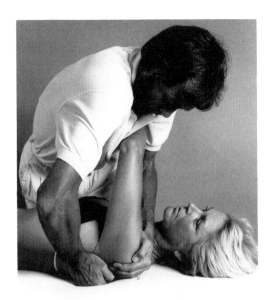

B

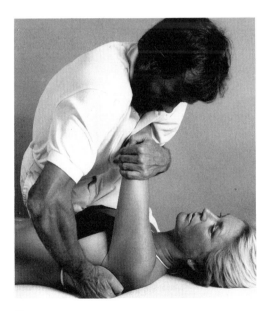

C

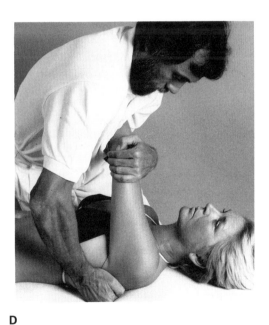

D

Figure 5–13 A, Initial position in stretching the supraspinatus and infraspinatus muscles; **B**, the scapula is fixed; **C**, while exerting axial pressure through the humerus, the shoulder is slowly brought into horizontal adduction; **D**, if necessary, slight internal rotation is added to increase the stretch.

increase the stretch (Figure 5–13). The therapist pays close attention to pain reactions or muscle splinting.

Various degrees of flexion may have to be positioned in order to determine where the best stretch can be felt.

Self-Stretching Exercise for Supraspinatus and Infraspinatus Tendopathies

The patient should perform the stretching exercise two or three times daily at home, particularly the first thing in the morning and before and after vigorous activities. An athlete should perform a more intensive stretching exercise program: stretching hourly is recommended during the first week of treatment, then every 2 hours in the second week of treatment. In the third week, the athlete should stretch two or three times per day.

Position of the Patient

The patient is instructed to bring the shoulder girdle into depression and retraction. The shoulder girdle must be actively held in this position during the entire stretch and is a way of fixing the scapula (Figure 5–14A).

If the patient's right side is affected, the right shoulder is flexed to approximately 90° with the right elbow also flexed 90°. The patient now grasps the right elbow with the left hand, whereby the right hand rests across, either on top of or underneath (Figure 5–14B), the opposite upper arm.

Performance

With the left hand, the patient gently pulls the right shoulder into horizontal adduction. Various degrees of flexion have to be tried in order to determine where the best stretch can be felt. If necessary, a slight amount of inter-

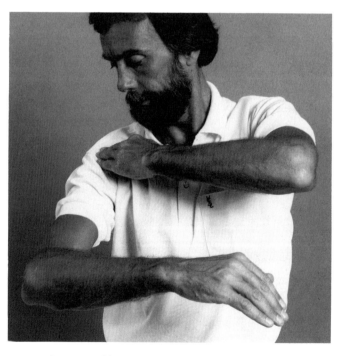

Figure 5–14A Home exercise: stretching the supraspinatus muscle of the right shoulder. First the shoulder girdle is brought into depression and retraction.

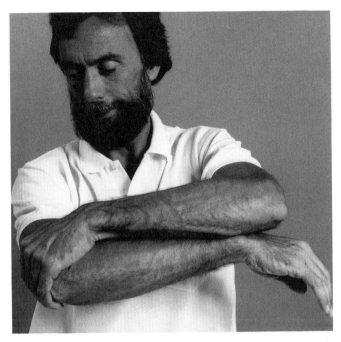

Figure 5–14B The arm then is brought into adduction, and if necessary internal rotation, in order to increase the stretch. Internal rotation can be performed by pushing the wrist gently downward with the elbow.

nal rotation can be added to increase the effect of the stretch.

Injection

In calcification of the tendon, or when six treatments of transverse friction massage and stretching bring minimal to no results, an injection of a local anesthetic is indicated (Table 5–2).

Position of the Patient

The patient sits on the treatment table, with the affected side as close to the edge of the table as possible, and leans back against the head of the table, which is inclined approximately 120°. In this position, the part of the greater tubercle where the supraspinatus inserts lies in the horizontal plane.

The patient places the forearm of the affected side behind the back (with this, the shoulder is in internal rotation and extension), whereby the shoulder rests in approximately 10° abduction. This position brings the insertion in front of the acromion, making it easier to localize.

Position of the Physician

The physician stands or sits at the affected side of the patient, next to the treatment table.

Performance

The insertion of the supraspinatus is located. A syringe is filled with 1 mL of local anesthetic (for instance, 1% lidocaine). If there is a calcium deposit in the tendon, a thick needle is used. In all other instances, a thin, 3-cm long needle is used for the injection.

The needle is inserted vertically; after passing through the skin, subcutaneous tissue, deltoid muscle, and bursa, the tough sturdy

Table 5–2 Treatment for Supraspinatus and Infraspinatus Insertion Tendopathies

Treatment	Number	Frequency	Results	Follow-Up

Transverse friction and stretching	Six	3–5 times per week	No improvement
			  Injection of local
			    anesthetic (two)
			Improvement
			  Continue with trans-
			    verse friction and
			    stretching
				Limit activities; continue home stretching exercise program, muscle strengthening, and treatment of primary cause (eg, instability)

Injection of local anesthetic	Three	1 time per week	No improvement
			  Injection of triamcino-
			    lone acetonide
			Improvement
			  At the most, two more
			    injections of a local
			    anesthetic
				Limit activities; continue stretching exercises

Injection of triamcino-lone acetonide, 10 mg/mL	One	1 time every 2 weeks	No improvement
			  Limit activities for a
			    long period (3–6 mo)
			    or arthroscopic
			    surgery
			Improvement
			  At the most, three
			    more injections
				3 days sling; limit activities for next 4 days

resistance of the tendon is reached (Figure 5–15A). As soon as the patient's pain is provoked, one drop of solution is injected. The needle is then further inserted until it contacts bone, at which point another drop is injected.

Now the needle is withdrawn to the subcutaneous tissue and reinserted in a slightly different direction, repeating the steps listed above (Figure 5–15B). In this way the needle is directed in several different spots, and the insertion is injected in a dropwise fashion corresponding to the patient's pain.

If the functional examination indicates pain at the end-range of passive elevation, the lesion is further medial and the needle should be directed more dorsally (under the acromion).

Follow-Up

The patient limits activities for 1 day and is reevaluated in 1 week. A second injection of a local anesthetic is given only if the patient's functional examination indicates significant improvement (Table 5–2). Usually in patients with a calcium deposit in the tendon, the improvement is remarkable.

If no further improvement is noted, an injection of triamcinolone acetonide is indicated. This injection is performed as described above. The patient then wears a sling for 3 days, limits activities for the following 4 days, and finally slowly returns to vigorous (or sports) activities after 10 days (Table 5–2).

After 2 weeks the patient should be seen again for follow-up. Depending on the find-

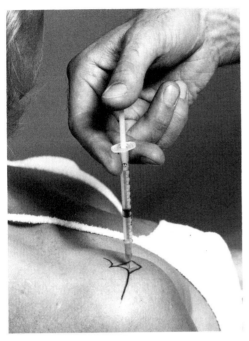

Figure 5–15A Injection of the supraspinatus insertion.

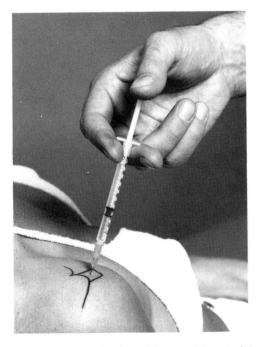

Figure 5–15B Injection of the medial part of the supraspinatus insertion.

ings from the functional examination, another injection may be performed. Even if the patient reports complete relief of pain, but the functional examination still shows some positive findings (such as pain on resisted abduction), a second injection is necessary. At this point, one likely needs only 0.5 mL of solution. The follow-up is the same as after the first injection.

Sometimes even a third injection (of corticosteroid) is necessary. Despite the injections and limiting activities for a longer period of time (3 to 6 months), if no significant improvement is noted, arthroscopic surgery (Neer acromioplasty) may be indicated.[34]

STRAIN OF THE SUPRASPINATUS MUSCULOTENDINOUS JUNCTION

Functional Examination

- Resisted abduction is painful.
- There is NO painful arc during active arm elevation, and end-range passive elevation is NOT painful.
- Sometimes passive internal rotation is painful (due to stretch).

Transverse Friction Massage

This lesion of the supraspinatus is seen much less often than the insertion tendopathy.

Position of the Patient

The patient sits next to the treatment table and rests the upper arm in a horizontal position on the table.

Note: With the arm in a neutral position, the musculotendinous junction is found underneath the acromion. By abducting the arm to 90°, the area that needs to be treated becomes palpable just medial to the acromion, between the scapular spine and the clavicle (Figure 5–16).

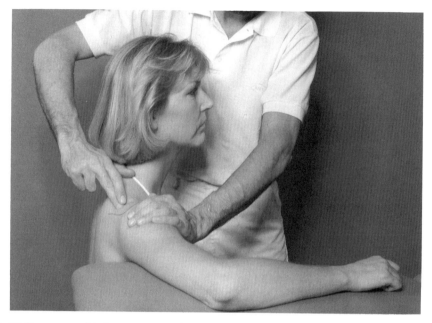

Figure 5–16 Transverse friction massage of the supraspinatus musculotendinous junction.

Position of the Therapist

The therapist stands next to the patient at the nonaffected side. If the right shoulder is affected, the therapist places the tip of the middle finger as lateral as possible between the clavicle and scapular spine (Figure 5–17A). With the left hand, the therapist supports the patient's shoulder from anterior.

Performance

Pressure exerted by the middle finger is reinforced with the tip of the index finger. The transverse friction occurs through a supination of the forearm. This supination movement must be performed to such a degree that, at the end of the motion, the therapist is able to see the palm of the hand (Figure 5–17B).

The middle finger is chosen for this treatment because it lies in line with the axis and therefore is an extension of the pronation and supination movement. The relaxation phase of the transverse friction massage occurs during the movement into pronation.

Duration of Treatment

The patient should be seen three times per week, and the transverse friction should last approximately 15 minutes. Stretching, particularly the home exercise, is also a necessary part of this treatment program (see Stretching for Supraspinatus and Infraspinatus Tendopathies). This treatment almost always leads to a full recovery within 6 to 10 sessions.

Note: An injection of this lesion with a local anesthetic offers no therapeutic benefit. However, it can help to confirm the diagnosis. *Corticosteroids are contraindicated.*

INFRASPINATUS INSERTION TENDOPATHY

Functional Examination

- Active elevation of the arm can be painful.
- Passive elevation of the arm can be painful at end-range.

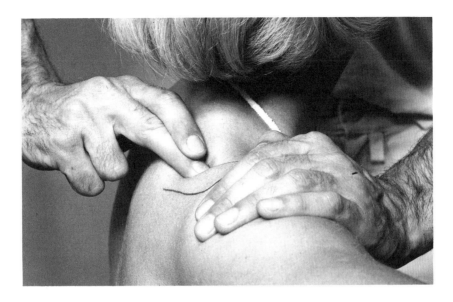

Figure 5–17A Transverse friction massage of the supraspinatus musculotendinous junction: initial position, and . . .

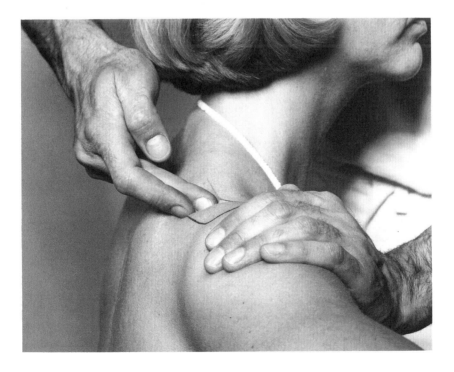

Figure 5–17B . . . end position.

- A painful arc can be encountered during active arm elevation.
- Passive internal rotation is often painful (due to stretch).
- Passive horizontal adduction can be painful (due to stretch).
- Resisted external rotation is painful and sometimes weak (partial tear).
- If the resisted test is repeated with a pull on the arm (in order to rule out involvement of the bursa), it is just as painful, if not more so.

Transverse Friction Massage

Differentiating from a lesion of the supraspinatus is not always easy, because the supraspinatus is also active during resisted external rotation. However, resisted abduction must also be painful in instances of supraspinatus tendinitis. If the *only* painful resisted test is external rotation, the lesion lies most likely in the infraspinatus.

Position of the Patient

The patient lies in a prone position, supporting the upper body on the elbows. There should be approximately 45° to 60° of flexion in the shoulders. The elbow of the affected side is placed approximately 10 cm from the edge of the table, and the patient grips the edge of the table with the hand (bringing the shoulder into slight external rotation). The patient then shifts the body over the elbow, thus bringing the shoulder into adduction.

The patient can also be positioned in a sitting position at the short end of the treatment table, as illustrated in Figure 5–18. The patient is instructed to place the elbows on the treatment table and lean far enough forward so that there is approximately 45° to 60° of flexion in the affected shoulder. As described above, the elbow rests approximately 10 cm from the edge of the table. The patient then grasps the edge of the table and shifts the upper body weight toward the edge of the

table. In this way the shoulder is in slight adduction and external rotation.

Note: If the patient's arm rests in a neutral position, the tendon of the infraspinatus cannot be reached by palpation; part of the insertion is now found underneath the acromion, and the entire tendon lies underneath. In the positions described above, the infraspinatus insertion is brought posteriorly out from under the acromion and is the most accessible for both palpation and injection.[42]

Position of the Therapist

The therapist stands next to the patient, at the affected side. The therapist's forearm is positioned in line with the running of the infraspinatus tendon, the thumb at the level of the lesion, and the fingers at the anterior aspect of the shoulder. If the left side is affected, the therapist uses the left hand.

The tendon is usually palpable directly distal to the angle formed between the scapular spine and the acromion. However, the lesion is most often located further lateral, at the insertion, than in the tendon itself.

Performance

The transverse friction can be performed in several different ways. One method is described as follows: The therapist places the tip of one thumb over the other; during the "friction" phase, both thumbs are adducted and both forearms are supinated (Figure 5–19A and B).

Duration of Treatment

The frequency of treatment can range from two to five times per week. Athletes should be seen daily for treatment. Each session of transverse friction should last approximately 15 to 20 minutes. Depending on the stage of the tendinitis, it may take 2 to 6 weeks for complete recovery.

The treatment of transverse friction should always be combined with stretching of the infraspinatus muscle. During the recovery period, activities should be reduced: in stage

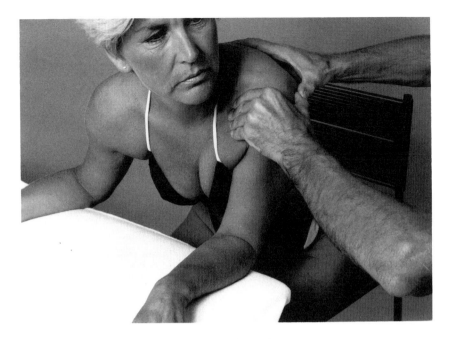

Figure 5–18 Transverse friction of the infraspinatus insertion.

2, by 50%; in stage 3 sports activities should be stopped temporarily. In cases where the treatment is unsuccessful or the patient has recurrent problems, an injection may be indicated.

As soon as the functional examination provokes no pain, a muscle-strengthening exercise program should be initiated. If the lesion is a consequence of a shoulder instability, emphasis is placed on strengthening the appropriate muscles for that particular type of instability.

Stretching

The treatment of transverse friction should always be combined with stretching during the recovery period (see Stretching for Supraspinatus and Infraspinatus Tendopathies).

Injection

If minimal to no results have been achieved with six treatments of transverse friction

massage, an injection of a local anesthetic is indicated.

Position of the Patient

The patient lies in a prone position, supporting the upper body on the elbows. There should be approximately 45° to 60° of flexion in the shoulders. The elbow of the affected side is placed approximately 10 cm from the edge of the table, and the patient grips the edge of the table with the hand (bringing the shoulder into slight external rotation). The patient then shifts the body over the elbow, thus bringing the shoulder into adduction.

The patient can also be positioned in a sitting position at the short end of the treatment table, as illustrated in Figure 5–18. The patient is instructed to place the elbows on the treatment table and lean far enough forward so that there is approximately 45° to 60° of flexion in the affected shoulder. As described above, the elbow rests approximately 10 cm from the edge of the table. The patient then grasps the edge of the table and shifts the

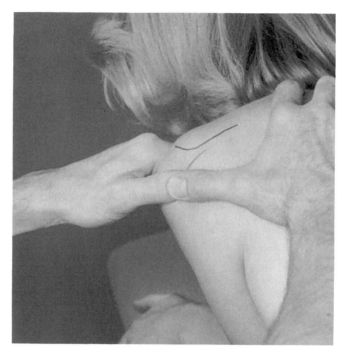

Figure 5–19A Initial position for the transverse friction of the infraspinatus insertion and . . .

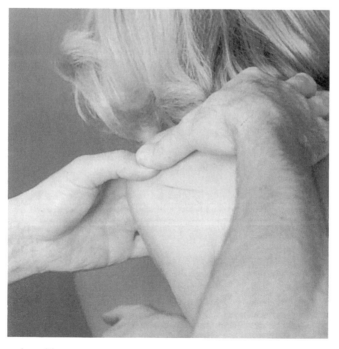

Figure 5–19B . . . end position.

upper body weight toward the edge of the table. In this way the shoulder is in slight adduction and external rotation.

Note: If the patient's arm rests in a neutral position, the tendon of the infraspinatus cannot be reached by palpation; part of the insertion is now found underneath the acromion, and the entire tendon lies underneath.

In the positions described above, the infraspinatus insertion is brought posteriorly out from under the acromion and is the most accessible for both palpation and injection.[42]

Position of the Physician

The physician sits or stands at the affected side of the patient, next to the treatment table (as described for supraspinatus injection).

The tendon is located directly distal to the angle formed between the scapular spine and the acromion. The most painful site of the lesion is usually found further lateral, at the insertion.

Performance

A 3- to 4-cm long needle with 1 mL of local anesthetic is used for the injection. The needle is inserted perpendicular to the skin. As soon as the patient's pain is provoked, one drop of solution is injected. The needle is then further inserted until it contacts bone, at which point another drop is injected (Figure 5–20).

Now the needle is withdrawn to the subcutaneous tissue and reinserted in a slightly different direction, repeating the steps listed above. In this way the needle is directed in several different spots, and the insertion is injected in a dropwise fashion corresponding to the patient's pain.

Follow-Up

The patient limits activities for 1 day and is reevaluated in 1 week.

A second injection of a local anesthetic is given only if the patient's functional examination indicates significant improvement.

If no further improvement is noted, an injection with triamcinolone acetonide is indicated. This injection is performed as described above. The patient then wears a sling for 3 days, limits activities for the following 4 days, and slowly returns to vigorous (or sports) activities after 10 days.

After 2 weeks the patient should be seen again for follow-up. Depending on the findings from the functional examination, an-

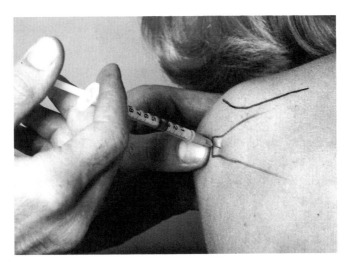

Figure 5–20 Injection of the insertion of the infraspinatus muscle.

other injection is performed. Even if the patient reports complete relief of pain, but the functional examination still shows some positive findings (such as pain on resisted external rotation), a second injection is necessary. At this point, one likely needs only 0.5 mL of solution. The follow-up is the same as that after the first injection.

SUBSCAPULARIS INSERTION TENDOPATHY

Functional Examination

- Active elevation of the arm can be painful.
- A painful arc is encountered during active arm elevation when the proximal part of the insertion is affected.
- Passive external rotation can be painful (due to stretch).
- Passive horizontal adduction is painful when the distal part of the insertion is affected.
- Resisted internal rotation is painful.
- If the resisted test is repeated with a pull on the arm (in order to rule out involvement of the bursa), the pain remains the same or even increases.

Transverse Friction Massage

In cases of irritation of the glenohumeral joint capsule and in instances of anterior shoulder instability, resisted internal rotation can be painful. This is likely due to the fact that the capsule and the subscapularis insertion are very closely connected. Contraction of the subscapularis muscle thus pulls on the irritated capsule.

Position of the Patient

The patient sits on the treatment table and leans back against the inclined head of the table. The affected shoulder is in the neutral (zero) position with the patient's hand resting in the lap (Figure 5–21).

In this position, the lesser tubercle is positioned directly forward and the entire insertion is accessible for both palpation and injection.

(To palpate the tendon, the shoulder is brought into approximately 80° external rotation. Palpation of the tendon is rarely necessary, however, because lesions in this region of the subscapularis are uncommon.)

Position of the Therapist

The therapist sits diagonally in front of the patient at the affected side. The lesser tubercle is palpated directly lateral to the coracoid process. If the right shoulder is to be treated, the therapist places the tip of the left thumb just distal to the lesion.

Performance

Technique 1. If the distal part of the insertion or the entire insertion is affected, the thumb is placed as far distal on the lesser tu-

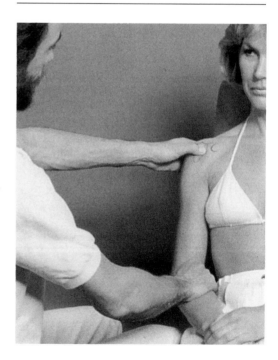

Figure 5–21 Transverse friction massage of the subscapularis.

bercle as possible (Figure 5–22A). If the lesion is located more in the proximal part of the insertion, the thumb is placed just distal to the proximal, most prominent part of the lesser tubercle.

The transverse friction phase occurs through adduction of the thumb, dorsal extension of the wrist, supination of the forearm

and slight adduction of the shoulder (Figure 5–22B).

Technique 2 (Not Pictured). The therapist stands behind the patient and places the tips of the index and middle fingers directly distal to the location of the lesion. The thumb rests against the scapula. The transverse fric-

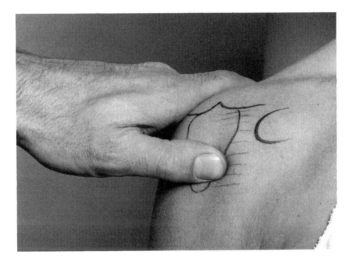

Figure 5–22A Initial position of the hand for the transverse friction of the proximal part of the subscapularis insertion.

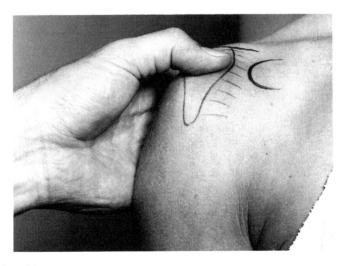

Figure 5–22B End position.

tion phase occurs through a dorsal extension of the wrist. The fingers themselves do not make a movement.

Follow-Up

Transverse friction massage along with stretching exercises for the subscapularis should be scheduled daily for athletes. Otherwise, the patient should be seen three times per week. The transverse friction massage should last 15 to 20 minutes per treatment session.

This lesion usually does not react as quickly to this treatment as the supraspinatus and infraspinatus tendopathies. After 10 treatment sessions significant improvement should be noted. If this is not the case, an injection of triamcinolone acetonide, 10 mg/mL, may be indicated.

Stretching

Stretching of the subscapularis muscle is indicated only if the lesion is *not* a consequence of an instability. Stretching is combined with the transverse friction treatment program. The patient is instructed to stretch several times daily at home.

Position of the Patient

The patient either lies in a supine position or sits inclined against the raised end of the treatment table.

Position of the Therapist

The therapist stands or sits next to the patient's affected side. The therapist positions the patient's shoulder in approximately 40° to 60° abduction and maximal external rotation. If the right shoulder is to be treated, the therapist grasps the patient's upper arm just proximal to the elbow. The other hand grasps the volar aspect of the patient's forearm, just proximal to the wrist.

Performance

Respecting the patient's pain and any muscle splinting, the therapist now slowly brings the patient's arm into extension and further into external rotation (Figure 5–23).

The patient should also perform self-stretching exercises several times daily at home. This can be performed by placing the hand on one side of a door frame, with the shoulder in approximately 40° to 60° abduction and maximal external rotation. By stepping forward slowly through the open door, the shoulder is brought into extension and more internal rotation.

Injection

A single injection with triamcinolone acetonide, 10 mg/mL, is so effective that sometimes one may choose to use this treatment method immediately rather than first performing transverse friction massage or giving an injection of a local anesthetic.

Position of the Patient

The patient sits on the treatment table and leans back against the inclined head of the table. The affected shoulder is in the neutral (zero) position with the patient's hand resting in the lap.

In this position, the lesser tubercle is positioned directly forward and the entire insertion is accessible for both palpation and injection.

Position of the Physician

The physician sits or stands diagonally in front of the patient at the affected side.

The lesser tubercle is palpated directly lateral to the coracoid process; the site of the lesion is located and marked.

Performance

The functional examination indicates which part of the insertion is affected.

A 2- to 3-cm long needle with a syringe of 0.5 to 1 mL of triamcinolone acetonide, 10 mg/mL, is used for the injection. The needle is inserted perpendicular to the skin. As soon as the patient's pain is provoked, one drop of

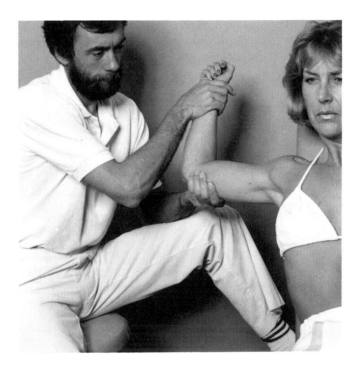

Figure 5–23 Stretch of the subscapularis muscle.

solution is injected. The needle is then further inserted until it contacts bone, at which point another drop is injected (Figures 5–24A and B).

Now the needle is withdrawn to the subcutaneous tissue and reinserted in a slightly different direction, repeating the steps listed above.

In this way the needle is directed in several different spots, and the insertion is injected in a dropwise fashion corresponding to the patient's pain.

Follow-Up

The patient should wear a sling for 3 or 4 days and limit activities for another week. Approximately 10 days after the injection, the patient may begin to increase activities slowly.

The patient should be rechecked after 2 weeks. Depending on the findings in the functional examination, a second injection may be necessary. Usually the patient has complete relief of pain after the first injection.

TENOSYNOVITIS OF THE LONG HEAD OF THE BICEPS

Functional Examination

- Active elevation of the arm is sometimes painful.
- Passive elevation of the arm, with overpressure in a posterior direction can be painful.
- A painful arc is sometimes encountered during active arm elevation.
- Very seldom, and generally only in very severe cases, is resisted elbow flexion (in combination with resisted forearm supination) painful.
- The stretch test is positive (with the scapula fixed, the shoulder is brought into physiological extension, the fore-

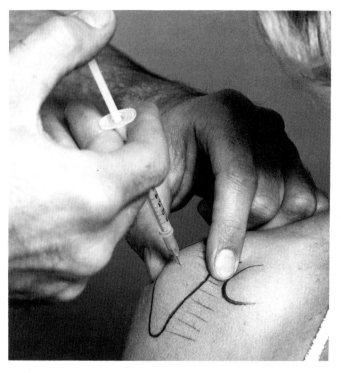

Figure 5–24A Injection of the proximal part of the subscapularis insertion. (Resisted internal rotation is painful, and a painful arc is encountered during active arm elevation.)

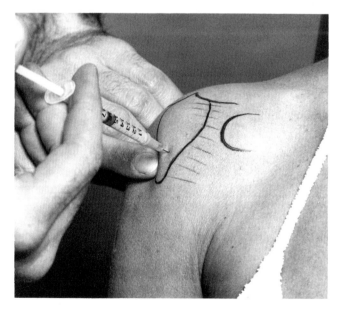

Figure 5–24B Injection of the distal part of the subscapularis insertion. (Resisted internal rotation is painful, and there is pain with horizontal adduction.)

arm is pronated, and then the elbow is extended).

Transverse Friction Massage

Based solely on palpation of local tenderness in the area of the long head of the biceps, the diagnosis of tendinitis or tenosynovitis is often *falsely* made. This local tenderness (referred tenderness) is often present in other lesions of the shoulder.

Position of the Patient

The patient sits on the treatment table and leans back against the inclined head of the table.

Position of the Therapist

The therapist sits at the affected side of the patient, next to the treatment table.

If the right shoulder is affected, the therapist grasps the patient's forearm with the right hand (the patient's forearm can be either in a neutral position or supinated) (Figure 5–25).

With the patient's shoulder in the physiological zero position, the tendon is located just lateral to the lesser tubercle. Usually the affected site is found directly below the acromion. The radial side of the left thumb is placed against the most tender spot on the tendon in the intertubercular sulcus (Figure 5–26A).

Performance

With the left thumb, the therapist exerts pressure against the tendon while bringing the patient's shoulder into approximately 30° external rotation; the tendon moves from medial to lateral underneath the thumb (Figure 5–26B). In the relaxation phase, the shoulder is returned to the zero position.

The friction can also be performed by moving from external rotation to the zero position. In this instance, the relaxation phase occurs during the external rotation movement.

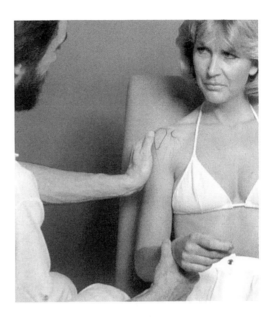

Figure 5–25 Transverse friction massage of the long head of the biceps.

Duration of Treatment

In most cases, complete recovery is achieved in six to eight treatment sessions of transverse friction massage.

Injection

Generally, the results of transverse friction are so good that only rarely is an injection of this lesion necessary.

Position of the Patient

The patient sits on the treatment table and leans back against the inclined head of the table.

Position of the Physician

The physician stands diagonally behind the patient's affected side next to the treatment table. The exact location of the lesion is determined by palpation. Usually the lesion lies in the tendon sheath directly distal to the acromion.

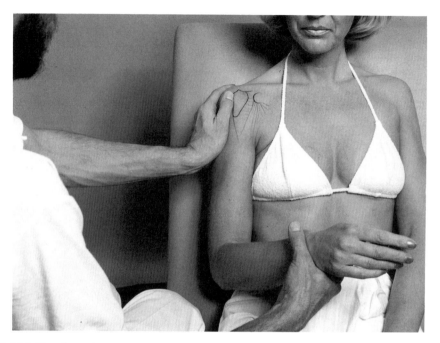

Figure 5–26A The therapist exerts pressure against the tendon of the long head of the biceps while bringing the patient's shoulder into approximately 30° external rotation. Initial position, and . . .

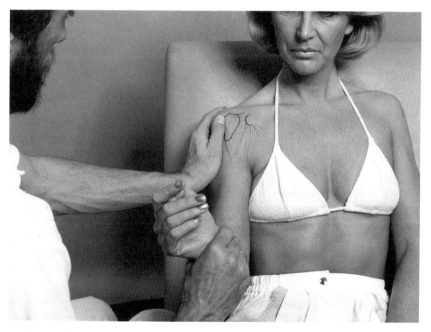

Figure 5–26B . . . end position. (This is the initial position if the therapist chooses to exert pressure against the tendon with the thumb, during movement into internal rotation.)

Performance

A 3-cm long needle and a syringe containing 1 mL of local anesthetic and 0.5 mL of triamcinolone acetonide, 10 mg/mL, are used for the injection.

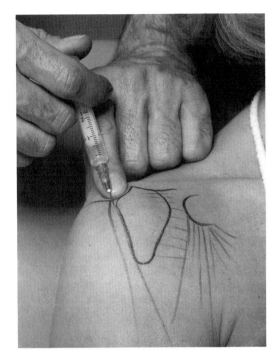

Figure 5–27 Injection between the tendon and the tendon sheath of the long tendon of the biceps.

The needle is inserted just distal to the acromion and slightly lateral to the lesser tubercle—directed parallel to the running of the lateral edge of the lesser tubercle. If a tough resistance is felt, the tendon has been reached. At this point, the needle is withdrawn slightly and reinserted in a slightly more anterior direction. The needle should now be lying between the tendon and its tendon sheath (Figure 5–27).

A small amount of solution is then injected, approximately 0.1 mL. If the needle is correctly positioned, a longitudinal swelling forms that is somewhat difficult to palpate. When the correct position of the needle has been confirmed using this method, the remainder of the solution is injected.

A few minutes after the injection, the tests from the functional examination that previously were positive should now be negative. This is true for all injections in which a local anesthetic has been used in the solution.

Follow-Up

The patient should support the arm in a sling for 3 or 4 days. Activities should be limited for another week. After that the patient can begin to increase activities slowly.

The patient should be rechecked after 2 weeks. Only seldom is a second injection necessary.

6

Peripheral Compression Neuropathies in the Shoulder Region

FUNCTIONAL ANATOMY

Although motor deficits do not occur in every compression syndrome of the upper extremity, an overview of the normal innervation of muscles should be kept on hand. Of course, these innervations are subject to significant variance, particularly distal in the extremity. In various anatomy books, descriptions of branching patterns and topography differ. Even the distribution of the segments is subject to interindividual differences. Therefore, the overview in Table 6–1 should be considered only a rough guide.

In regard to sensory innervation, there is even greater variance between individuals. Thus, in making a diagnosis, the examiner should not hold rigidly to one diagram. Regarding innervation of the hand, however, the following rules generally apply:

- The fifth finger and the ulnar aspect of the fourth finger are supplied entirely by the ulnar nerve.
- The other parts of the fingers are supplied dorsally by the radial nerve and palmarly by the median nerve.

SUPRASCAPULAR NERVE

The suprascapular nerve (C5-C6) arises from the upper trunk of the brachial plexus.

At the level of the posterior scalenic port, the nerve branches off from the plexus in the direction of the suprascapular notch (Figure 6–1). The suprascapular nerve runs laterally and deep to the trapezius until it reaches the suprascapular notch, where it runs under the superior transverse scapular ligament and enters the supra- and infraspinous fossae. The nerve innervates the supraspinatus and infraspinatus muscles, as well as parts of the glenohumeral and acromioclavicular joint capsules.

Trauma or extreme adduction movements in front of the body (cross-body actions) can cause the nerve to be pulled taut against the transverse ligament. This can result in the so-called sternal notch syndrome: a compression neuropathy of the suprascapular nerve.

Compression Neuropathy

Functional Anatomy

Compression neuropathies of the suprascapular nerve (C5-C6) generally are located in the scapular notch under the superior transverse scapular ligament. The cause is usually an acute trauma in the shoulder region. This can involve an indirect trauma such as a fall on the outstretched arm or an adduction trauma whereby the upper arm crosses in

Table 6–1 Overview of Normal Innervation of Muscles

Muscle	Nerve	Segments
Trapezius	Accessory nerve	Cranial nerve XI
Latissimus dorsi	Thoracodorsal	C6 to C8
Rhomboids	Dorsal scapular	C4, C5
Levator scapula	Cervical roots	C3, C4
	Dorsal scapular	C5
Pectoralis major	Lateral and medial pectoral	C5 to T1
Pectoralis minor	Lateral and medial pectoral	C5 to C8
Subclavius	Branch from the brachial plexus	C5, C6
Serratus anterior	Long thoracic	C5 to C7
Deltoid	Axillary	C5, C6
Subscapularis	Upper and lower subscapular	C5, C6
Supraspinatus	Suprascapular	C4 to C6
Infraspinatus	Suprascapular	C4 to C6
Teres minor	Axillary	C4 to C6
Teres major	Lower subscapular	C6, C7
Coracobrachialis	Musculocutaneous	C5 to C7

front of the body. Often the compression neuropathy is a complication after a Colles fracture (distal radius fracture) or a fracture of the scaphoid. Chronic compression, such as is sometimes seen in gymnasts, can also lead to a neuropathy.

In many cases, a capsular pattern of limited motions occurs in the shoulder as a result of pain due to the injured suprascapular nerve. In the clinic, the patient presents with a traumatic arthritis of the glenohumeral joint; however, the primary cause does not lie in the glenohumeral joint.

Differential Diagnosis

- arthritis of the glenohumeral joint
- tendopathy or (partial) rupture of the infraspinatus and supraspinatus muscles
- acromioclavicular pathology

Clinical Findings

- The patient complains of burning pain at the lateral and posterior aspect of the shoulder. Sometimes there is severe pain at the anterior aspect of the acro-

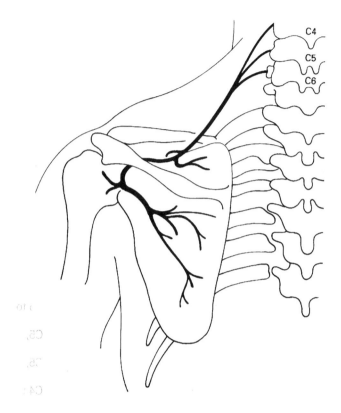

Figure 6–1 Trajectory of the suprascapular nerve.

mioclavicular joint. The pain is experienced deeply and the patient is unable to describe clearly the location of the pain. Often there is deep radiating pain in the upper arm, along the trajectory of the radial nerve. Active movements of the shoulder increase the pain. At night the pain can also be severe, especially in the acute stage.

- In long-standing lesions, there is loss of strength of the supraspinatus and infraspinatus muscles. Later, atrophy is also visible (Figure 6–2).
- Passively performed horizontal adduction of the shoulder can provoke extreme pain in the acute stage, due to the stretch on the nerve. Stretch is increased further by adding cervical rotation and sidebending away from the affected side.

Treatment

The treatment of choice is a perineural injection of corticosteroid in the suprascapular notch. The injection is administered at intervals of 2 weeks, and usually two to four injections are required to achieve complete relief of pain. (Caution must be taken not to pierce the suprascapular artery.)

If the result with injection therapy is unsatisfactory, the superior transverse scapular ligament can be removed surgically.

LONG THORACIC NERVE

The long thoracic nerve arises from the roots of C5 to C7. The C5 and C6 nerve fibers pierce through the middle scalene before coming together to form the main branch of the long thoracic nerve, which descends dorsal to the brachial plexus. The fibers from C7 run somewhat lower through the posterior scalenic triangle and join the main branch at the level of the superior border of the serratus anterior. The nerve as a whole runs further distally over the lateral surface of the serratus anterior. Separate branches supply each of the digitations of the serratus anterior.

Compression Neuropathy

Functional Anatomy

Lesions of the long thoracic nerve are fairly common, and are usually the result of carrying something heavy on the shoulder or of carrying a heavy backpack for long periods. Sometimes this lesion is also seen in people who perform heavy labor. Compression of the long thoracic nerve leads to weakness of the serratus anterior muscle.

Clinical Findings

- Symptoms usually consist only of vague pain in the neck-scapula region.
- During examination of the active shoulder motions, the patient is unable to per-

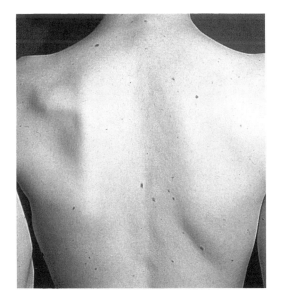

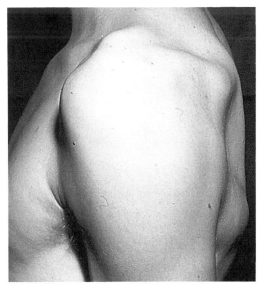

A   **B**

Figure 6–2 A patient with compression of the suprascapular nerve. Significant atrophy of both the supraspinatus and infraspinatus muscles is noted. **A**, Posterior view; **B**, side view.

form full elevation of the arm; however, passively the motion is normal.

- If the patient leans with both hands against the wall (with elbows extended), a scapula alata (usually unilateral) is evident. The medial edge of the scapula on the affected side lifts away from the thorax. In addition, the scapula is positioned too close to the vertebral column, with the inferior angle lying most medial.

Treatment

Therapeutic measures do not have any effect on recovery. The ultimate prognosis is usually good; however, complete recovery sometimes takes up to 2 years.

7

Thoracic Outlet Syndrome

Thoroughness during the functional examination is essential in differentiating thoracic outlet syndrome from other compression neuropathies of the upper extremity. Therefore, this syndrome is discussed in a chapter of its own. For differential diagnosis in regard to cervical nerve root syndromes, refer to *Diagnosis and Treatment of the Spine*, Chapter 6, Cervical Spine.

In the term *thoracic outlet syndrome*, disturbances of the thoracic inlet are also included. The syndrome involves compression of nerves and/or blood vessels that lie close to the skeleton and/or run through narrow openings in the shoulder girdle region. Symptoms are nonradicular in nature. Seen more frequently in women than in men, the syndrome can also be found particularly in people who perspire easily or become dizzy. Individuals in the latter group who develop thoracic outlet syndrome often complain that the fingers feel "thick." However, actual evidence of swelling in the fingers is not found.

FUNCTIONAL ANATOMY OF THE THORACIC OUTLET REGION

Generally, in thoracic outlet syndrome, there is a problem with the passage of nerves and/or blood vessels through one or more of the following sites (Figure 7–1):

- the anterior and/or posterior scalenic triangle
- the space between the first rib and the clavicle (costoclavicular space)
- the space dorsal to the pectoralis minor (coracothoracopectoral space)

Structures That Can Cause Compression

Anterior Scalenic Triangle.
- Muscle bellies or insertions of the sternocleidomastoid and anterior scalene (rare)

Posterior Scalenic Triangle.
- Hypertrophy of the anterior and middle scalenes (eg, in patients with bronchial asthma or hyperventilation, or in some types of sports)
- Abnormally wide insertions of the anterior and middle scalenes, or fusion of both insertions on the first rib

Costoclavicular Space.
Compression of the neurovascular structures in the thoracic outlet occurs most often in the costoclavicular space. Usually a functional disturbance of the clavicular joints is involved: during arm elevation, the clavicle reaches its end position too early. In many instances, this is due to an often long-standing periarticular shoulder problem. Other possibilities for a narrowing of this space are as follows:

- callus formation, pseudarthrosis, or angulation after a clavicle fracture
- exostosis of the first rib
- significantly enlarged C7 transverse process (megatransversus), with or without

157

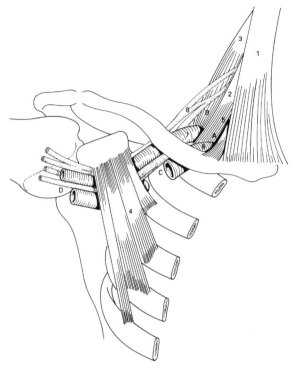

Figure 7–1 Possible sites of compression in the thoracic outlet region. **A**, Anterior scalenic triangle; **B**, posterior scalenic triangle; **C**, costoclavicular space; **D**, coracothoracopectoral space; **1**, sterno-cleidomastoid; **2**, anterior scalene; **3**, middle scalene; **4**, pectoralis minor; **5**, phrenic nerve; **6**, subclavian vein; **7**, subclavian artery; **8**, brachial plexus.

---

collagenous tissue connections to the first rib (cervical bands)
- complete cervical rib
- collagenous tissue connections from a rudimentary first rib to the second rib
- Pancoast tumor (pulmonary sulcus tumor)

Coracothoracopectoral Triangle.
- Shortening or hypertonia of the pectoralis minor
- Apparent shortening of the pectoralis minor in a rigid thorax

Structures That Can Become Compromised

Anterior Scalenic Triangle.
- Subclavian vein

- Phrenic nerve
- Large lymph vessels

Posterior Scalenic Triangle.
- Subclavian artery
- Brachial plexus

Costoclavicular Space.
- Subclavian vein
- Lymph vessels
- Subclavian artery
- Brachial plexus (problems occur primarily in the microcirculation, affecting mainly the sympathetic nerve fibers)

Coracothoracopectoral Space.
- Subclavian artery
- Subclavian vein
- Brachial plexus

Subclavian Artery and Vein

The right subclavian artery arises from the brachiocephalic trunk; the left arises directly from the aorta.

Initially, the subclavian artery runs cranially in the direction of the scalene muscles. At the apex of its course, the artery lies approximately 1.5 cm above the clavicle. The artery then runs through the posterior scalenic triangle and curves slightly downward to the lateral edge of the first rib, where its name changes to axillary artery.

The subclavian vein is a continuation of the axillary vein. The vein runs from the lateral edge of the first rib to the anterior scalenic triangle, where it joins with the internal jugular vein to form the brachiocephalic vein. The latter empties into the superior vena cava.

Brachial Plexus

In the formation of the brachial plexus (Figure 7–2), rearrangement of the nerve fibers takes place at three sites.

First Arrangement

- Ventral rami of spinal nerves from the cervical spine unite to form three trunks:
  1. upper trunk (C5, C6)
  2. middle trunk (C7)
  3. lower trunk (C8, T1)
- Contribution from the T4 and T1 segments varies significantly.

Second Arrangement

The trunks bifurcate into divisions, which go on to form the so-called cords:

cord	trunk	segments
lateral	upper & middle	C5 to C7
medial	lower	C7 to T1
posterior	upper, middle & lower	C5 to T1

Third Arrangement

Nerves that innervate the upper extremities branch off from the cords. In regard to symptomatology of the compression syndromes, the most important nerves are as follows:

nerve	cord	segments
radial	posterior	C5 to T1
median	lateral & medial	C5 to T1
ulnar	medial	C8 to T1

The radial, median, and ulnar nerves belong to the "infraclavicular" part of the brachial plexus. Other infraclavicular branches are as follows:

nerve	cord
medial cutaneous nerve of the forearm	medial
medial cutaneous nerve of the arm	medial
medial pectoral	medial
lateral pectoral	lateral
upper and lower subscapular	posterior
thoracodorsal	posterior
axillary	posterior
musculocutaneous	lateral

Branches from the "supraclavicular" part of the brachial plexus include the following:

- long thoracic nerve
- dorsal scapular nerve
- suprascapular nerve
- subclavian nerve

Scalenic Triangles

The triangular space between the anterior scalene and the sternocleidomastoid is called the anterior scalenic triangle. Also triangular in shape, the space between the anterior and middle scalenes is called the posterior

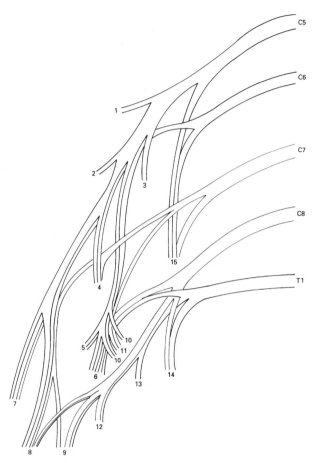

Figure 7–2 Simplified illustration of the right brachial plexus. **1**, Dorsal scapular nerve; **2**, suprascapular nerve; **3**, subclavian nerve; **4**, lateral pectoral nerve; **5**, axillary nerve; **6**, radial nerve; **7**, musculocutaneous nerve; **8**, median nerve; **9**, ulnar nerve; **10**, subscapular nerve; **11**, thoracodorsal nerve; **12**, medial cutaneous nerve of the forearm; **13**, medial cutaneous nerve of the arm; **14**, medial pectoral nerve; **15**, long thoracic nerve.

scalenic triangle. The base of each triangle is formed by the first rib.

Running through the anterior scalenic triangle are the subclavian vein, phrenic nerve, and several lymph vessels. Compression of these structures can occur primarily as a result of hypertrophy of the sternocleidomastoid and/or anterior scalene muscles.

Running through the posterior scalenic triangle is the subclavian artery, surrounded by the three cords of the brachial plexus. Compression of these structures can occur as a

result of hypertrophy or abnormal development of the anterior and middle scalenes.

Costoclavicular Space

Both the brachial plexus and the subclavian artery and vein have to pass through the space between the clavicle and the first rib. Various pathological processes and/or congenital deviations can narrow this space, leading to disturbances in the microcirculation. In addition, long-lasting postural deviations in which the clavicle is maintained in depression can also lead to compression of structures within the costoclavicular space.

Coracothoracopectoral Space

The pectoralis minor is a thin triangular muscle that runs from the cartilage of the third to the fifth ribs, over the thorax, and ends in a flat tendon at the coracoid process. The muscle is entirely covered by the pectoralis major.

Dorsal to the pectoralis minor, a space is located through which the axillary neurovascular structures run. The roof of this space is formed by the coracoid process. Thus, this region is called the coracothoracopectoral space (Figure 7–1).

Shortening or hypertonia of the pectoralis minor can lead to a narrowing of the coracothoracopectoral space, resulting in increased pressure on the blood vessels and/or nerves.

OVERVIEW OF EXAMINATION OF THE THORACIC OUTLET

General Inspection

The examiner should note the position of the patient's head, shoulders, and arms. Significant information can be gained from how the patient shakes hands.

History

Specific questions regarding location and occurrence of the symptoms should be asked. In thoracic outlet syndrome, symptoms often occur only at night.

Nerve root compression syndromes in the cervical spine and peripheral compression neuropathies in the upper extremities (including the shoulder area) should be ruled out. Localized loss of strength, atrophy, and sensory disturbances are of significant diagnostic importance.

Specific Inspection

Discoloration of the hand can occur in thoracic outlet syndrome. If the subclavian artery is involved, the hand is pale. If the vein is involved, the hand is blue and swollen.

Atrophy is sometimes evident, particularly in the hand region.

If the patient has a cervical rib, the supraclavicular fossa may appear to be full.

Palpation

Visible swelling and atrophy are palpated for consistency. The patient's hands are palpated for temperature and moistness.

Functional Examination

During the functional examination, the nonaffected side is always tested first in order to make a comparison with the affected side.

In suspecting a thoracic outlet problem, the cervical spine and shoulder should also be examined. If the cervical spine and shoulder examinations are negative, tests are performed in order to determine involvement of the thoracic outlet region. If these tests are also negative, a peripheral compression neuropathy should be suspected.

Tests for Determining Involvement of the Thoracic Outlet

7.1. Roos test[43]
7.2. Adson test[44]
7.3. Eden test[45]
7.4. Wright test[46]
7.5. Median nerve stretch test
7.6. Radial nerve stretch test
7.7. Ulnar nerve stretch test
7.8. Cervicothoracic rotation test
7.9. Clavicle test
7.10. Scalene muscle test
7.11. Upper and midthoracic mobility test
7.12. Pectoralis minor length test
7.13. Pectoralis major length test
7.14. First rib test

Palpation

If the functional examination indicates that compression is occurring in one of the scalenic triangles, coracothoracopectoral space, or costoclavicular space, the corresponding site is palpated.

Supplementary Examination

Radiological Examination

On radiological examination, a "panoramic" view of the upper thorax aperture is performed. The following findings may be demonstrated:

- megatransversus C7
- cervical rib
- connective tissue connections between a rudimentary first rib and the second rib (only the rudimentary first rib is visible on radiograph)
- exostosis of the first rib
- clavicle fracture
- Pancoast tumor

Laboratory (Blood and Urine) Tests

For differential diagnosis refer to Pathology of the Thoracic Outlet.

Electromyography (EMG)

Because the compression is usually intermittent, paresis rarely occurs. Moreover, the problem generally lies too proximal to be able to perform a valid and reliable EMG evaluation. In a very small number of patients, delayed conduction of the ulnar nerve is found.

Arteriography and Phlebography

To diagnose vascular compression, arteriography and/or phlebography can be performed. A series of images is made with the patient at rest as well as in positions that provoke the symptoms.

Although this examination is not indicated in the presence of primarily uncomplicated symptoms, it is definitely indicated when thrombosis or microemboli are suspected. Sometimes this examination is repeated after resection of a rib, when severe symptoms remain. In this way, postoperative vascular problems can be diagnosed.

Doppler Ultrasound

Evaluation of arterial pulsation by ultrasonography can be performed if stenosis is suspected. Ultrasonographic registration of venous flow can be performed to rule out thrombus formation.

Plethysmography

Plethysmography is photoelectric examination of capillary flow in an organ or body part. In thoracic outlet syndrome, plethysmography can be performed on the nail bed of the thumb.

Neurological Examination

Reflexes are rarely abnormal in thoracic outlet syndrome. Sometimes there is mild hypoesthesia (fine tactile sense, pain) in one or more of the dermatomes from C2 to T1. Generally, loss of strength cannot be objectified. Because of pain and decreased circulation, however, the patient often demonstrates apparent weakness during provocation of the symptoms.

In approximately 5% of all cases, increased perspiration is noted.

FUNCTIONAL EXAMINATION IN THE THORACIC OUTLET SYNDROME

Before beginning the examination, the examiner determines whether the patient is experiencing symptoms of the thoracic outlet syndrome. Per test, the examiner notes any change in the symptoms.

7.1. Roos Test

The patient is instructed to bring the shoulder girdle into depression and retraction. The

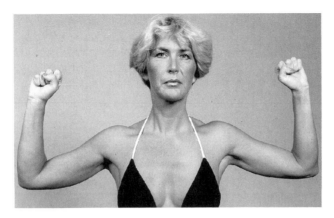

Test 7.1A

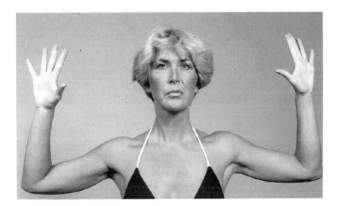

Test 7.1B

upper arms are positioned in approximately 80° abduction and the elbows in approximately 90° flexion. The patient is then asked to make a fist slowly and firmly, alternating with spreading and extending the fingers. Generally, this procedure is performed for 3 minutes.

The test is positive if the patient's symptoms are provoked. In most cases, when the test is positive, the patient quickly indicates that opening and closing the hand becomes slower and more difficult. Sometimes, discoloration of the hand(s) is noted. One hand can become either pale or blue. The radial pulse often remains unchanged.

The Roos test[43] is the most significant, specific, and sensitive test for thoracic outlet syndrome. If the test is positive, there is definitely a thoracic outlet syndrome. If the test is negative, the chance is less likely that this disorder is present.

If the test is positive, there is irritation of the brachial plexus 98% of the time. In 1.5% of cases there is compression of the subclavian vein; in 0.5% the subclavian artery is involved.[43]

7.2. Adson Test

In sitting, the patient is instructed to make the neck as long as possible and either rotate

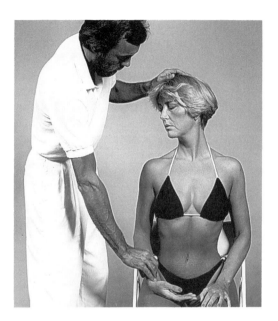

Test 7.2

the head to the side being tested (the scalenes approach each other) or rotate the head to the opposite side (the scalenes contract). Then the patient is told to inhale deeply.

In the first instance (head rotated to the side being tested), the scalenic triangles are tested: during deep inspiration the scalenic triangles become more narrow and the first rib is lifted up. Consequently, the costoclavicular space diminishes in size.

The examiner places one hand on the patient's head to facilitate the position of making the neck as long as possible. With the other hand, the examiner palpates the patient's radial pulse. For the sake of comparison, the test is then repeated on the other side.

The test is positive when the patient's symptoms are provoked.

Although Adson and Coffey[44] describe palpating the radial pulse during this test, in our opinion disappearance of the radial pulse is usually not clinically relevant.

With a stethoscope, the examiner can determine the presence of a supraclavicular and/or infraclavicular souffle (vascular murmur of a blowing quality).

7.3 Eden Test

The examiner sits next to the patient at the side to be tested. The patient stands with the leg on the side being tested placed against the examiner's leg. The patient is instructed to depress and retract the shoulder girdle, and to sidebend the upper body away from the examiner. The examiner grasps the patient's arm at the elbow with one hand and exerts an inferior axial pull on the arm. The other hand palpates the patient's radial pulse while the patient inhales deeply. The test is positive when the specific complaints of the patient are provoked.

This maneuver tests mainly the costoclavicular space.

As with the Adson test, diminishing or disappearance of the radial pulse is not clinically relevant. Attention can be given to the pres-

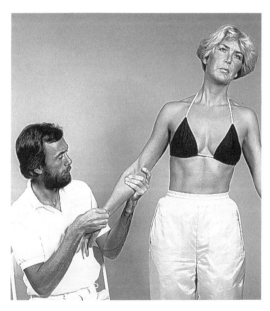

Test 7.3

ence of a supraclavicular and/or infraclavicular souffle.

7.4. Wright Test

The patient sits with both arms relaxed and the hands resting in the lap. The examiner stands on the side to be tested and slowly brings the patient's arm passively into elevation through abduction. At the same time, the examiner palpates the patient's radial pulse.

As with the other tests, this test is positive when the patient's symptoms are provoked. It is important to note how quickly the symptoms arise; diminishing or disappearance of the radial pulse is not clinically relevant.

In this test, mainly the coracothoracopectoral space is narrowed.

7.5. Median Nerve Stretch Test

While stabilizing the patient's shoulder in depression and retraction, the examiner brings the patient's arm into 90° abduction with an extended and supinated elbow. The wrist is brought into full extension, followed

by extension of the fingers. In this way the median nerve is stretched.

During the second phase of this test, the patient's head is positioned passively in contralateral sidebending in order to put an even greater stretch on the median nerve through tension on the brachial plexus.

This test is important in differentiating thoracic outlet syndrome from a lesion of the median nerve. The rationale behind the test is similar to that for the tests according to Lasègue and Bragard (discussed in *Diagnosis and Treatment of the Spine*, Chapter 4, Lumbar Spine).

Tests 7.5, 7.6, and 7.7 do *not* provide *absolute* information regarding differentiation.

7.6. Radial Nerve Stretch Test

The radial nerve is tested in a manner similar to that described for the median nerve. While stabilizing the patient's shoulder in depression and retraction, the examiner brings the patient's arm into 90° abduction with an extended elbow and pronated forearm. The wrist is brought into full flexion, allowing the

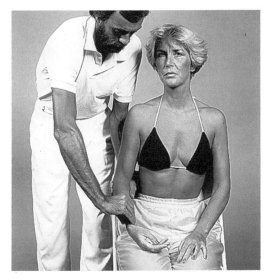

Test 7.4A Initial position.

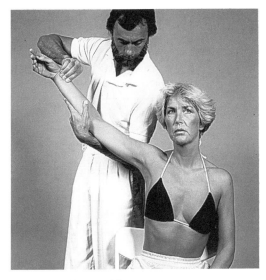

Test 7.4B End position.

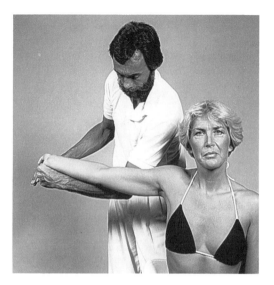

Test 7.5A

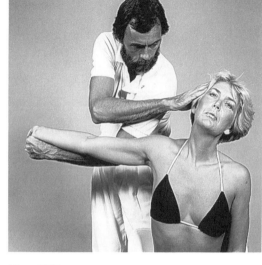

Test 7.5B

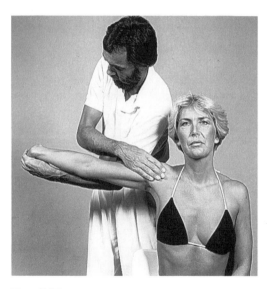

Test 7.6A

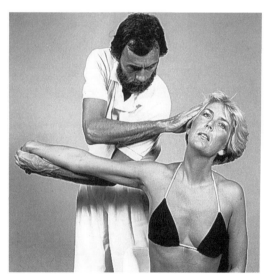

Test 7.6B

fingers to remain in extension. In the second phase, the cervical spine is positioned passively in contralateral sidebending.

This test is important in differentiating thoracic outlet syndrome from a lesion of the radial nerve.

7.7. Ulnar Nerve Stretch Test

While stabilizing the patient's shoulder in depression and retraction, the examiner brings the patient's arm into 90° abduction with a flexed elbow and pronated forearm.

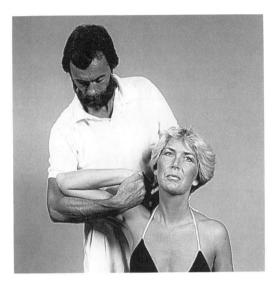

Test 7.7A

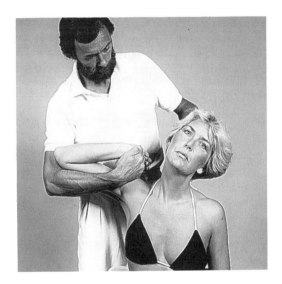

Test 7.7B

This test is important in differentiating thoracic outlet syndrome from a lesion of the ulnar nerve.

7.8. Cervicothoracic Rotation Test

During passive elevation of the arm over approximately 160°, an ipsilateral rotation of C7 to T4 occurs. Per segment, this rotation can be tested as described below.

The examiner fixes the segment's caudal vertebra by placing the thumb against the lateral aspect of the spinous process on the contralateral side; the tip of the thumb lies in the interspinous space. As the patient's arm is brought passively into end-range elevation, the examiner registers the movement of the cranial spinous process over the tip of the thumb. The C7 to T4 segments are tested successively from cranial to caudal.

In thoracic outlet syndrome, rotation of the cervicothoracic junction is often found to be

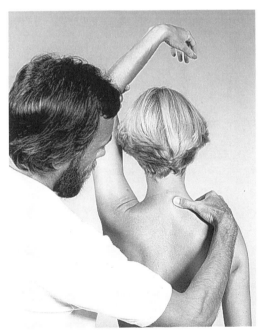

The wrist is then brought passively into full extension. In the second phase, the cervical spine is positioned passively in contralateral sidebending.

Test 7.8

limited. As a result of this limitation, the clavicle reaches its end position too early during arm elevation. This can lead to compression of the structures in the costoclavicular space.

7.9. Clavicle Test

With one finger placed on the cranial aspect of the clavicle as close as possible to the sternoclavicular joint, the examiner palpates the movement of the clavicle while bringing the patient's arm passively (Test 7.9A) into approximately 45° elevation (Test 7.9B).

During the first phase of this passive motion, the clavicle moves slightly forward, making more room for the palpating finger. This is the beginning of a half-ellipsoid movement pattern that ensures that sufficient room remains between the clavicle and the first rib during arm elevation.

Limited range of motion in the acromioclavicular and/or sternoclavicular joint can lead to an abnormal trajectory in the movement pattern of the clavicle. The clavicle moves too quickly in a dorsal direction and reaches its end position too early during elevation, resulting in a narrowing of the costoclavicular space.[47]

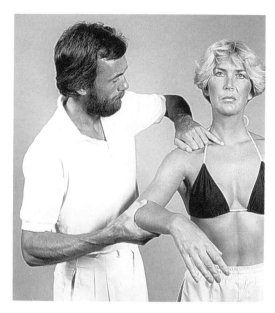

Test 7.9B End position.

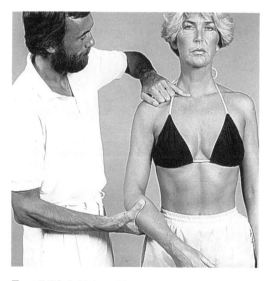

Test 7.9A Initial position.

7.10. Scalene Muscle Test

The patient is instructed to pull the chin in, flatten the cervical spine as much as possible, and exhale maximally. When the patient exhales, the scalenes lengthen and narrowing of the posterior scalenic triangle results (Test 7.10).

In hypertrophy of the scalenes, such as in some athletes (weight lifters) as well as in patients with chronic obstructive pulmonary disease (in pronounced cases), compression of the structures in the posterior scalenic triangle occurs. In addition, if the first rib is positioned too high, the costoclavicular space is also diminished during this maneuver.

7.11. Upper and Midthoracic Mobility Test

The patient lies in a prone position, and the examiner tests the mobility of the upper and

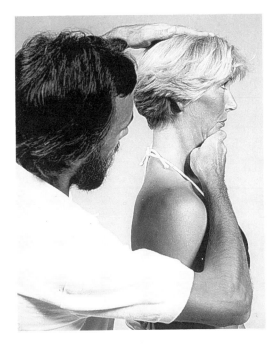

Test 7.10

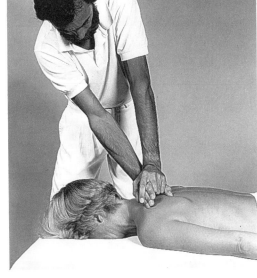

Test 7.11A

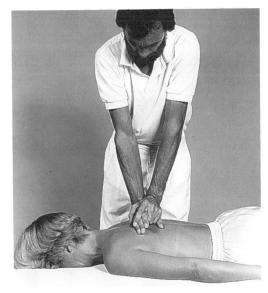

Test 7.11B

midthoracic segments from cranial (Test 7.11A) to caudal (Test 7.11B).

The examiner exerts ventral pressure against the segment's cranial spinous process in a direction perpendicular to the local curvature of the spine. The examiner then returns to the initial position and repeats this maneuver several times to determine the amount of motion. During the last ventral translation at each segment, the patient is asked to exhale. At the end of the exhalation, the examiner exerts overpressure. In this way, the end-feel is determined. (For more detailed information regarding this test as well as abnormal thoracic kyphosis, refer to *Diagnosis and Treatment of the Spine*, Chapter 5, Thoracic Spine.)

Due to a rigid thorax, scapular elevation can be slightly limited. Subsequently, arm elevation is also limited. The clavicle attempts to compensate partially for this loss of motion and reaches its end-position too early. Narrowing of the costoclavicular space results.

Usually in a rigid thorax, the pectoralis minor is too short. This leads to a narrowing of the coracothoracopectoral space during arm elevation.

7.12. Pectoralis Minor Length Test

The patient lies in a supine position with the knees flexed to approximately 90°. The patient is instructed to make the neck as long as possible and exhale as deeply as possible. At the end of the exhalation, the patient tries to bring the shoulder girdle into depression and retraction (Test 7.12). Generally, the patient should be able to touch the table with both shoulders. If this is not the case, shortening of the pectoralis minor muscle(s) is indicated.

In such instances, the shoulders remain in protraction. A consequence of this shortening is limited arm elevation, which is compensated to a certain degree by movement of the clavicle. During this compensatory motion, the clavicle reaches its end-range too soon, and the costoclavicular space is diminished.

Shortening of the pectoralis minor also leads to a narrowing of the coracothoracopectoral space during arm elevation.

7.13. Pectoralis Major Length Test

The patient lies in a supine position and places one foot on the knee of the other leg, which is positioned in 45° hip flexion. In this position, the lumbar spine is completely flattened.

The patient is instructed to elevate maximally both extended arms and then exhale as deeply as possible. At the end of exhalation, the patient tries to touch the table with the upper arms without allowing a compensatory lordosis in the cervical and lumbar spines (Test 7.13). During this maneuver, the abdominal part of the pectoralis major is tested.

If there is tightness of the pectoralis major muscles, the patient is unable to reach the table with the upper arms. Tight pectoralis major muscles lead to a functional disturbance of the shoulder girdle in arm elevation, during which both costoclavicular and coracothoracopectoral compressive moments can occur.

7.14. First Rib Test

In medical literature, various positions for testing the first rib are described. Each position has different advantages and disadvantages; for instance, when the head is positioned in an ipsilateral rotation, the rib is easier to palpate, but the tension from the trapezius is greater.

For this test the patient is examined with the head in a neutral position, supported by a small pillow if necessary (depending on the patient's thoracic kyphosis). The arms rest alongside the body.

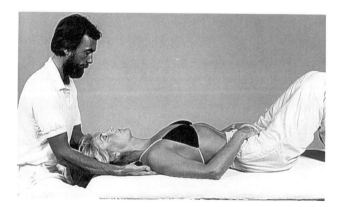

Test 7.12

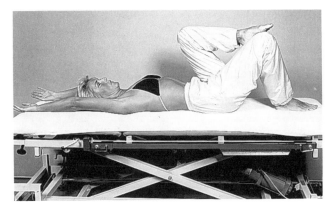

Test 7.13

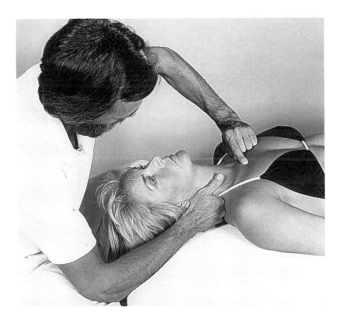

Test 7.14

The examiner stands or sits at the head of the treatment table. The spinous process of T1 and the superior angle of the scapula are localized. If the right side is to be tested, the examiner places the radial aspect of the right index finger's proximal phalanx on the cranial aspect of the first rib at the level of the C7-T1 interspinous space and cranial to the superior angle of the scapula. The first rib is palpated through the trapezius.

The index finger of the other hand can palpate the cartilage of the first rib just caudal to the sternal end of the clavicle. This is not a testing finger, however; palpation of this area offers only a confirmation that the first rib is moving.

The amount of movement is determined during relaxed breathing of the patient. With the cranial hand, the examiner moves the rib in a caudal, ventral, and contralateral direction (Test 7.14). The optimal direction of movement varies significantly; the examiner may have to change the direction of motion slightly to find the optimal direction.

The end-feel is determined by slight overpressure, performed at the end of a deep exhalation. The amount of movement and end-feel are always compared with those of the other side.

PATHOLOGY OF THE THORACIC OUTLET

General Functional Anatomy

The thoracic outlet compression syndrome is a nonradicular disorder caused by compression of nerves and/or blood vessels within the shoulder girdle due to a narrowed passageway.

When a thoracic outlet syndrome is suspected, a tumor of the sulcus of the lung (Pancoast tumor) should always be ruled out (Figure 7–3).

Under the collective term *thoracic outlet syndrome*, the following syndromes are included:

- Scalene syndrome—symptoms result from compression in one or both scalenic triangles.
- Costoclavicular compression syndrome—symptoms result from compression in the costoclavicular space.
- Pectoralis minor syndrome—symptoms result from compression in the coracothoracopectoral space.

DIFFERENTIAL DIAGNOSIS

Cervical Spine

- (Bilateral) disc protrusion C6-C7, C7-T1
- Traumatic injury

- Neurofibromas at the levels of C2 to T1
- Nerve root compression as a result of spondylosis, spondylarthrosis, or uncarthrosis
- Poliomyelitis
- Tuberculosis
- Syringomyelocele
- Intra- or extramedullary inflammatory processes

Upper Extremity

- Traumatic injury of the brachial plexus
- Compression neuropathies
- Disorders of the arm, forearm, or hand

Other Disorders

- Raynaud's disease
- Vascular migraine
- Hyperventilation

GENERAL CLINICAL FINDINGS

When Symptoms Are Primarily Due to Neurogenic Compression

- Tingling can occur at the beginning, during, and after the compressive moments. Tingling during activities is often drowned out by the activity itself, or by the accompanying pain that has been provoked; tingling at rest can persist several minutes and then gradually disappear again (release phenomenon[48]).
- Paresthesia often wakes the patient at night, due to either the release phenomenon or new compressive moments, such as when the individual lies on the arm or lies with the arm over the head.

When Symptoms Are Primarily Due to Venous Compression

- The hand(s) becomes blue and thick; veins are more visible.
- The patient complains of pain, sluggishness, and a heavy feeling in the arm and

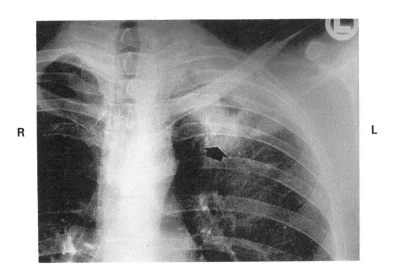

Figure 7–3 Conventional radiograph of a Pancoast tumor *(arrow)* with compression of the phrenic nerve (the diaphragm is in an elevated position on the left). Clinically, the patient presented with a thoracic outlet syndrome: compression of the phrenic nerve and of the subclavian vein.

has difficulty carrying objects. Sometimes pressure from the bra straps is uncomfortable.

- Complications include thrombosis, ulceration, and gangrene (rare).

When Symptoms Are Primarily Due to Arterial Compression

- The skin is pale and blue.
- Paralyzing pain arises during vigorous activities. The patient has difficulty with activities in which the arms have to be held overhead, such as washing windows, blow-drying hair, playing the violin, or working under an automobile.
- An arterial obstruction can lead to a transient "dropping hand."
- Tingling disappears after a period of rest and/or after changing positions, for instance, positioning the shoulder girdle in elevation by sitting with the arms supported on armrests.

Thoracic outlet syndrome should be suspected particularly in the presence of the following symptoms:

- pain in the arm(s), sometimes with radiating pain to the hand, often only in the little finger, and sometimes radiating up the back of the head
- tingling in the dermatomes (C2 to C7), C8 and T1
- feeling of weakness during or after performing certain movements

Primarily responsible for the pain, tingling, and feeling of weakness is a decrease in the microcirculation of the brachial plexus with resultant irritation of the sympathetic nerve fibers. Because the compression is temporary, complications such as paresis, thrombosis, emboli, ulcerations, and gangrene are seen rarely.

The Roos test is the most significant and specific test in diagnosing thoracic outlet syndrome.

GENERAL TREATMENT

In principle, treatment is based on causal factors. The various disturbances found during the functional examination have to be resolved. Because thoracic outlet syndrome can occur in a number of different situations and disorders, treatment is always different.

In Conjunction with Sports Activities

Functional Anatomy. In certain athletes, such as weight lifters and wrestlers, hypertrophy and hypertonia of the scalenes can occur. The syndrome can also arise as a result of unilateral shoulder activities, for example, as in playing tennis.

Clinical Findings. Refer to General Clinical Findings.

Treatment.
* Stretch the scalenes.
* Begin a muscle-strengthening exercise program for the nonaffected arm to improve symmetry of the shoulder girdle.

In Conjunction with Chronic Obstructive Pulmonary Disease

Functional Anatomy. In chronic obstructive pulmonary disease (COPD), incorrect breathing patterns can lead to hypertrophy of the scalenes, coupled with an inspiration position of the thorax.

Clinical Findings. Refer to General Clinical Findings.

Treatment.
* Institute respiratory therapy.
* Stretch the scalenes.
* Mobilize the first rib into expiration.

In Conjunction with Scheuermann Disease

Functional Anatomy. Due to the increased thoracic kyphosis, shortening of the pectoralis major and minor muscles can occur.

Note: A similar shortening of these muscles can also occur in individuals who hold the shoulder girdle in prolonged protraction and have an increased thoracic kyphosis.

Clinical Findings. Refer to General Clinical Findings.

Treatment.
* Restore the muscle balance by means of stretching exercises for the pectoral muscles.
* Begin strengthening exercises for the thoracic spine extensors.
* When appropriate, mobilize the thoracic spine.

In Conjunction with Shoulder Problems in General

Functional Anatomy. Whenever a shoulder problem has been present for a long period of time, secondary dysfunction of the clavicular joints occurs. Because of the often-restricted shoulder function, the clavicle reaches its end position too early and costoclavicular compression can occur.

Clinical Findings. Refer to General Clinical Findings.

Treatment.
* Treat the shoulder problem primarily.
* If necessary, mobilize the clavicular joints.

In Conjunction with Pathology of the Acromioclavicular or Sternoclavicular Joint

Functional Anatomy. As mentioned above for general shoulder problems, pathology of the acromioclavicular or sternoclavicular joint can lead to compression of the structures found between the clavicle and first rib. After a dislocation of the acromioclavicular joint, the coracoclavicular ligaments sometimes calcify and may also lead to compression (Figure 7–4).

Clinical Findings. Refer to General Clinical Findings.

Treatment.
* Mobilize to restore joint function.

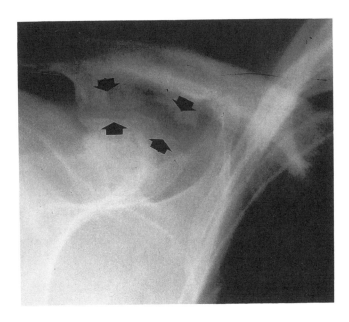

Figure 7–4 Conventional radiograph of a patient with thoracic outlet syndrome due to abnormal calcification of the costoclavicular ligaments *(arrows)* after a dislocation of the acromioclavicular joint with a fracture of the coracoid process.

In Conjunction with a Limitation of Motion in the Cervicothoracic Junction of the Spine

Functional Anatomy.

- Ipsilateral rotation of the cervicothoracic junction is necessary to obtain full elevation range of motion of the arm. As with pathology of the acromioclavicular and sternoclavicular joints, when there is limited or insufficient rotation of the cervicothoracic junction, the shoulder girdle reaches its end-position too early during arm elevation. As a result, narrowing of the costoclavicular space can occur.

Clinical Findings. Refer to General Clinical Findings.

Treatment.

- Mobilize the cervicothoracic junction to restore rotation range of motion.
- If necessary, stretch the scalene muscles and mobilize the first rib.

Post-Traumatic

Functional Anatomy.

- After an acceleration (whiplash) trauma, compression in the scalenic triangles can occur as a result of hypertonia of the sternocleidomastoid and scalenes.
- After fracture of the clavicle or first rib, callus formation can lead to costoclavicular compression (Figure 7–5).

Clinical Findings. Refer to General Clinical Findings.

Treatment.

- Treatment depends on the findings of the functional examination. Often in the acute phase, a cervical collar is given. In addition, pain-relieving and muscle-relaxing modalities can be applied, possibly in conjunction with analgesic medication.

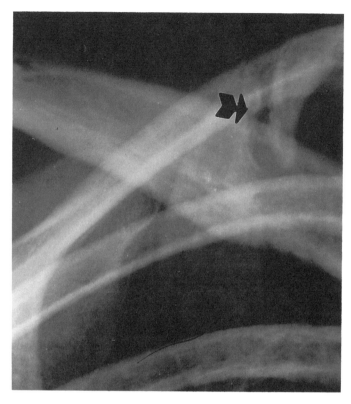

Figure 7–5 Conventional radiograph showing pseudarthrosis of the first rib, possibly the consequence of a stress fracture *(arrow)*, in a 28-year-old Olympic handball athlete with clinical presentation of a thoracic outlet syndrome.

- Treatment is not necessary; the symptoms disappear as the callus formation diminishes.

In Conjunction with Sloping Shoulders and Heavy Breasts

Functional Anatomy. Due to the weight of the breasts and often too-narrow bra straps, constant slight compression of the neurovascular structures occurs. Symptoms arise only after the compression is relieved, for instance at night (release phenomenon).

Clinical Findings. Refer to General Clinical Findings.

Treatment.
- Increase the width of the bra straps, for instance, with felt pads.

- Restore the muscle balance by means of stretching exercises for the pectoral muscles.

- Begin strengthening exercises for the thoracic spine extensors.

- When appropriate, mobilize the thoracic spine.

- Give instruction in proper posture, including teaching the patient to maintain slight contraction of the trapezius muscles.

Before going to bed at night, the patient should sit in a chair with the elbows fully supported whereby the shoulder girdle is positioned in elevation and remain in that position until the symptoms arise. Initially it takes a long time for the paresthesia to occur (it may take 2 to 3 hours). If this technique is performed on a daily basis, the time span before the onset of paresthesia gradually decreases.

It is extremely important that the patient remain in this position until the paresthesia has disappeared. Sometimes this takes only a few minutes, but most often it takes much longer. The patient has the tendency to want to let the arm(s) hang down as soon as the hand(s) start to tingle. This must not be allowed to happen. Thorough explanation to the patient along with the reasoning behind this technique is very important. The patient has to be well motivated during this treatment.

Usually the result is noticeable immediately. Instead of waking up in the middle of the night with paresthesia, the patient now wakes up several hours later. After 1 to 2 weeks, the patient can sleep through the night without problems.

In Conjunction with Congenital Collagenous Bands and/or Cervical Ribs

Functional Anatomy. Usually congenital collagenous bands and/or cervical ribs cause problems only in certain positions, such as during activities in which the hands are held over the head. Individuals with congenital bands and/or cervical ribs who have to work frequently with the hands overhead are prone to experiencing symptoms during such activities as well as after a trauma.

Clinical Findings. Refer to General Clinical Findings.

Treatment.
- Treatment depends on findings of the functional examination.
- Treatment can consist of any of the previously mentioned programs.
- In severe cases, surgery may be indicated.

8

Treatment—Compression Neuropathies of the Shoulder Region

THORACIC OUTLET SYNDROME

The thoracic outlet is the region where blood vessels and nerves run from the uppermost aperture of the thorax to the axilla. In about 98% of thoracic outlet syndrome cases, the brachial plexus is compressed. However, the large blood vessels are rarely involved in this compression: the subclavian vein in approximately 1.5% and the subclavian artery in approximately 0.5% of the cases.[43] Compression of the structures in this area can have many possible causes. Effective treatment depends on accurate diagnosis.

The Roos test is the most important "specific" test in diagnosing a thoracic outlet syndrome. In making this diagnosis, and subsequently determining the most appropriate treatment, results of the Roos test are considered along with findings from the functional examination of the cervical and thoracic spines, and the shoulder.

The Roos test is performed by positioning the shoulder girdle in depression and retraction, with arms in approximately 60° to 90° elevation, and elbows in 90° flexion. The fingers are then slowly opened and closed for a period of up to three minutes or until the symptoms have been provoked.

Treatment of the thoracic outlet syndrome (TOS) focuses on the cause of the problem and thus consists of techniques aimed at alleviating the disturbances found during the functional examinations. Several examples are listed in Table 8–1.

Stretch of the Scalene Muscles (Anterior, Middle, and Posterior)

During bilateral contraction, the function of the scalene muscles is flexion of the cervical spine. If the cervical spine is fixed, the muscles function to lift both of the first ribs.

In unilateral contraction of the scalene muscles, a contralateral rotation, ipsilateral sidebending, and slight flexion of the cervical spine occur.

Position of the Patient

The patient sits or lies supine.

Position of the Therapist

The therapist stands or sits behind the patient. The therapist grasps the patient's head in such a way that the hand and forearm form one unit with the head. With the other hand, the therapist fixes the patient's thorax via the shoulder of the side to be stretched.

Performance

The therapist brings the patient's cervical spine in ipsilateral rotation, contralateral sidebend, and extension. In other words, if the right side is being stretched, the therapist brings the patient's cervical spine into right rotation, left sidebend, and extension (Figure 8–1). This motion is performed very slowly. If pain occurs, the therapist either holds that position for a few seconds or slightly reduces the stretch.

Table 8–1 Causes, Results, and Treatment of Thoracic Outlet Syndrome*

Cause	Result	Treatment
Sports examples		
Weight lifting	Hypertrophy and hypertonia of the scalene muscles occur.	Begin stretching the scalene muscles.
Tennis	Unilateral shoulder-arm activity, such as in playing tennis, can result in TOS.	Begin strengthening exercises of the other arm to improve symmetry.
Chronic obstructive pulmonary disease (TOS due to poor breathing habits [chest breathing])	Hypertrophy of the scalene muscles occurs along with an inspiration position of the thorax.	Instruct in proper abdominal breathing; stretch the scalene muscles; mobilize the first rib into expiration.
Scheuermann's disease	Shortening of the pectoral muscles occurs.	Improve the muscle imbalance by stretching and strengthening exercises.
Shoulder problems in general	Whenever shoulder problems have been present for a long time, secondary dysfunction of the clavicular joints arises. Because of the often limited shoulder function, the clavicle reaches its end position too early, and costoclavicular compression can occur.	Treat the primary shoulder problem; if necessary, mobilize the acromioclavicular and sternoclavicular joints.
Primary lesion of the acromioclavicular joint or sternoclavicular joint	Compression between the clavicle and first rib can also occur in this instance.	Mobilize the limited joint function(s).
Limitation of motion of the cervical spine	Because of limited or inadequate rotation of the cervicothoracic junction, the rest of the shoulder girdle reaches its end position too early during arm elevation.	Mobilize the cervicothoracic spine; sometimes, stretching the scalene muscles and mobilization of the first rib are also necessary.
Post-traumatic examples		
Whiplash trauma	Hypertonia of the sternocleidomastoid and scalene muscles can cause compression in the scalenic triangles to occur.	Depending on findings in the functional examination, a cervical collar is often worn during the acute phase. In addition, pain-relieving modalities, possibly in combination with analgesics, can be administered.

continues

Table 8–1 continued

Cause	Result	Treatment
Post-traumatic examples (cont'd)		
After clavicle fracture	Callus formation can cause costoclavicular compression.	Generally, no treatment is necessary; the symptoms subside as the callus formation decreases. In rare cases, surgery is required.
Rounded shoulders and heavy breasts	The weight of the breasts and, often, too-narrow bra straps can cause constant slight compression of the blood vessels and nerves. When the compression is alleviated (for instance at night), symptoms can arise due to the release phenomenon.	• Improve the muscle imbalance by stretching and strengthening exercises. • Increase the width of the bra straps, with felt pads for example. • Instruct in proper posture, including teaching the patient to maintain slight contraction of the trapezius muscles. • Instruct the patient to do this: Before going to bed at night, the patient should sit in a chair in such a way that the shoulder girdle is in elevation and the elbows are fully supported on armrests. The patient should remain in this position until the symptoms arise. Initially it takes a long time for the paresthesia to occur (it may take 2 to 3 hours). If this technique is performed on a daily basis, the time span before the onset of paresthesia gradually decreases. It is extremely important that the patient remain in this position until the paresthesia has disappeared. Sometimes this only takes a few minutes, but most often it takes much longer. The patient has the tendency to want to let the arm(s) hang down as soon as the hand(s) start to tingle. This must not be allowed to happen. Thorough explanation to the patient along with the reasoning behind this technique is very important. The patient has to be well motivated during this treatment. Usually the result is immediately noticeable. Instead of waking up in the middle of the night with paresthesia, the patient now wakes up several hours later. After 1 to 2 weeks, the patient can sleep through the night without problems.

continues

Table 8–1 continued

Cause	Result	Treatment
Congenital collag-enous bands and/or cervical rib(s)	Usually congenital collag-enous bands and/or cervical ribs cause problems only in certain positions, such as during activities in which the hands are held over the head. Individuals with congenital bands and/or cervical ribs who have to work frequently with the hands overhead are prone to experiencing symptoms during such activities, as well as after a trauma.	Refer to aforementioned conditions for recommended treatment. In severe cases, surgery is indicated.

*The above-described situations and pathology all have a different cause, yet in each of these instances, thoracic outlet syndrome can occur. Note that the treatment is always different.

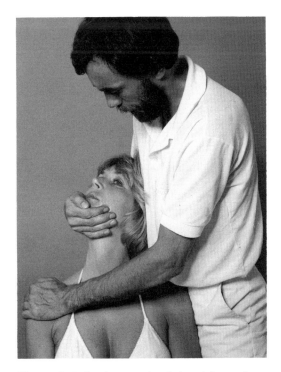

Figure 8–1 Static stretch of the right scalene muscles.

As soon as pain and muscle splinting decrease, the stretch is increased. If stretching further is not possible, the patient is instructed to exhale slowly and as deeply as possible. In so doing, caudal movement of the first rib causes even more stretch to occur.

Even though the symptoms may be unilaterally localized, both sides should be stretched. This static stretching technique can be performed from approximately 30 seconds to several minutes. The patient is instructed to perform bilateral self-stretching at home, several times a day. For description of the home exercise, as well as an alternative performance of this technique (in which the first rib is also mobilized), refer to *Diagnosis and Treatment of the Spine*, Chapter 5, Thoracic Spine, Treatment.

Note: Caution should be exercised with elderly patients to ensure that symptoms of vertebral artery compression do not arise because of too much pressure on those structures.

Stretch of the Pectoralis Major

Functions of the pectoralis major include adduction and internal rotation of the humerus. With the arm fixed in abducted elevation, the muscle assists in elevation of the thorax (accessory breathing muscle). The muscle is also active during forced inhalation, such as in certain sports activities and in some cases of chronic obstructive pulmonary disease (COPD).

Functions of the various parts of the muscle are as follows:

- *pars abdominalis:* depression of the shoulder girdle and adduction of the humerus in the direction of the opposite hip
- *pars sternocostalis:* adduction of the humerus in the direction of the fourth and fifth ribs on the opposite side
- *pars clavicularis:* horizontal adduction of the humerus

Position of the Patient

The patient lies in a supine position with the side to be stretched as close as possible to the edge of the treatment table. One leg is positioned with the hip and knee slightly flexed and the foot resting on the table. The hip and knee of the other leg are brought into even more flexion, whereby the foot of that leg is placed just proximal to the knee of the leg resting on the table. This positioning prevents the lumbar spine from lordosing during the stretching. The patient's arm lies in abducted elevation and external rotation. The amount of abduction depends on which part of the pectoralis major is to be stretched.

Position of the Therapist

The therapist stands at the head of the table next to the patient's affected side.

If the right side is to be stretched, the therapist uses the left hand to fix the right aspect of the patient's thorax (pars abdominalis) or the sternum (pars sternocostalis and pars clavicularis) (Figures 8–2A–C). The right hand grasps the patient's arm just proximal to the elbow, and the patient's forearm is held between the therapist's forearm and trunk.

Performance

Very gradually the patient's arm is brought further into elevation and external rotation, with respect for pain and muscle splinting:

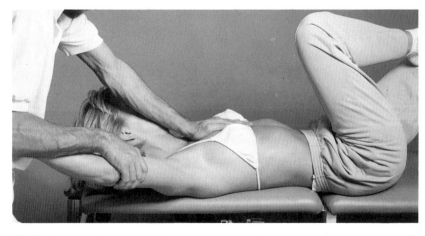

Figure 8–2A Static stretch of the right pectoralis major muscle, pars abdominalis and pars sternocostalis: initial position (see also Figure 8–2B).

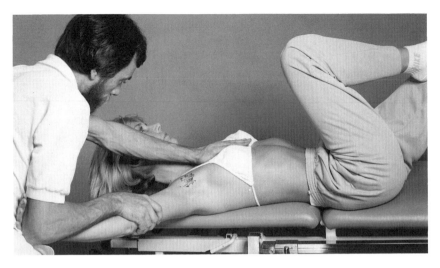

Figure 8–2B End position.

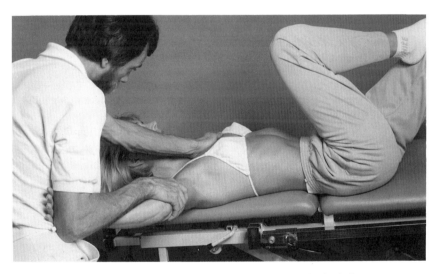

Figure 8–2C Static stretch of the pectoralis major, pars clavicularis.

- In maximal elevation, the pars abdominalis is stretched.
- In approximately 125° elevation, the pars sternocostalis is stretched.
- In approximately 90° elevation, the pars clavicularis is stretched.

Note: During the stretching, some patients experience paresthesia in parts of the hand.

This is probably due to compression of part of the brachial plexus underneath and against the coracoid process. Generally, it is beneficial to stretch the pectoralis major on both sides. The therapist can perform a bilateral stretch by fixing the patient's thorax to the treatment table with a mobilization belt. In this instance, the therapist stands behind the supine patient at the head of the table. The patient should also stretch several times per day at home.

Stretch of the Pectoralis Minor

The function of the pectoralis minor with a fixed thorax is chiefly a tipping of the scapula. If the scapula is fixed, the muscle assists in lifting the thorax (accessory breathing muscle).

Position of the Patient

The patient lies in a supine position with the shoulder (scapula) over the edge of the table.

Position of the Therapist

The therapist stands next to the patient's affected side.

The therapist grasps the patient's forearm just proximal to the wrist. If the right side is to be stretched, using the right hand, the therapist brings the patient's arm into internal rotation, slight adduction, and approximately 70° flexion.

The left hand is placed on the coracoid process and anterior aspect of the patient's right shoulder (Figure 8–3).

Performance

The patient's shoulder is slowly brought into a craniodorsal direction. At the end of the range of motion, the stretch can be increased by instructing the patient to exhale deeply.

Both the right and left sides should be stretched. The patient should also stretch several times per day at home. When the patient stretches at home, both sides should be stretched simultaneously.

COMPRESSION NEUROPATHY OF THE SUPRASCAPULAR NERVE

Functional Examination

- Active arm elevation can be slightly limited.

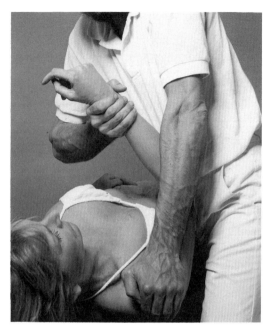

Figure 8–3 Static stretch of the pectoralis minor.

- Passive horizontal adduction is painful and limited in the acute stage. Pain increases significantly when the arm is held in horizontal adduction and the head is brought into contralateral sidebending and rotation.
- In the chronic stage, resisted external rotation and abduction are weak.

Injection

A perineural injection of the suprascapular nerve is both diagnostic and therapeutic. If the symptoms resolve after one or more injections, strength of the supraspinatus and infraspinatus muscles should return. If the injection does not have any effect, surgical treatment (resection of the transverse scapular ligament) may be indicated. If the most significant symptom is weakness rather than pain, an injection is worthless. In this case, the self-healing process is awaited or surgery is considered.

Position of the Patient

The patient sits on the treatment table and leans against the inclined end of the table.

Position of the Physician

The physician stands next to or behind the patient's affected side.

Performance

A 2-mL syringe is filled with 1 mL of local anesthetic and 1 mL of corticosteroid. An 8-cm long thin needle is inserted at the midpoint of a sagittal line running from the lateral third of the clavicle to the scapular spine. First, the needle is inserted at a 70° angle (from the horizontal) until it contacts bone (scapula) (Figures 8–4 and 8–5). From here,

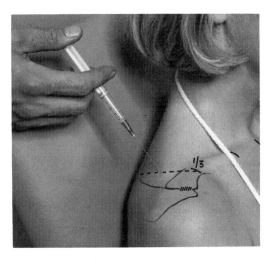

Figure 8–4 Perineural injection of the suprascapular nerve.

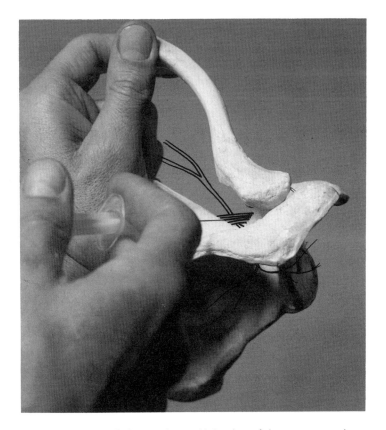

Figure 8–5 The position of the needle in a perineural injection of the suprascapular nerve.

the needle is withdrawn slightly and reinserted at an angle of 50° to 60° in a ventrocaudal direction. After approximately 5 cm, when bone is again contacted, the 2 mL of solution (after first aspirating) is injected.

Aspiration is particularly important here because at the scapular notch, the suprascapular artery usually runs just cranial to the nerve, not under, but over the transverse scapular ligament.

General considerations when giving injections

Before injecting the solution, aspiration should always be performed. Aspiration is important to ensure that the injection is not accidentally given into a blood vessel. If this occurs, there is risk of toxic side effects and false-negative results.

When giving an intra-articular injection, the first drop of solution should always be injected into the subcutaneous tissue. In this way, the danger of a bacterial arthritis is diminished; the possibly nonsterile plug of skin that may be in the opening of the needle is not brought into the joint.

PART I—SHOULDER REVIEW QUESTIONS

1. With an insertion tendopathy of the supraspinatus, what findings are possible in the functional examination?

2. Why is passive internal rotation of the shoulder painful with an insertion tendopathy of the infraspinatus?

3. Explain why passive horizontal adduction of the shoulder is sometimes painful with an insertion tendopathy of the subscapularis.

4. Explain why passive horizontal adduction of the shoulder is sometimes painful with a compression neuropathy of the suprascapular nerve.

5. Which muscles are innervated by the suprascapular nerve?

6. From the functional examination, which tests can be positive with a tenosynovitis of the tendon from the long head of the biceps brachii?

7. Explain why an insertion tendopathy of the teres minor does not cause a painful arc.

8. How can one differentiate an insertion tendopathy of one of the cuff muscles from a chronic subacromial-subdeltoid bursitis?

9. Name the five most common lesions that can cause a painful arc.

10. How can one differentiate an acute subacromial-subdeltoid bursitis from chronic bursitis?

11. Which joints and junctions are involved in active arm elevation?

12. Name the three most important causes for the frequent occurrence of cuff lesions.

13. The shoulder-hand syndrome belongs to which "clinical picture," and which clinical stages does it discern?

14. Which lesions of the acromioclavicular joint occur most frequently, and where is the pain localized?

15. Which lesions of the sternoclavicular joint occur most frequently, and where is the pain localized?

16. List, from proximal to distal, the structures that lie between the roof of the shoulder and the humeral head.

17. What is the treatment of choice for an idiopathic arthritis of the shoulder?

18. Name some sports whereby a high risk of anterior shoulder instability exists.

19. Which part of the shoulder joint capsule is most frequently affected in an anterior instability? Name the ligaments that make up this part of the capsule.

20. What finding occurs most often with a lesion of the long thoracic nerve, and what causes this to happen?

21. Describe schematically the therapeutic possibilities for a patient who has both a history of anterior subluxation of the shoulder and a lesion of the supraspinatus.

22. What are the most important structures for the stability of the acromioclavicular joint?

23. How can one differentiate an acute bursitis from an acute arthritis in the shoulder joint?

24. Describe the third clinical stage of a traumatic arthritis of the shoulder.

25. During the functional examination of the shoulder, when, among other tests, resisted extension of the elbow is painful, one thinks in first instance of a . . . ?

26. Which of the following lesions are self-limiting, and what is the average duration of the problem? Acute subacromial-subdeltoid bursitis, Traumatic arthritis, Idiopathic arthritis.

27. How can one differentiate between an acute subacromial-subdeltoid bursitis and a total rupture of the supraspinatus?

28. What is meant by the "wringing out" phenomenon of the supraspinatus?

29. Why can resisted external rotation be painful with an insertion tendopathy of the supraspinatus?

30. Explain why, in arthritis of the shoulder, sometimes one or more resisted tests are positive.

PART I—SHOULDER REVIEW ANSWERS

1. Sometimes, pain during active arm elevation.

   Sometimes, pain during passive arm elevation.

   Sometimes, painful arc.

   Usually painful passive internal rotation.

   Always painful resisted abduction.

   Frequently painful resisted external rotation.

   Sometimes painful resisted elbow extension.

2. Due to stretching.

3. Due to compression of the distal part of the insertion at the lesser tubercle against the coracoid process.

4. Due to stretch of the nerve.

5. Supraspinatus and infraspinatus.

6. Sometimes active arm elevation.

   Sometimes passive arm elevation with overpressure to the posterior.

   Sometimes flexion of the elbow against resistance.

   Always the stretch test.

7. The insertion lies too far distally to cause an impingement against the roof of the shoulder.

8. In both cases resisted tests can be painful; with a bursitis the pain diminishes or disappears when the resisted tests are repeated with a simultaneous downward pull on the arm.

9. —Insertion tendopathy of the supraspinatus, infraspinatus, and subscapularis.

   —Tendinitis and/or tenosynovitis of the tendon of the long head of the biceps brachii.

   —Chronic subacromial-subdeltoid bursitis.

10. With an acute bursitis one finds a significant noncapsular pattern of limitation, whereas a chronic bursitis often causes no limitation of motion. With an acute bursitis, the limitation is usually so great that no painful arc exists, whereas a painful arc with a chronic bursitis is almost always present.

11. The shoulder joint (glenohumeral joint), the acromio- and sternoclavicular joints, the scapulothoracic junction, the cervicothoracic junction, and the first three (or four) ribs.

12. —The fact that there is little room between the head of the humerus and the roof of the shoulder.

    —The overall moderate to poor vascularization of the supraspinatus tendon and insertion.

    —The relative lack of stability of the shoulder joint, through which (particularly with an instability) an overload on the cuff muscles quickly occurs.

13. Sympathetic reflex-dystrophy, the hypertrophic and the atrophic stages.

14. Traumatic arthritis (overstretching of the joint capsule); subluxation; dislocation (piano key phenomenon) (also classified by Allman[50] and Tossy et al.[25]: I, II, III); osteolysis; nontraumatic arthritis. In all cases, the pain is localized in the C4 dermatome.

15. Subluxation and dislocation; arthrosis; subacute degeneration. In all cases, the pain is localized in the area of the joint.

16. Inferior acromioclavicular ligaments (partially); subacromial-subdeltoid bursa; supraspinatus tendon; glenohumeral joint capsule.

17. Intra-articular injection of corticosteroid.

18. —All throwing and racquet sports.

    —Swimming, particularly front crawl, backstroke, and the butterfly stroke.

19. The anterior capsule: middle and inferior glenohumeral ligaments.

20. Winging scapula due to a deficit of the serratus anterior muscle.

21. —Treatment of local pain, for example, by means of transverse friction massage and muscle stretching.

    —As soon as resisted abduction is negative, selective muscle strengthening of the adductors with internal rotators as well as the adductors with external rotators.

    —Causal treatment, such as improvement of throwing, smashing, or swimming technique.

    —Patient must perform stretching exercises daily.

22. The coracoclavicular ligaments.

23. An acute bursitis causes limited range of motion in a noncapsular pattern, and an acute arthritis causes limited range of motion in a capsular pattern.

24. —The pain radiates distally from the elbow.

    —The patient cannot lie on the shoulder.

    —There is pain at rest.

25. . . . a lesion of one of the structures between the humeral head and the roof of the shoulder. The pain occurs as a result of compression. Lesions of the triceps brachii, in the area of the shoulder, are rare.

26. —Acute subacromial-subdeltoid bursitis; approximately 2 to 4 weeks.

    —Traumatic arthritis; approximately 1 year.

    —Idiopathic arthritis; approximately 1.5 to 2.5 years.

27. With an acute bursitis, as well as with a total rupture of the supraspinatus, the patient is unable to elevate the arm actively. However, passive elevation is possible with the supraspinatus rupture, whereas with an acute bursitis it is impossible because of pain.

28. When the arm is adducted, the already poorly vascularized area is further compromised due to the increased compression of the head of the humerus against the supraspinatus insertion.

29. Against resistance, the supraspinatus muscle also assists in external rotation.

30. The cuff muscle insertions have a firm connection with the joint capsule.

PART I—REFERENCES

1. Sugahara R. Electromyographic study on shoulder movements. *Rehab Med Japan.* 1974;11:41–52.

2. De Luca CJ, Forest WJ. Force analysis of individual muscles acting simultaneously on the shoulder joint during isometric abduction. *J Biomech.* 1973; 6:385–393.

3. Glousman R, Jobe F, Tibone J, Moynes D, Antonelli D, Perry J. Dynamic electromyographic analysis of the throwing shoulder with glenohumeral instability. *J Bone Joint Surg [Am].* 1988;70A:220–226.

4. Freedman L, Munro RR. Abduction of the arm in the scapular plain: a roentgenographic study. *J Bone Joint Surg [Am].* 1966;48:1503–1510.

5. Inman VT, Saunders JB, Abbott LC. Observation on the function of the shoulder joint. *J Bone Joint Surg [Am].* 1944;26:1–30.

6. Poppen NK, Walker PS. Forces at the glenohumeral joint in abduction. *Clin Orthop.* 1978;135:165–170.

7. Poppen NK, Walker PS. Normal and abnormal motion of the shoulder. *J Bone Joint Surg [Am].* 1976;58:195–201.

8. McCarty DJ, ed. *Arthritis and Allied Conditions: A Textbook of Rheumatology.* 11th ed. Philadelphia: Lea & Febiger; 1989.

9. Schwartzman RJ, McLellan TL. Reflex sympathetic dystrophy. *Arch Neurol.* 1987;44:555–561.

10. Kopell HP, Thompson WAL. Pain and the frozen shoulder. *Surg Gynecol Obstet.* 1959;109:92–96.

11. Murnaghan JP. Frozen shoulder. In: Rockwood CA, Matsen FA III, eds. *The Shoulder.* Philadelphia: Saunders; 1989:837–862.

12. Neviaser RF, Neviaser TJ. The frozen shoulder diagnosis and management. *Clin Orthop.* 1987;233: 59–64.

13. Sattar MA, Lugman WA. Periarthritis: another duration-related complication of diabetes mellitus. *Diabetes Care.* 1987;8:507–510.

14. Andren L, Lundberg BJ. Treatment of rigid shoulders by joint distension during arthrography. *Acta Orthop Scand.* 1965;36:45–53.

15. Older MWJ. Distension arthrography of the shoulder joint. In: Bayley, Kessel, eds. *Shoulder Surgery.* Stuttgart: Springer Verlag; 1982:123–127.

16. DePalma AF. Loss of scapulohumeral motion (frozen shoulder). *Ann Surg.* 1952;135:193–204.

17. Leffert RD. The frozen shoulder. *Instructional Course Lectures 34.* 1985:199–203.

18. Mumenthaler M. *Der Schulter-Arm-Schmerz.* Bern: Hans Huber; 1982.

19. Garancis JC, Cheung HS, Halverson PD, McCarty DJ. "Milwaukee shoulder": association of microspheroids containing hydroxyapatite crystals, active collagenase, and neutral protease with rotator cuff defects. *Arthritis Rheum.* 1981;24:484–491.

20. Neer CS II, Craig EV, Fukuda H. Cuff tear arthropathy. *J Bone Joint Surg [Am].* 1983;65:1232–1244.

21. Brownlee C, Cofield MD. *Shoulder replacement in cuff tear arthropathy.* Presented at American Society of Orthopaedic Surgeons meeting, 1986, New Orleans.

22. Harryman DT, Sidles JA, Clark JM, McQuade KJ, Gibb TD, Matsen FA. Translation of the humeral head on the glenoid with passive glenohumeral motion. *J Bone Joint Surg [Am].* 1990;72:1334–1343.

23. Howell SM, Galinat BJ, Renzi AJ, Marone PJ. Normal and abnormal mechanics of the glenohumeral joint in the horizontal plane. *J Bone Joint Surg [Am].* 19;70:227–232.

24. Grant JCB. *Method of Anatomy.* 7th ed. Baltimore: Williams & Wilkins; 1965.

25. Tossy JD, Mead NC, Sigmond HM. Acromioclavicular separations: useful and practical classification for treatment. *Clin Orthop.* 1963;28:111–119.

26. Allman FL. Fractures and ligamentous injuries of the clavicle and its articulation. *J Bone Joint Surg [Am].* 1967;49:774–784.

27. Post M. Current concepts in the diagnosis and management of acromioclavicular dislocations. In: *Sports Injuries: Proceedings of the Fifth International Jerusalem Symposium.* London: Freund Publishing House Ltd; 1989:77–81.

28. Rockwood CA, Young C. Disorders of the acromioclavicular joint. In: Rockwood CA, Matsen FA III, eds. *The Shoulder.* Philadelphia: Saunders; 1989.

29. Bannister GC, Wallace WA, Stableforth PG, Hutson MA. The management of acute acromioclavicular dislocation: a randomized prospective controlled trial. *J Bone Joint Surg [Br].* 1989;71:848–850.

30. Dias JJ, Steingold RF. Richardson RA, Tesfayohannes B, Gregg PJ. The conservative treatment of acromioclavicular dislocation. *J Bone Joint Surg [Am].* 1987;69:719–722.

31. Wojtys EM, Nelson G. Conservative treatment of grade III acromioclavicular dislocations. *Clin Orthop.* 1991;268:112–119.

32. Cahill BR. Osteolysis of the distal clavicle in male athletes. *J Bone Joint Surg [Am].* 1982;64:1053–1058.

33. Cooper D, Cutter R. Traumatic osteolysis in women. In: Rockwood CA, Matsen FA III, eds. *The Shoulder.* Philadelphia: Saunders; 1989.

34. Neer CS II. Anterior acromioplasty for the chronic impingement syndrome in the shoulder. *J Bone Joint Surg [Am].* 1972;54:41–50.

35. Matsen FA III, Arntz CT. Subacromial impingement. In: Rockwood CA, Matsen FA III, eds. *The Shoulder.* Philadelphia: Saunders; 1989:647–677.

36. Neer CS II. Impingement lesions. *Clin Orthop.* 1983;173:70–77.

37. Wilson CL, Duff GL. Pathologic study of degeneration and rupture of the supraspinatus tendon. *Arch Surg.* 1943;47:121–135.

38. Petersson CJ, Gentz CF. Ruptures of the supraspinatus tendon: the significance of distally pointing acromioclavicular osteophytes. *Clin Orthop.* 1983;174:143–148.

39. Matsen FA III, Arntz CT. Rotator cuff tendon failure. In: Rockwood CA, Matsen FA III, eds. *The Shoulder.* Philadelphia: Saunders; 1989:647–677.

40. Herrlinger R. *Geschichte der Medizinischen Abbildung von der Antike bis um 1600.* 2nd ed. München: Heinz Moos Verlag; 1973.

41. Manes HR. A new method of shoulder reduction in the elderly. *Clin Orthop.* 1980;147:200–202.

42. Vaes PH, Annaert JM, Claes P, OpdeCam P. Anatomische en kinesiologische studie van de rotatorcuffpezen. *Ned Tijdschr Manuele Ther.* 1992;2,1:2–11.

43. Roos DB. New concepts in the etiology, diagnosis and surgical treatment of the thoracic outlet syndrome. In: Greep JM, Lemmens HAJ, Roos DB, Urschel HC, eds. *Developments in Surgery,* Vol 1: *Pain in Shoulder and Arm.* Den Haag: Martinus Nijhoff; 1979:201–210.

44. Adson WA, Coffey JR. Cervical rib, method of anterior approach for relief of symptoms by division of scalenus anticus. *Ann Surg.* 1927;85:839–857.

45. Eden JC. Vascular complication of cervical rib and first thoracic rib abnormalities. *Br J Surg.* 1939;27:105–111.

46. Wright IS. The neurovascular syndrome produced by hyper-abduction of the arm. *Am Heart J.* 1945;29:1.

47. Stenvers JD, Overbeek WJ. *Het Kissing Coracoid.* Lochem: De Tijdstroom; 1981.

48. Cyriax J. *Textbook of Orthopedic Medicine*, Vol 1: *Diagnosis of Soft Tissue Lesions.* London: Baillière Tindall; 1978.

49. Allman F. Impingement, biceps, and rotator cuff lesions. In: Zarins B, Andrews JR, Carson WG, eds. *Injuries to the Throwing Arm.* Philadelphia: Saunders; 1985:159–171.

Part I—SUGGESTED READING

Amstutz HC, Thomas BJ, Kabo JM, Jinnah RH, Dorey FJ. The Dana total shoulder arthroplasty. *J Bone Joint Surg [Am].* 1988;708:1174–1181.

Andrews JR, Gillogly S. Physical examination of the shoulder in throwing athletes. In: Zarins B, Andrews JR, Carson WG, eds. *Injuries to the Throwing Arm.* Philadelphia: Saunders; 1985:51–65.

Ansink BJJ, Meerwijk GM van, et al. *Neurologie voor Paramedische Beroepen.* Utrecht: Bunge; 1982.

Bach BR, O'Brien SJ, Warren RF, Leighton M. An unusual neurological complication of the Bristow procedure: a case report. *J Bone Joint Surg [Am].* 1988;70:458–460.

Bach BR, Warren RF, Fonek J. Disruption of the lateral capsule of the shoulder. *J Bone Joint Surg [Br].* 1988;70:274–276.

Baker CL, Thornberry R. Neurovascular syndromes. In: Zarins B, Andrews JR, Carson WG, eds. *Injuries to the Throwing Arm.* Philadelphia: Saunders; 1985:177–187.

Barker ME. Manipulation in general medical practice for thoracic pain syndromes. *Br Osteop J.* 1983;15:95–97.

Barrett WP, Franklin JL, Jackins SE, Wyss CR, Matsen. Total shoulder arthroplasty. *J Bone Joint Surg [Am].* 1987;69:865–872.

Barry TP, Lombardo SJ, Kerlan RK, Jobe FW, et al. The coracoid transfer for recurrent anterior instability of the shoulder in adolescents. *J Bone Joint Surg [Am].* 1985;67:383–387.

Bayley JC, Cochran TP, Sledge CB. The weight-bearing shoulder: the impingement syndrome in paraplegics. *J Bone Joint Surg [Am].* 1987;69:676–678.

Belder KRJ de. Excision of the clavicle: a review of the nineteenth-century literature. *J Bone Joint Surg [Br].* 1985;67:282–285.

Benoehr HC. Polymyalgia rheumatica with arteritis temporalis Horton. *Internist.* 1983;24:285.

Biesinger E. Die Schulterluxation: funktionelle Ergebnisse, Rezidivhäufigkeit, Prinzipien und Bediutung der krankengymnastischen Behandlung. *Z Krankengymnastik.* 1984;7:417–423.

Bohlman HH, Freehafer A, Dejak J. The results of treatment of acute injuries of the upper thoracic spine with paralysis. *J Bone Joint Surg [Am].* 1985;67:360–369.

Booth RE, Marvel JP. Differential diagnosis of shoulder pain. *Orthop Clin North Am.* 1975;6:353–379.

Braunstein EM, O'Connor G, Arbor A. Double-contrast arthrotomography of the shoulder. *J Bone Joint Surg [Am].* 1982:192–195.

Britt LP. Non-operative treatment of the thoracic outlet syndrome symptoms. *Clin Orthop.* 1976;51:45–48.

Buckerfield CT, Castle ME. Acute traumatic retrosternal dislocation of the clavicle. *J Bone Joint Surg [Am].* 1984;66:379–385.

Büge E. Einführung in die funktionelle Bewegungslehre am Beispiel der Schulterbehandlung. *Z Krankengymnastik.* 1984;36:434–441.

Bulgen DY, Binder AI, Haxleman BL, Dutton J, Roberts S. Frozen shoulder: prospective clinical study with an evaluation of three treatment regimens. *Ann Rheum Dis.* 1984;43:353–360.

Carmichael SW, Hart DL. Anatomy of the shoulder joint. *J Orthop Sports Phys Ther.* 1985;6:225–228.

Chung SMK, Nissenbaum MM. Congenital and developmental defects of the shoulder. *Orthop Clin North Am.* 1975;6:381–391.

Clain A, ed. *Hamilton Bailey's Demonstrations of Physical Signs in Clinical Surgery.* Bristol: John Wright & Sons; 1965.

Cofield RH. Total shoulder arthroplasty with the Neer prosthesis. *J Bone Joint Surg [Am].* 1984;66:899–906.

Cofield RH. Current concepts review of rotator cuff disease of the shoulder. *J Bone Joint Surg [Am].* 1985;67:974–979.

Cofield RH, Irving JF. Evaluation and classification of shoulder instability: with special reference to examination under anesthesia. *Clin Orthop.* 1987;223:32–42.

Colvin PC. The frozen shoulder. *Br Osteop J.* 1982;4:87–95.

Cook PC, Horowitz M. Bipolar clavicular dislocation: a case report. *J Bone Joint Surg [Am]*. 1987;69:145–147.

Crawford Adams J. *Outline of Orthopaedics*. 6th ed. London: Churchill Livingstone; 1967.

Dahmen G, Gärtner J. Ergebnisse der Drehosteotomie nach Weber bei der Behandlung der habituellen Schulterluxation. *Z Orthop*. 1983;121:541–546.

DeOrio JK, Cofield RH. Results of a second attempt at surgical repair of a failed initial rotator cuff repair. *J Bone Joint Surg [Am]*. 1984;66:563–567.

Dunant JH. The diagnosis of thoracic outlet syndrome. In: Greep JM, Lemmens HAJ, Roos DB, Urschel HC, eds. *Developments in Surgery*, Vol 1: *Pain in Shoulder and Arm*. Den Haag: Martinus Nijhoff; 1979:153–164.

Ebraheim NA, An HS, Jackson WT, Pearlstein SR, et al. Scapulothoracic dissociation. *J Bone Joint Surg [Am]*. 1988;70:428–432.

Elias N. *Über den Prozeß der Zivilisation*. 5th ed. Baden-Baden: Suhrkamp; 1978.

Fauls D. General training techniques to warm up and cool down the throwing arm. In: Zarins B, Andrews JR, Carson WG, eds. *Injuries to the Throwing Arm*. Philadelphia: Saunders; 1985:267–276.

Ferretti A, Cerullo G, Russo G. Suprascapular neuropathy in volleyball players. *J Bone Joint Surg [Am]*. 1987;69:260–262.

Fickenscher D. Habituelle und rezidivierende Schulterluxationen. *Physikal Ther*. 1987;8:76–82.

Fidler MW, Goedhart ZD. Excision of prolapsed thoracic intervertebral disc: a transthoracic technique. *J Bone Joint Surg [Br]*. 1984;66:518–522.

Foo CL, Swann M. Isolated paralysis of the serratus anterior: a report of 20 cases. *J Bone Joint Surg [Br]*. 1983;65:552–556.

Garcia G, McQueen D. Bilateral suprascapular nerve entrapment syndrome: case report and review of the literature. *J Bone Joint Surg [Am]*. 1981;63:491–492.

Gardner E, Gray DJ, O'Rahilly R. *Anatomy*. Philadelphia: Saunders; 1975.

Gelberman RH. Pyogenic arthritis of the shoulder in adults. *J Bone Joint Surg [Am]*. 1980;62:550–553.

Gerber C, Ganz R. Clinical assessment of instability of the shoulder: with special reference to anterior and posterior drawer tests. *J Bone Joint Surg [Br]*. 1984;66:551–556.

Gerber C, Rockwood CA. Subcoracoid dislocation of the lateral end of the clavicle: a report of three cases. *J Bone Joint Surg [Am]*. 1987;69:924–927.

Gerber C, Terrier F, Ganz R. The role of the coracoid process in the chronic impingement syndrome. *J Bone Joint Surg [Br]*. 1985;67:703–708.

Gerber C, Terrier F, Ganz R. The trillat procedure for recurrent anterior instability of the shoulder. *J Bone Joint Surg [Br]*. 1988;70:130–134.

Gibson KR. Rheumatoid arthritis of the shoulder. *Phys Ther*. 1986;66:1920–1929.

Gibson T. Een diagnose die niet mag worden gemist (polymyalgia rheumatica). *Mod Med*. 1978:1005–1007.

Gilliatt RW. The classical neurological syndrome associated with a cervical rib and band. In: Greep JM, Lemmens HAJ, Roos DB, Urschel HC, eds. *Developments in Surgery*, Vol 1: *Pain in Shoulder and Arm*. Den Haag: Martinus Nijhoff; 1979:173–183.

Gray H, Williams PL, Warwick R. *Gray's Anatomy*. 36th ed. London: Churchill Livingstone; 1980.

Greenman PE. Manipulative therapy for the thoracic cage. *Osteop Ann*. 1977;140:63–73.

Greep JM, Lemmens HAJ, Roos DB, Urschel HC. *Pain in Shoulder and Arm*. Den Haag: Martinus Nijhoff; 1979.

Haak A, Steendijk R, de Wijn IF. *De samenstelling van het menselijk lichaam*. Assen: Van Gorcum; 1968.

Ha'eri GB, Wiley AM. Advancement of the supraspinatus muscle in the repair of ruptures of the rotator cuff. *J Bone Joint Surg [Am]*. 1981;63:232–237.

Hafferl A. *Lehrbuch der topographischen Anatomie des Menschen*. Berlin: Springer Verlag; 1957.

Halverson PB, Cheung HS, McCary DJ. "Milwaukee shoulder": association of microspheroids containing hydroxyapatite crystals, active collagenase, and neutral protease with rotator cuff defects. II: Synovial fluid studies. *Arthritis Rheum*. 1981;24:474–483.

Hamilton WJ, Simon G, Hamilton SGI. *Surface and Radiological Anatomy*. 5th ed. London: The Macmillan Press Ltd; 1976.

Hart DL, Carmichael SW. Biomechanics of the shoulder. *J Orthop Sports Phys Ther*. 1985;6:229–234.

Hawkins RJ, Brock RM, Abrams JS, Hobeika P. Acromioplasty for impingement with an intact rotator cuff. *J Bone Joint Surg [Br]*. 1988;70:795–797.

Hawkins RJ, Koppert G, Johnston G. Recurrent posterior instability (subluxation) of the shoulder. *J Bone Joint Surg [Am]*. 1984;66:169–174.

Hawkins RJ, Neer CS, Pianta RM, Mendoza FX. Locked posterior dislocation of the shoulder. *J Bone Joint Surg [Am]*. 1987;69:9–18.

Haymaker W, Woodhall B. *Peripheral Nerve Injuries*. 2nd ed. Philadelphia: Saunders; 1956.

Healy EJ, Seybold WD. *A Synopsis of Clinical Anatomy*. Philadelphia: Saunders; 1969.

Heerkens YF, Meijer OG. *Tractus-anatomie*. Interfaculty Physical Education. Amsterdam; 1980.

Hoppenfeld S. *Physical Examination of the Spine and Extremities.* New York: Appleton-Century-Crofts; 1976.

Hovelius L. Anterior dislocation of the shoulder in teenagers and young adults: five year prognosis. *J Bone Joint Surg [Am].* 1987;69:393–399.

Hovelius L, Körner GL, Lundberg B, Akermark GC, Herberts P, Wredmark T, Berg E. The coracoid transfer for recurrent dislocation of the shoulder: technical aspects of the Bristow-Latarjet procedure. *J Bone Joint Surg [Am].* 1983;65:926–934.

Huaux JP. Reumatische schouderaandoeningen. *Spectrum Int.* 1983;26:1–4.

Ikeda T, Awaya G, Suzuki S, Okada Y, Tada H. Torn acetabular labrum in young patients: arthroscopic diagnosis and management. *J Bone Joint Surg [Br].* 1988;70:13–16.

Jägermann V. Die frische AC-Gelenksprengung Tossy III operieren oder nicht? *Sportverletzungen-Sportschaden.* 1991;5:51–52.

Jain AS. Traumatic floating clavicle: a case report. *J Bone Joint Surg [Br].* 1984;66:560–561.

Janis JL, Mahl GF, Kagan J, Holt RR. *Personality, Dynamics, Development, and Assessment.* New York: Harcourt, Brace and World, Inc; 1969.

Janson M, Rasker JJ. Polymyalgia rheumatica. *Ned Tijdschr Fysiother.* 1984;94,9:184–187.

Jobe CM. Gross anatomy of the shoulder. In: Rockwood CA, Matsen FA III, eds. *The Shoulder.* Philadelphia: Saunders; 1989:34–97.

Jörgens H. Das Schulter-Arm-Schmerz-Syndrom aus internistischer Sicht. *Z Krankengymnastik.* 1976;28:408–415.

Jupiter JB, Leffert RD. Non-union of the clavicle: associated complications and surgical management. *J Bone Joint Surg [Am].* 1987;69:753–760.

Jurik AG, Graudal H, Carvalho A de. Monarticular involvement of the manubriosternal joint. *Skeletal Radiol.* 1985;14:99–103.

Katznelson A. Rupture of ligaments about the acromioclavicular joint and reconstruction. In: *Sports Injuries: Proceedings of the Fifth International Jerusalem Symposium.* London: Freund Publishing House Ltd; 1989:87–89.

Kay SP, Yaszemski MJ, Rockwood CA. Acute tear of the rotator cuff masked by simultaneous palsy of the brachial plexus: a case report. *J Bone Joint Surg [Am].* 1988;70:611–612.

Kennedy JC, Hawkins RJ. Swimmer's shoulder. *Phys Sports Med.* 1974;2:34–38.

Kerlan RK. The treatment of common throwing injuries to the shoulder. In: Zarins B, Andrews JR, Carson WG, eds. *Injuries to the Throwing Arm.* Philadelphia: Saunders; 1985:113–120.

Kessel L. *Clinical Disorders of the Shoulder.* New York: Churchill & Livingstone; 1982.

Kessel L, Watson M. The painful arc syndrome. *J Bone Joint Surg [Br].* 1977;59:166–172.

Kingma MJ. Schouderpijn. *Ned Tijdschr Geneeskd.* 1976;120:325–337.

Klein Rensink GJ, Smits M. Entrapment neuropathieën. *Tijdschr Ned Belg Vereniging Orthop Geneeskd.* 1983;3:33–48.

Korst JK van der. Periarthritis humeroscapularis beschouwd vanuit de reumatologie. *Ned Tijdschr Fysiother.* 1980;9:260–276.

Korst JK van der, Cats A. Het schouder-hand-syndroom: een retrospectief onderzoek van 75 gevallen. *Ned Tijdschr Geneeskd.* 1967;111:723–728.

Krämer J, Seibel R. Funktionell anatomische Grundlagen zur operativen Behandlung der Periarthropathia humero scapularis. *Zeitschr Orthop.* 1983;121:98–101.

Kruger GD, Rock MG, Munro TG. Condensing osteitis of the clavicle: a review of the literature and report of three cases. *J Bone Joint Surg [Am].* 1987;69:550–557.

Kumar VP, Balasubramaniam P. The role of atmospheric pressure in stabilizing the shoulder: an experimental study. *J Bone Joint Surg [Br].* 1985;67:719–721.

Lankenner PA, Michell LJ. Stress fracture of the first rib: a case report. *J Bone Joint Surg [Am].* 1985;67:159–160.

Lascelles RG. The thoracic outlet syndrome. *Brain.* 1979;100:601–612.

Laude M, Kénési C, Patte D, Riggs E. Abduction and horizontal extension of the arm. *Anat Clin.* 1978;1:65–72.

Leach RE. The impingement syndrome. In: Zarins B, Andrews JR, Carson WG, eds. *Injuries to the Throwing Arm.* Philadelphia: Saunders; 1985:121–127.

Leach RE. Tennis serving compared with baseball pitching.. In: Zarins B, Andrews JR, Carson WG, eds. *Injuries to the Throwing Arm.* Philadelphia: Saunders; 1985:307–310.

List M. Untersuchung und Behandlung von Schultergürtel und Schultergelenk. *Z Krankengymnastik.* 1984;36:424–433.

Lohman AGM. *Vorm en beweging. Leerboek van het bewegingsapparaat van de mens.* 4th ed. Utrecht: Bohn, Scheltema & Holkema; 1977.

Lundberg BJ. The frozen shoulder. *Acta Orthop Scand [Suppl].* 1969;119:1–59.

Lunseth PA, Chapman KW, Frankel VH. Surgical treatment of chronic dislocation of the sternoclavicular joint. *J Bone Joint Surg [Br].* 1975;57:193–196.

Macnab I. Rotator cuff tendinitis. *Ann Roy Coll Surg Engl.* 1973;53:271–287.

Marcove RC. Neoplasms of the shoulder girdle. *Orthop Clin North Am.* 1975;6:541–552.

Mayba II. Non-union fractures of the sternum. *J Bone Joint Surg [Am].* 1985;67:1091–1093.

McAuliffe TB, Dowd GS. Avulsion of the subscapularis tendon: a case report. *J Bone Joint Surg [Am].* 1987;69:1454–1455.

McCue FC III, Gieck JH, West JO. Throwing injuries to the shoulder. In: Zarins B, Andrews JR, Carson WG, eds. *Injuries to the Throwing Arm.* Philadelphia: Saunders; 1985:95–111.

McLeod WD. The pitching mechanism. In: Zarins B, Andrews JR, Carson WG, eds. *Injuries to the Throwing Arm.* Philadelphia: Saunders; 1985.

McMinn RMH, Hutching RT. *A Color Atlas of Human Anatomy.* London: Wolfe Medical Publications Ltd; 1977.

Meerwijk GM van. *Syllabus Onderzoeken en Behandelen.* Amsterdam: Stichting Akademie voor Fysiotherapie Amsterdam; 1979; chap 16.

Mitzkat K, Eulert J. Sur Diagnostik der Sehnentunnelsyndrom im Bereich des Schultergürtels. *Orthopadische Praxis.* 1982; 12:947–949.

Mowery CA, Garfin SR, Booth RE, Rothman RH. Recurrent posterior dislocation of the shoulder: treatment using a bone block. *J Bone Joint Surg [Am].* 1985;67:777–781.

Moynes DR, Perry J, Antonelli DJ, Jobe FW. Electromyography and motion analysis of the upper extremity in sports. *Phys Ther.* 1986;66:1905–1911.

Mudge MK. Rotator cuff tears associated with os acromiale. *J Bone Joint Surg [Am].* 1986;66:427–429.

Müller-Faßbender H. Der Schulter-Arm-Schmerz aus internistischer Sicht. *Physikalische Ther.* 1986;7:454–459.

Mumenthaler M, Schliack H. *Läsionen peripherer Nerven.* Stuttgart: Georg Thieme Verlag; 1977.

Neer CS II. Anterior acromioplasty for the chronic impingement syndrome in the shoulder: a preliminary report. *J Bone Joint Surg [Am].* 1972;54:41–50.

Neviaser JS. A study of the pathological findings in periarthritis of the shoulder. *J Bone Joint Surg.* 1945;17:211–222.

Neviaser RJ, Neviaser TJ, Neviaser JS. Concurrent rupture of the rotator cuff and anterior dislocation of the shoulder in the older patient. *J Bone Joint Surg [Am].* 1988;70:1308–1311.

Norwood LA. Posterior shoulder instability. In: Zarins B, Andrews JR, Carson WG, eds. *Injuries to the Throwing Arm.* Philadelphia: Saunders; 1985:153–157.

O'Brien SJ, Arnoczky DVM, Warren RF, Rozbruch SR. Developmental anatomy of the shoulder and anatomy of the glenohumeral joint. In: Rockwood CA, Matsen FA III, eds. *The Shoulder.* Philadelphia: Saunders; 1989:1–33.

Oostendorp RAB. Fysiotherapeutische benadering van het schouderprobleem. *Ned Tijdschr Fysiother.* 1976;12:309–315.

Oostra DJ, Schrijer FJJM. Thoracic outlet syndrome. *Ned Tijdschr Manuele Ther.* 1984;3:16–26.

Ozaki J, Fujimoto S, Nakagawa Y, Masuhara K, Tamai S. Tears of the rotator cuff of the shoulder associated with pathological changes in the acromion: a study in cadavers. *J Bone Joint Surg [Am].* 1988;70:1124–1230.

Paar O, Bernett P. Das sogenannte Schulter-Arm-Syndrom: Diagnostik aus der Sicht des Sporttraumatologen. *Physikalische Ther.* 1986;7: 404–414.

Penny JN, Welsh RP. Shoulder impingement syndromes in athletes and their surgical management. *Am J Sports Med.* 1981;9:11–15.

Pettronee FA. Shoulder problems in swimmers. In: Zarins B, Andrews JR, Carson WG, eds. *Injuries to the Throwing Arm.* Philadelphia: Saunders; 1985:318–330.

Prakke PC, Kirk RS. Bursitis subacromialis: fact or fiction? *Beneeskd Sport.* 1989;22:24.

Pratt NE. Neurovascular entrapment in the regions of the shoulder and posterior triangle of the neck. *Phys Ther.* 1986;66:1894–1900.

Priest JD, Nagel DA. Tennis shoulder. *Am J Sports Med.* 1976;4,1:28–42.

Protzman RR. Anterior instability of the shoulder. *J Bone Joint Surg [Am].* 1980;62:909–918.

Rathbun JB, Macnab I. The microvascular pattern of the rotator cuff. *J Bone Joint Surg [Br].* 1970;52:540–553.

Refior HJ, Melzer C. Läsionen der langen Bizepssehne: Diagnostik und Therapie. *Praktische Sport Traumatol Sportmedizin.* 1987;4:42–47.

Richardson JB, Ramsay A, Davidson JK, Kelly IG. Radiographs in shoulder trauma. *J Bone Joint Surg [Br].* 1988;70:457–460.

Rockwood CA, Matsen FA III, eds. *The Shoulder.* Philadelphia: Saunders; 1989.

Rothman RH, Marvel JP, Heppenstall RB. Anatomic considerations of the glenohumeral joint. *Orthop Clin North Am.* 1975:341–352.

Rowe CR. Anterior subluxation in the throwing shoulder. In: Zarins B, Andrews JR, Carson WG, eds. *Injuries to the Throwing Arm.* Philadelphia: Saunders; 1985:144–151.

Rowe CR. Recurrent transient subluxation of the shoulder: the "dead arm" syndrome. *Clin Orthop.* 1987;223:11–19.

Rowe CR, Zarins B. Recurrent transient subluxation of the shoulder. *J Bone Joint Surg [Am].* 1981;63:863–871.

Rowe CR, Zarins B, Ciullo JV. Recurrent anterior dislocation of the shoulder after surgical repair: apparent causes of failure and treatment. *J Bone Joint Surg [Am].* 1984;66:159–168.

Russe O, Gerhardt JJ, King PS. *An Atlas of Examination, Standard Measurements and Diagnosis in Orthopaedics and Traumatology.* Bern: Hans Huber Verlag; 1972.

Sahlstrand T, Säve-Söderbergh J. Subacromial bursitis with loose bodies as a cause of refractory painful arc syndrome: a case report. *J Bone Joint Surg [Am].* 1980;62:1194–1196.

Sain J, Andrews JR. Proper pitching techniques. In: Zarins B, Andrews JR, Carson WG, eds. *Injuries to the Throwing Arm.* Philadelphia: Saunders; 1985:30–37.

Samilson RL, Prieto V. Dislocation arthropathy of the shoulder. *J Bone Joint Surg [Am].* 1983;65:456–460.

Scavenius M, Iversen BF, Stürup J. Resection of the lateral end of the clavicle following osteolysis, with emphasis on non-traumatic osteolysis of the acromial end of the clavicle in athletes. *Injury.* 1987;18:261–263.

Schinze W, Heise U, Dahmen G. Engpaßsyndrom des Nervus suprascapularis bei einem Leistungssportler. *Dtsc Zeitschr Sportmedizin.* 262–264.

Schneider A. Beitrag zur physikalische-therapeutischen Behandlung des Schulter-Arm-Schmerz-Syndroms. *Zeitschr Krankengymnastik.* 1976;28:412–413.

Selesnick FJ, Jablon M, Frank C, Post M. Retrosternal dislocation of the clavicle: report of four cases. *J Bone Joint Surg [Am].* 1984;66:287–291.

Serratrice G. De pijnlijke schouder. *Tempo Med Ned.* 1981;6:47–62.

Simeone FA. Neurological complications of closed shoulder injuries. *Orthop Clin North Am.* 1975;6:499–505.

Simon WH. Soft tissue disorders of the shoulder: frozen shoulder, calcific tendinitis, and bicipital tendinitis. *Orthop Clin North Am.* 1975:6:521–539.

Skurja M, Monlux JH. Case studies: the suprascapular nerve and shoulder dysfunction. *J Orthop Sports Phys Ther.* 1985;6:254–257.

Sobotta J, Becher PH. *Atlas of Human Anatomy.* Vol 1, 2 and 3. 9th English ed. Berlin: Urban & Schwarzenberg; 1975.

Stanley D, Trowbridge EA, Norris SH. The mechanism of clavicular fracture: a clinical and biomechanical analysis. *J Bone Joint Surg [Br].* 1988;70:461–464.

Stenvers JD, Overbeek WJ. Bestaat bij de frozen shoulder toch ook een benige beperking? *Ned Tijdschr Geneeskd.* 1978;122:1081–1087.

Strizak AM, Danzig TL, Jackson DW, Resnick D, Staple T. Subacromial bursography: an anatomical and clinical study. *J Bone Joint Surg [Am].* 1982;64:196–201.

Thetter O, Steckmeier B, Schmölder A, Rolle A. Das Thoracic-Outlet-Syndrom. *Orthopade.* 1987;16:441–447.

Thompson WAL, Kopell HP. Peripheral entrapment neuropathies of the upper extremity. *N Engl J Med.* 1959;260:1261–1265.

Tyson RR, Kaplan GF. Modern concepts of diagnostics and treatment of the thoracic outlet syndrome. *Orthop Clin North Am.* 1975;6:507–519.

Uhthoff HK, Piscopo M. Anterior capsular redundancy of the shoulder: congenital or traumatic? An embryological study. *J Bone Joint Surg [Br].* 1985;67:363–366.

Varriale PL, Adler ML. Occult fracture of the glenoid without dislocation: a case report. *J Bone Joint Surg [Am].* 1983;65:688–689.

Verhoef J, Verplanke L. De "frozen shoulder": een uniek fenomeen? *Ned Tijdschr Manuele Ther.* 1985;85/5,3:46–65.

Visser JD, Konings JG. Pijnlijk bewegingstraject van het schoudergewricht. *Ned Tijdschr Geneeskd.* 1981;125,26:1035–1038.

Vleeming A, Stoeckart R, Klein HW, Volkers ACW. Misverstanden betreffende bursae van de schouder. *Ned Tijdschr Geneeskd.* 1987;131,41:1807–1809.

Wadsworth CT. Frozen shoulder. *Phys Ther.* 1986;66:1878–1883.

Warren-Smith CD, Ward MW. Operation for acromioclavicular dislocation: a review of 29 cases treated by one method. *J Bone Joint Surg [Br].* 1987;69:715–718.

Weisman JA von, Matison JA. Zur Röntgendiagnostik der habituellen Luxation des Oberarmgelenks. *Fortschr Rontgenst.* 1977;126:29–35.

Wells R. Suprascapular nerve entrapment. In: Zarins B, Andrews JR, Carson WG, eds. *Injuries to the Throwing Arm.* Philadelphia: Saunders; 1985.

Welter HF, Thetter O, Schweiberer L. Kompressionssyndrome der oberen Thoraxapertuur. *Münchener Med Wochenschr.* 1984;126:1122–1125.

White GM, Riley LH. Isolated avulsion of the subscapularis insertion in a child: a case report. *J Bone Joint Surg [Am].* 1985;67:635–636.

Wilhelm A. Unklare Schmerzzustände an der oberen Extremität. *Orthopade.* 1987;16:458–464.

Williams PL, Warwick R, eds. *Gray's Anatomy.* 36th ed. Edinburgh: Longman; 1980.

Winkel D, Fisher S. *Schematisch handboek voor onderzoek en behandeling van weke delen aandoeningen van het bewegingsapparaat.* 6th ed. Delft: Nederlandse Akademie voor Orthopedische Geneeskunde; 1982.

Wyke B. Morphological and functional features of the innervation of the costovertebral joints. *Folia Morphol.* 1975;23:296–305.

Wyke B. The neurological basis of thoracic spinal pain. *Rheumatol Phys Med.* 1970;10:356–367.

Part II

The Elbow

9

Functional Anatomy of the Elbow

The elbow joint is an excellent example of a compound joint (articulatio composita). Within the joint capsule are located the distal part of the humerus, radial head, and proximal part of the ulna. In a sense, the elbow consists of three separate joints: the humeroulnar, the humeroradial, and the proximal radioulnar. These three joints are enclosed by the capsule of the cubital articulation.

Movements in the elbow joint are closely related to those in the wrist. This is particularly true for the pronation and supination movement in both proximal and distal radioulnar connections. Numerous muscles in the forearm have a function both in the elbow and in the wrist joints.

JOINT MORPHOLOGY

Humeroulnar Joint

The head of the humeroulnar joint is formed by the trochlea of the humerus. The socket is formed by the trochlear notch of the ulna. These joint surfaces are not completely congruent. In full extension the trochlear notch does not have contact with the medial part of the trochlea, and in full flexion it does not have contact with the lateral part.

The trochlea is angulated approximately 45° anteriorly in relation to the longitudinal axis of the ulna. This results in an increased possibility of flexion range of motion.

The trochlear notch of the ulna is also anteriorly angulated 45°. A ridge is found between the medial and lateral parts of the notch. It ends in the tip of the coronoid process at its anterior aspect. A part of the joint surface often is not covered with joint cartilage. This absence of cartilage can be seen between the part of the trochlear notch that forms the anterior aspect of the olecranon and the part that, in the anatomical position, is almost horizontally positioned (Figure 9–1).

Humeroradial Joint

The capitulum of the humerus forms the head of the humeroradial joint. The concave surface on the radial head forms the socket. One can see it as a ball and socket joint (articulatio spheroidea). Because of the radius' relationship with the ulna (the proximal radioulnar joint) and the humeroulnar joint, however, there is a much smaller functional range of motion than in other ball and socket joints.

Proximal Radioulnar Joint

The articular circumference of the radius articulates with the radial notch of the ulna as well as with the annular ligament. The annular ligament encloses the radial circumference. Its function is to maintain contact between the ulna and radius. At its inner aspect, the ligament is covered with cartilage. It is funnel shaped, with the wide part of the funnel proximal and the small part distal. The

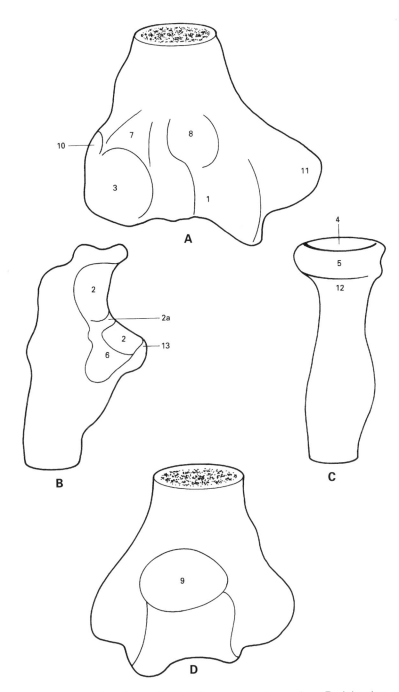

Figure 9–1 Different aspects of the elbow. **A**, Right humerus, anterior view; **B**, right ulna, radial view; **C**, right radius, anterior view; **D**, right humerus, posterior view; **1**, humeral trochlea; **2**, trochlear notch; **2a**, part of the notch that is often not covered with cartilage; **3**, humeral capitulum; **4**, fovea (facet) of the head of the radius; **5**, circumference of the head of the radius; **6**, radial notch of the ulna; **7**, radial fossa; **8**, coronoid fossa; **9**, olecranon fossa; **10**, lateral humeral epicondyle; **11**, medial humeral epicondyle; **12**, neck of the radius; **13**, coronoid process.

proximal part of the ligament is connected to the cubital joint capsule; the distal part is connected to the radius.

Distal Radioulnar Joint

The movements in the proximal radioulnar joint cannot take place independently from motions in the distal radioulnar joint. Functionally, both joints form a kinematic unit.

The head of the distal radioulnar joint is formed by the ulnar articular circumference and the socket is formed by the ulnar notch of the radius. Because of the intimate connection with the triangular fibrocartilaginous complex, the distal radioulnar joint can be seen to have an articular disc. The capsule of the joint is thickened at its dorsal and volar aspects; however, one cannot speak of real ligaments here.

Radius and ulna are also connected to each other by means of a fibrous joint, the interosseus membrane. This membrane forms the site for the attachment of numerous forearm muscles.

Joint Capsule

Anteriorly, the joint capsule of the elbow runs from just above the radial and coronoid fossae to just below the radial articular circumference and coronoid process of the ulna. At the posterior aspect of the elbow, the capsule runs from the proximal border of the olecranon fossa to below the radial articular circumference and, with a fold, to the olecranon. (This fold unfolds in flexion.) Both humeral epicondyles are extra-articular.

The capsule has a thin fibrous membrane that is reinforced by ligaments (Figures 9–2, 9–3, and 9–4). Within the capsule, two collateral ligaments are found. The ulnar (medial) collateral ligament runs from the medial epicondyle, in three parts, toward the ulna. The anterior and posterior bands are the strongest. The oblique band often is not well developed. The anterior band is the primary restraint of passive extension.

The radial (lateral) collateral ligament is a strong triangular band that runs from the lateral epicondyle toward the radius and annular ligament. This ligament also is very closely connected to the insertions of the supinator and extensor carpi radialis brevis muscles.

MUSCULATURE

Flexion and extension, pronation and supination are the active movements in the elbow joint (Figure 9–5). The muscles that are involved in each active motion are as follows:

- for flexion
  1. brachialis
  2. biceps
  3. brachioradialis
  4. pronator teres
  5. to a lesser extent, extensors carpi radialis longus and brevis
- for extension
  1. triceps
  2. anconeus (only against resistance)
- for pronation
  1. pronator quadratus
  2. pronator teres
  3. with fast movements and against resistance: flexor carpi radialis
- for supination
  1. supinator
  2. biceps (in 90° flexion of the elbow its activity is maximal)
  3. with fast movements and against resistance: extensors carpi radialis longus and brevis

OTHER STRUCTURES

Attachment of the Extensors Carpi Radialis Longus and Brevis

Only a very small part of the extensor carpi radialis longus originates from the lateral epicondyle (Figure 9–6). Its main origin is along a crest on the humerus, directly

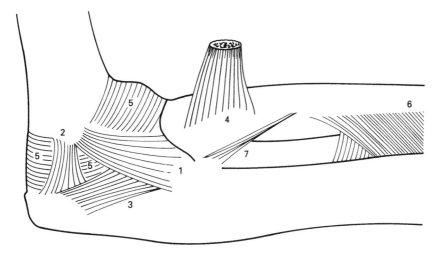

Figure 9–2 Joint capsule, medial view. **1**, Anterior band of the ulnar collateral ligament; **2**, posterior band of the ulnar collateral ligament; **3**, oblique band of the ulnar collateral ligament; **4**, tendon of the biceps; **5**, fibrous capsule; **6**, interosseus membrane; **7**, oblique cord.

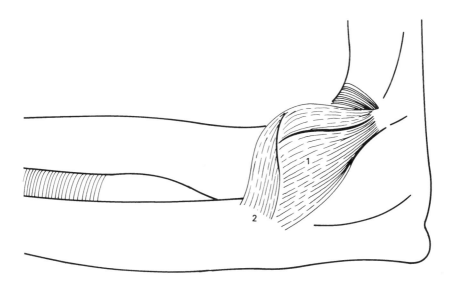

Figure 9–3 Joint capsule, lateral view. **1**, Radial collateral ligament; **2**, annular ligament.

proximal to the lateral epicondyle. The muscle also has an attachment to the lateral intermuscular septum.

The extensor carpi radialis brevis attaches to the lateral epicondyle through a tendon that is shared with the extensor digitorum.

The extensor carpi radialis brevis also has an origin at the radial collateral ligament as well as to a thickening in the fascia that covers this muscle. In particular, this last connection could play an important role in the transfer of loads generated by the extensor

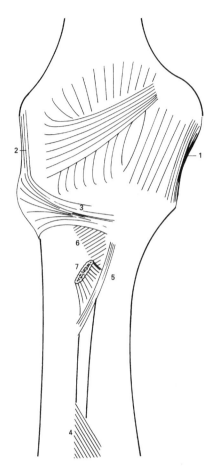

Figure 9–4 Joint capsule, anterior view. **1**, Ulnar collateral ligament; **2**, radial collateral ligament; **3**, annular ligament; **4**, interosseus membrane; **5**, oblique cord; **6**, quadrate ligament; **7**, tendon of the biceps.

aponeurosis runs over the pronator teres. The bicipital aponeurosis is the connection of the biceps with the antebrachial fascia. This strong, bandlike structure sometimes hinders the occurrence of swelling in instances of pronator teres hypertrophy. Eventually, increased pressure on the nerve is the result (pronator teres syndrome).

The ulnar nerve runs along the medial epicondyle in a groove between the medial epicondyle and the olecranon. The roof of this groove is formed by the antebrachial fascia, forming a tunnel (cubital tunnel). If the groove is too shallow and the fascia weakens, the ulnar nerve can subluxate out of the groove during elbow flexion.

Directly distal to the cubital tunnel, the nerve runs through the muscle belly of the flexor carpi ulnaris. Compression neuropathies can occur at this site if, for example, the flexor carpi ulnaris is hypertrophied.

As the radial nerve courses through the cubital region, it can become compressed at various sites. A recurrent ramus of the radial nerve, described by Kopell and Thompson,[1] innervates the periosteum of the lateral epicondyle. In instances of hypertonia of the supinator, the recurrent ramus can become compressed as it runs through this muscle. A syndrome strongly resembling that of a tennis elbow develops. Furthermore, the deep branch of the radial nerve, the posterior interosseous nerve, can become compressed in its track underneath the supinator.

BIOMECHANICS

Movements around two axes are possible in the cubital articulation. From full extension of the elbow (in a lateral view, the longitudinal axis of the upper arm is in line with the longitudinal axis of the forearm), active flexion can be performed to approximately 145°. Passive flexion is possible to approximately 160°.

The elbow is considered to be in the zero position when the upper arm and forearm are in line with each other. In many individuals

carpi radialis brevis. By way of this fascia, part of the load can be diverted away from the epicondyle.

Nerves in the Cubital Region

Several factors can be responsible for a compression of the median, radial, or ulnar nerves as they pass through the cubital region (Figure 9–7).

In the cubital region, the median nerve runs through, in between, or underneath the heads of the pronator teres. In addition, the bicipital

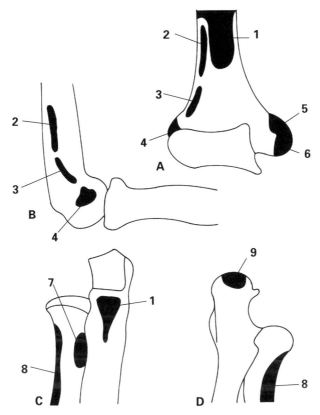

Figure 9–5 Muscle attachments at the elbow. **A**, Right humerus, anterior view; **B**, right humerus and radius, lateral view; **C**, right humerus and ulna, anterior view; **D**, right radius and ulna, posterior view; **1**, brachialis; **2**, brachioradialis; **3**, extensor carpi radialis longus; **4**, extensor carpi radialis brevis (plus the extensor digitorum, extensor carpi ulnaris, and supinator); **5**, pronator teres; **6**, origin of the hand flexors; **7**, biceps; **8**, supinator; **9**, triceps.

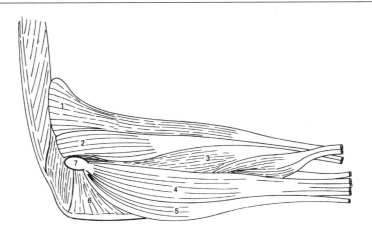

Figure 9–6 Musculature at the lateral aspect of the elbow. **1**, Brachioradialis; **2**, extensor carpi radialis longus; **3**, extensor carpi radialis brevis; **4**, extensor digitorum; **5**, extensor carpi ulnaris; **6**, anconeus; **7**, lateral epicondyle.

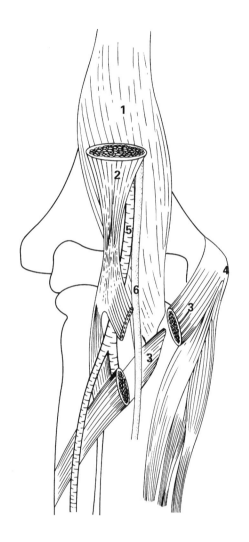

Figure 9–7 Anterior aspect of the elbow. **1**, Brachialis; **2**, biceps; **3**, pronator teres; **4**, origin of the wrist flexors; **5**, brachial artery; **6**, median nerve.

(especially women), however, more extension is possible (hyperextension). With the elbow in the zero position, the angle between the arm and forearm does not equal 0° in the frontal plane: there is a physiological valgus of 10° to 15° in men and one of 20° to 25° in women.

Pronation and supination range of motion amounts to approximately 90° (from the midposition); usually pronation is slightly less than supination. Pronation and supination are mainly restricted by the capsuloligamentous structures of the distal radioulnar joint. The dorsal structures restrict primarily pronation; the volar structures limit supination.

Outside forces on the elbow joint result in reactive forces *within* the joint. An estimation of these forces can be made by accepting a few simplifications in the calculation. In order to keep the elbow bent, it has been calculated that there must be a reaction force within the joint of approximately 30 newtons (N). With a weight of 1 kg in the hand, the reaction force amounts to 80 N.[2] During extension against gravity, the reaction force amounts to approximately 110 N. These estimates are for static loads.

Nicol et al. (cited by Frankel et al.[2]) estimate the reaction forces during daily activities to be as much as approximately half of body weight. If an individual rises from a chair by pushing up with the arms, the reaction force is estimated to be more than 1700 N (more than twice the body weight in a person weighing 70 kg). Therefore, even simple movements cause significant forces to stress the elbow joint.

10

Surface Anatomy of the Arm, Elbow, and Forearm

Palpation of the arm, elbow, and forearm is performed with the subject in a sitting or standing position and is directed at localizing specific structures. The structures to be localized are sequenced in a way that is best for the practical study of surface anatomy. Thus, the following method of classification deviates from the usual systematic or topographic anatomical descriptions. First, the palpable bony and ligamentous structures, organized per region, are discussed, followed by the palpable muscles and other soft tissue structures. An overview is provided to describe the blood vessels and neurological structures of the shoulder girdle and arm, emphasizing their topographic relationships (refer to Appendix A).

Because of the emphasis on *surface* anatomy, the relevant structures are classified and sequenced based on two main considerations: (1) the ability to palpate the structure and (2) its practical application in the clinic. Thus, if some structures are not mentioned, either they are not easily palpable (usually they are located too deeply or are covered by other structures) or palpation of the structures is not clinically significant. The sequence in which the various structures are discussed is based on orientation. For instance, during examination of a certain region, characteristic structures ("reference points" or "landmarks") are found before more specific palpation is performed.

Every palpation is preceded by inspection of the region. If the inspection is not performed, an "anatomy book knowledge" is often projected onto the body without having established a basis in fact. After the inspection, palpation of the relaxed structures follows. *For the purpose of study, as well as in the clinic, it is advisable to outline the palpated structures with a marker or skin pencil.* In this way, the examiner is forced to *see* the results of the palpation and can avoid gross mistakes.

In the framework of joint examination, every inspection and palpation at rest is followed by inspection and palpation during motion. When examining muscles, inspection and palpation during contraction is also desirable. (This contraction can be static or dynamic.) Thus, the following sequence is applied during a session of surface anatomy:

1. specific inspection at rest
2. palpation at rest
3. inspection during movement or contraction
4. palpation during movement or contraction

Of course, the entire sequence does not have to be followed when palpating every structure, but in evaluating joints and muscles it can be very helpful. Phenomena such as "misleading tenderness" and "referred pain" confuse every examiner who does not follow a logical palpation sequence.

PALPATION OF BONY AND LIGAMENTOUS STRUCTURES

Initial Position: Sitting or Standing

To identify anomalies of bony and ligamentous structures, one has to be familiar with the characteristic palpation of normal bony and ligamentous structures. For instance, a bony structure feels "hard" on palpation. Uncovered bony structures are not encountered in surface anatomy; bones and their prominences are surrounded by periosteum and usually by muscles. In addition, palpation is always made through subcutaneous and cutaneous layers. Ligamentous structures generally feel "firm." Joint lines also tend to be firm on palpation and to lie between two structures that are hard on palpation.

PALPATION OF MUSCLES AND OTHER SOFT TISSUE STRUCTURES OF THE ARM

Biceps

Observing this muscle is very simple (Figures 10–1A–D and 10–2). Place the elbow in flexion and forearm in supination, and then exert isometric resistance against these motions. Sometimes both muscle bellies are visible.

With a skin marker, outline the contours of the coracoid process, lesser tubercle, and greater tubercle. (Refer to Part I, The Shoulder, for details on localizing these structures through palpation.) With the help of these structures, the origin of the short head of the biceps can be located at the coracoid process (together with the coracobrachialis muscle).

The long head of the biceps is not palpable at its origin, but it can be palpated in the intertubercular sulcus. Bring the arm into abduction in order to inspect both muscle bellies.

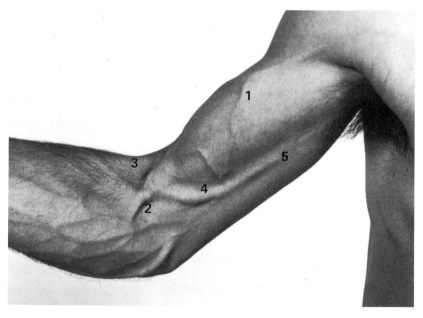

Figure 10–1A 1, Biceps brachii muscle; **2**, bicipital aponeurosis; **3**, brachioradialis muscle; **4**, basilic vein; **5**, basilic hiatus.

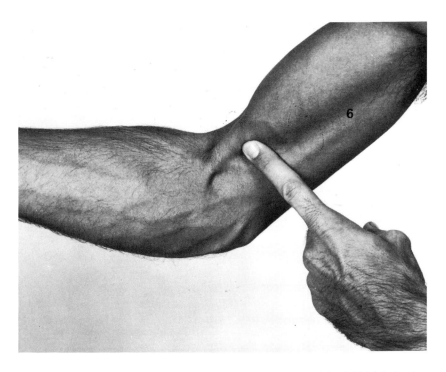

Figure 10–1B Palpation of the biceps musculotendinous junction. **6**, Medial bicipital sulcus.

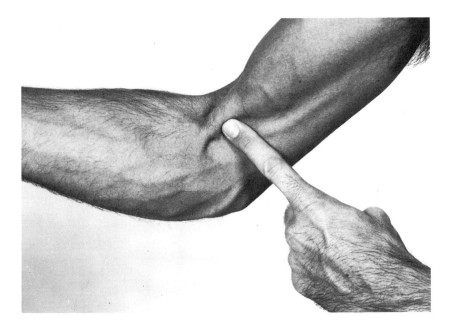

Figure 10–1C Palpation of the biceps tendon.

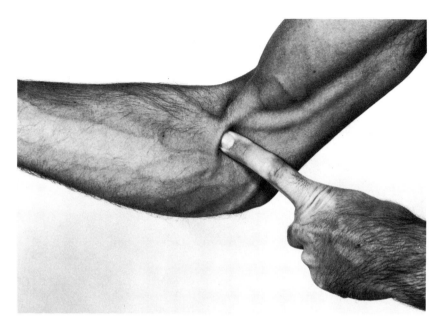

Figure 10–1D Palpation of the bicipital aponeurosis.

Sometimes a long groove can be palpated between both bellies.

At the dorsomedial aspect of the biceps, the medial bicipital sulcus can be found. In this sulcus, the brachial artery and basilic vein can be palpated. Here the basilic vein is subcutaneous before it becomes the brachial vein within the basilic hiatus. Depending on the amount of subcutaneous fat, the median and the ulnar nerves are usually palpable just medial to the musculotendinous junction of the biceps.

The lateral bicipital sulcus is located dorsolaterally between the biceps and the brachialis. In this groove (or directly ventromedial to the groove) the cephalic vein can be palpated along its course to the infraclavicular fossa.

The biceps ends with a main tendon at the radial tuberosity, located deeply within the cubital fossa. Its other insertion radiates medially into a flat superficial tendinous expansion, the bicipital aponeurosis.

Lesions of the biceps are indicated when resisted flexion and supination of the elbow are painful. If the biceps is affected more proximally, the pain is experienced diffusely in the shoulder. In lesions at the elbow region, the pain is usually felt more locally.

Brachialis

The brachialis can be palpated dorsal to the deltoid tuberosity. From the deltoid tuberosity, the muscle runs distally, parallel to the triceps. Although it runs underneath and parallel to the biceps, the division between both is easy to palpate (lateral bicipital sulcus) (Figure 10–2).

The brachialis can also be palpated for a short distance medially, from the musculotendinous junction of the biceps to the proximal border of the bicipital aponeurosis.

Coracobrachialis

The coracobrachialis can be palpated at the lateral border of the axillary fossa with the

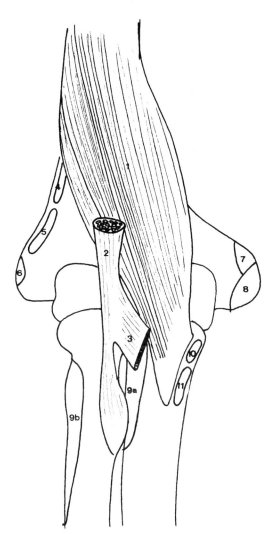

Figure 10–2 1, Brachialis muscle; **2**, biceps brachii muscle; **3**, bicipital aponeurosis; **4**, origin of the brachioradialis muscle; **5**, origin of the extensor carpi radialis longus muscle; **6**, origin of the extensor carpi radialis brevis muscle; **7**, origin of the pronator teres muscle; **8**, common origin of the wrist flexors; **9a**, origin of the supinator muscle; **9b**, insertion of the supinator muscle; **10**, origin of the flexor digitorum superficialis muscle, ulnar head; **11**, origin of the pronator teres muscle, ulnar head.

arm in abduction. The course of the muscle, together with the neurovascular bundle, can be followed along the arm (Figures 2–20A and 2–20B).

In athletes who participate in sports that require throwing motions, the origin of this muscle can be injured at the coracoid process.

Triceps

Weight-bearing movements, such as pushing the body up with the hands on the armrests of a chair, will reveal the contours of the triceps. Location of the several heads of the triceps is often confusing. Depending on the position of the arm, the long head can be clearly observed medially. The lateral head is actually located more proximal than lateral, to the medial head.

Usually, only the long head and the lateral head of the triceps are visible. Start the palpation of the long head in the middle of the dorsal aspect of the upper arm and follow it proximally until it runs between the teres major and minor. The palpation can be simplified by bringing the arm into 90° abduction and performing active dorsal movement of the arm against resistance.

The lateral head of the triceps borders directly on the brachial muscle. The medial head of the triceps runs underneath both the long and lateral heads of the triceps. It can be felt at the dorsomedial and dorsolateral aspects of the arm, where it runs out from underneath the long and lateral heads. Palpate both heads of the triceps until their common tendinous insertion at the olecranon.

Lesions of this muscle are rarely seen in the clinic.

Anconeus

The anconeus is a continuation of the lateral head of the triceps. Although the function of the anconeus has not been clearly determined, it is called the capsular "tightener" of the elbow joint. Between the olecranon, the posterior border of the ulna, and the lateral epicondyle, a small muscular triangle can be palpated. This is the anconeus (Fig-

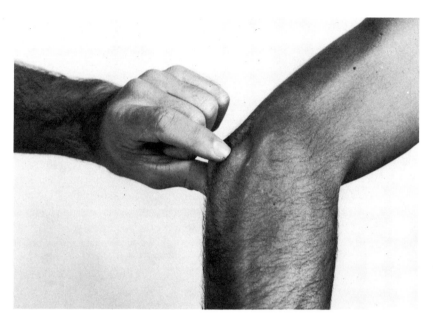

Figure 10–3 Anconeus, lateral view, right arm.

ure 10–3). Its contraction is obvious during elbow extension.

Medial Bicipital Sulcus

Just dorsomedial to the biceps (Figure 10–1B), look for pulsation of the brachial artery. This artery lies on top of a clearly palpable "cord," the median nerve. The median nerve can be palpated from this site to an area just proximal to the bicipital aponeurosis.

In the upper half of the arm, the ulnar nerve runs behind the brachial artery. In the lower half, it runs more dorsally until it reaches the sulcus for the ulnar nerve, which is the groove between the olecranon and the medial epicondyle. The nerve can be palpated easily along the entire arm. (Palpate with gentle pressure!) Irritation of the nerve in its groove often occurs.

The basilic vein is also located at the level of the medial bicipital sulcus. Usually it is visible until it reaches the basilic hiatus. At the hiatus, it disappears into the depths of the arm,

where it flows into the brachial vein (Figure 10–1A).

Lateral Bicipital Sulcus

At the level of the lateral bicipital sulcus, the cephalic vein is located. It runs toward the infraclavicular fossa through the Mohrenheim groove. (The topography of this vein is highly variable.)

PALPATION OF THE BONY AND LIGAMENTOUS STRUCTURES

Cubital Joint (Articulatio Cubiti)

Mark the round medial epicondyle of the humerus (Figures 10–2, 10–4, and 10–5A), and palpate the humerus proximally as far as possible. Note possible lymph node swelling within the medial bicipital sulcus. Also note any thickening of the epicondyle which could influence the function of the ulnar nerve.

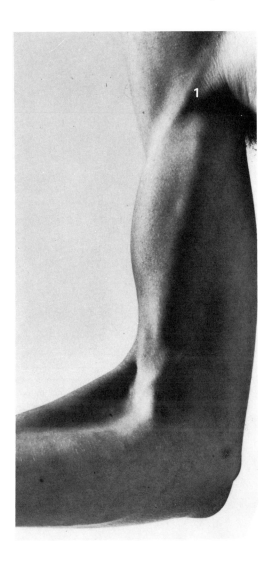

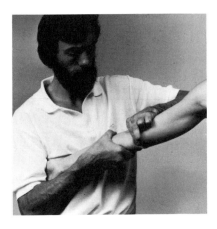

Figure 10–5A Palpation of the origin of the wrist flexors, at the right elbow, on the medial epicondyle.

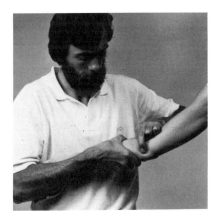

Figure 10–5B Palpation of the musculotendinous junction of the wrist flexors, at the right side.

Figure 10–4 Right arm, medial view. **1**, Cephalic vein; **2**, tendon of the biceps brachii muscle; **3**, bicipital aponeurosis; **4**, cubital fossa; **5**, brachioradialis muscle; **6**, medial epicondyle; **7**, pronator teres muscle.

Next, the olecranon can be palpated and outlined. Remember, between the olecranon and the skin, there is a bursa. The olecranon ends distally in a point. From this point, the posterior border of the ulna can be palpated along its entire length, down to the ulnar styloid process at the level of the carpus.

Now locate and mark the less obvious lateral epicondyle of the humerus. When the elbow joint is in 90° flexion, the three bony prominences just mentioned (medial and lateral epicondyles and the olecranon) form an isosceles triangle. If the arm is extended, these three points lie in line with each other. In the presence of fractures and other elbow joint lesions, the normal form of this triangle can be disturbed. Especially at the medial side, supracondylar fractures often occur in children and the elderly.

Inspection of the extended and supinated elbow from behind allows a small groove, visible at the radial side of the olecranon, to be seen. This is the entrance to the humeroradial joint. Palpation of the radial head is described below.

Radial Head (Caput Radii)

Palpation of the radial head and humeroradial joint can be done by standing in front of the subject (Figures 10–6A, B and 10–7). Both the forearms are grasped from behind and each index finger is placed at the lateral humeral epicondyles. The index fingers then slide dorsally and distally between the humerus and the radial head. The size of each joint can be compared. During pronation and supination, both radial heads can be more easily palpated. Often a flat structure running from the radial head toward the lateral epicondyle can be felt; this is the radial collateral ligament.

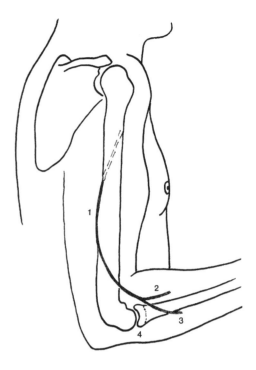

Figure 10–7 Course of the right radial nerve in relation to the radial head. This location is important to note when giving injections or friction massages in the elbow region. **1**, Radial nerve; **2**, radial nerve, superficial ramus; **3**, radial nerve, deep ramus (posterior interosseus nerve); **4**, radial head.

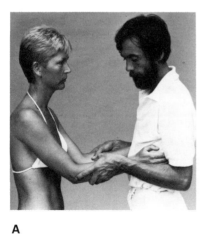

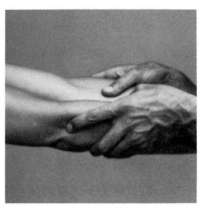

A   **B**

Figure 10–6A and B Palpation of the radial heads with flexion and extension of the elbows.

This technique can also be used to assess thickening of the joint capsule at the level of the radial head (such as in rheumatoid arthritis).

The annular ligament, which runs over the radial head, can also be palpated. This ligament will feel less hard than the surrounding structure, which will feel bony. Proximal to the radial head, the humeral capitulum can be palpated. This structure is often mistaken for the lateral epicondyle.

PALPATION OF THE MUSCLES AT THE DORSORADIAL ASPECT OF THE FOREARM

Brachioradialis

The brachioradialis is clearly visible as the radial border of the cubital fossa (Figures 10–8 and 10–9). It is brought into view by flexing the elbow against resistance with 90°

flexion in the elbow, and the forearm in a position between supination and pronation.

Although the muscle is an elbow flexor, topographically it belongs to the dorsolateral group of the forearm. In addition, together with the pronator teres, it forms the border between the wrist extensors (located more dorsally) and flexors (located more volarly).

Start palpating the brachioradialis at the radial aspect of the cubital fossa and move in a proximal direction to where the muscle can be found between the brachialis and biceps. Next, palpate in a distal direction, holding the muscle belly between thumb and index finger. The muscle can be followed down to the hand, where its tendon inserts at the radial styloid process.

Supinator

The supinator is discussed here, although it does not belong to the forearm extensors. Its borders within the cubital fossa are formed by

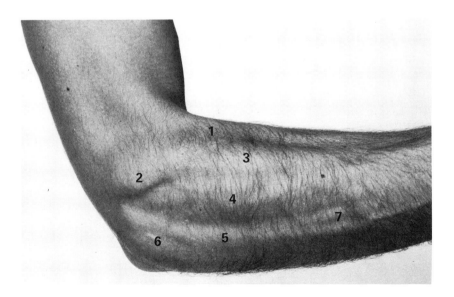

Figure 10–8 Right arm, lateral view. **1**, Brachioradialis muscle; **2**, extensor carpi radialis longus muscle; **3**, extensor carpi radialis brevis muscle (during contraction, its muscle belly is in line with the short belly of the extensor carpi radialis longus); **4**, extensor digitorum muscle; **5**, extensor carpi ulnaris muscle; **6**, anconeus muscle; **7**, extensor digiti minimi muscle.

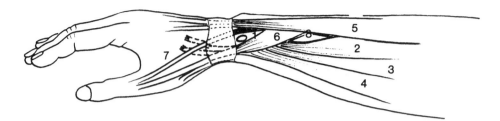

Figure 10–9 Forearm and hand, right side, radial view. **1**, Lister's tubercle; **2**, extensor carpi radialis brevis muscle; **3**, extensor carpi radialis longus muscle; **4**, brachioradialis muscle; **5**, extensor digitorum muscle; **6**, abductor pollicis longus and extensor pollicis brevis muscles; **7**, extensor pollicis longus muscle; **8**, radius.

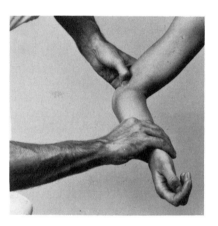

Figure 10–10A Palpation of the origin of the right extensor carpi radialis longus.

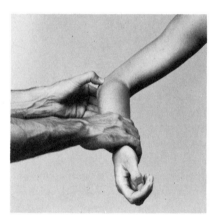

Figure 10–10B Palpation of the origin of the right extensor carpi radialis brevis.

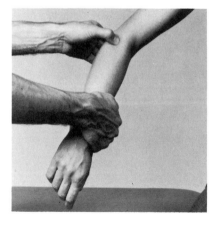

Figure 10–10C Palpation of the tendon of the right extensor carpi radialis brevis.

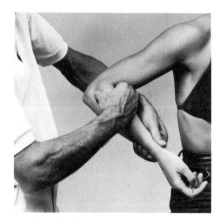

Figure 10–10D Palpation of the musculotendinous junction and proximal muscle belly of the right extensor carpi radialis brevis.

the brachioradialis (radially), pronator teres (ulnarly), and tendon of the biceps (proximally) (Figure 10–2).

During forceful supination against resistance, a small part of the supinator can be felt by palpating just ulnar to the brachioradialis.

Extensor Carpi Radialis Longus

The extensor carpi radialis longus becomes visible by firmly making a fist with the wrist in slight extension (Figures 10–8 and 10–9). Its muscle belly is seen directly distal to the brachioradialis. When palpating, the muscle can be followed between the epicondyle and brachioradialis by means of an alternating palpation (index and middle fingers).

Occasionally, the extensor carpi radialis longus insertion is affected in the so-called tennis elbow. Palpation helps to confirm the diagnosis. The tip of the thumb is placed just superior to the lateral epicondyle and against the anterior aspect of the humeral supracondylar ridge. In so doing, the examiner's forearm is in line with the patient's forearm. By means of an adduction movement, the thumb palpates transverse to the fibers (Figure 10–10A).

Extensor Carpi Radialis Brevis

Palpation of the extensor carpi radialis brevis starts at the lateral epicondyle. From this point, the muscle runs diagonally in a radial direction toward the brachioradialis and the extensor carpi radialis longus (Figures 10–8, 10–9, and 10–10B–D).

In the frequently seen lateral tennis elbow, the extensor carpi radialis brevis is the most often affected structure. Therefore, palpation of various predilection sites should be done precisely.

The origin of this muscle is best palpated by positioning the subject's shoulder in 45° abduction. In so doing, the corresponding part of the lateral epicondyle is brought into a horizontal plane. Furthermore, by bringing the elbow into 90° flexion and the forearm

into full supination, the muscle is relaxed and more accessible to palpation. If a position other than this is taken, the palpation is sometimes not painful despite a lesion of the muscle's teno-osseous transition.

To determine whether the insertion of the extensor carpi radialis brevis is affected, the examiner supinates the patient's forearm with the ipsilateral hand and uses the thumb of the other hand to palpate the epicondyle. The other fingers of the palpating hand support the patient's elbow while maintaining the position of the arm. The tip of the palpating thumb, flexed at the interphalangeal joint, is placed on the edge of the lateral epicondyle. At the same time, the grip between the thumb and the fingers that support the dorsomedial aspect of the elbow is increased. Without changing the amount of pressure, the examiner moves the thumb (by moving the entire arm) 0.5 cm medially. This movement is repeated from proximal to distal in order to palpate different aspects of the lateral epicondyle (Figure 10–10B).

The proximal tendon of the extensor carpi radialis brevis is best palpated with the subject's elbow in 45° flexion and maximally pronated. In this position, the tendon runs over the radial head and is easy to palpate. Place the flattened end phalanx of the thumb over the tendon and perform the palpation through a radial deviation movement of the wrist (Figure 10–10C). Pathology is seldom encountered at this site.

To palpate the musculotendinous junction and the proximal part of the muscle belly, position the subject's elbow in 100° flexion and maximal supination. Palpation is performed with a grasping motion between thumb and index finger, in which the thumb is at the level of the radial neck and the index finger is lateral to the biceps tendon (Figure 10–10D).

Extensor Digitorum Communis

In a thin, muscular person, the extensor digitorum communis can be observed easily by asking for extension of the hand with extended fingers (see Figures 10–8, 16–7, and 16–10). With the help of the following technique, the extensor digitorum can be distinguished easily from the extensor carpi radialis brevis.

First, Lister's tubercle is located (a small bony protuberance at the distal end of the radius) (Figures 10–9 and 16–7). With the forearm in the zero position, a diamond-shaped area can be found one finger length proximal to this tubercle; in this region the radius is not covered by soft tissue (Figures 10–9 and 10–11). The extensor digitorum is palpable directly ulnar to this diamond-shaped area. Radial to it, the extensor carpi radialis brevis is located. At the distal aspect of the diamond, the abductor pollicis longus and extensor pollicis brevis can be found.

Another method for locating the extensor digitorum communis is first to locate the extensor carpi ulnaris. Between this muscle and the extensor carpi radialis brevis, the extensor digitorum communis can be outlined. The extensor indicis runs with the extensor digitorum communis through the same extensor tunnel at the wrist.

Extensor Digiti Minimi

The extensor digiti minimi is easy to palpate at the middle and distal third of the forearm (Figures 16–7 and 16–19). Ask for resisted pronation of the forearm with simultaneous resisted extension of the little finger. Palpate the extensor digiti minimi tendon directly radial to the ulnar head and proximal to the extensor retinaculum. Then follow it as far as possible proximally and distally. The location of this tendon at the level of the ulnar head is an important reference point in finding the distal radioulnar joint.

Extensor Carpi Ulnaris

Palpating the extensor carpi ulnaris can be made simple by first finding the posterior border of the ulnar (this is the border of the ulna that is clearly palpable along its entire length, from the olecranon to the styloid process). The extensor carpi ulnaris is located dorsal to the posterior border of the ulna, and runs parallel to it. Follow the muscle distally to its tendon. By slightly resisting wrist extension and ulnar deviation, the tendon can be palpated from the base of the fifth metacarpal to about 2 inches proximally (Figures 10–8 and 16–7).

Abductor Pollicis Longus and Extensor Pollicis Brevis

At the distal aspect of the forearm, the muscle bellies of the abductor pollicis longus and extensor pollicis brevis superficially cross over the dorsal aspect of the tendons of the brachioradialis and extensors carpi radialis longus and brevis (Figures 10–9, 16–7, and 16–19). Both run further to the thumb, forming the radial border of the anatomical snuff box (radial fossa).

Extensor Pollicis Longus

The extensor pollicis longus also crosses over the extensors carpi radialis longus and brevis. Its tendon forms the ulnar border of the anatomical snuff box (Figure 10–9).

PALPATION OF THE FLEXORS OF THE FOREARM

Cubital Fossa

The cubital fossa serves as the starting point for palpation and localization of structures in the volar forearm region (Figure 10–4).

The cubital fossa can be defined easily by resisting elbow flexion with the forearm in the neutral position between supination and pronation. The cubital fossa is triangular in shape, with its apex distally. The brachioradialis is found on the radial side of the triangle, and the pronator teres on the ulnar side. At the base of the triangle, the round cord-like main tendon and the flat superficial tendon (aponeurosis) of the biceps can be palpated. The brachial artery first runs medial to, then underneath, the bicipital aponeurosis. The median nerve runs distally, either dorsal to or crossing over the artery. This nerve disappears between the two heads of the pronator teres.

Superficially in the fossa the median cubital vein is found. This vein is often used for taking blood samples.

Pronator Teres

The pronator teres muscle is very easy to see in a thin or muscular person during resisted flexion and simultaneous pronation with the elbow in 90° flexion.

Palpate the medial epicondyle. Approximately one fingerwidth radial to the epicondyle is the origin of the pronator teres. This muscle forms the medial border of the cubital fossa as it runs to the end of the proximal third of the forearm. Deep palpation during contraction is difficult because of the antebrachial fascia, which covers the cubital fossa and into which the radiating fibers from the bicipital aponeurosis are anchored (Figures 10–11 and 16–10).

Flexor Carpi Radialis

With active flexion (15°) and simultaneous radial deviation of the hand, two or sometimes three tendons can be seen in the middle of the volar aspect of the forearm.

The radial tendon is the flexor carpi radialis, which is the only part of this muscle that can be seen. The muscle can be further palpated along an imaginary line between its tendon and the medial epicondyle. If this is difficult, the tendon can be palpated and followed proximally by using two fingers and alternating the palpation (Figures 10–10 and 16–10).

Palmaris Longus

If present, the palmaris longus tendon can be palpated directly ulnar to the flexor carpi radialis (the palmaris longus is absent in 10% to 15% of cases). Palpation can be made easier by asking for forceful opposition of the tips of the thumb and little finger with the wrist slightly flexed. In the middle of the volar aspect of the hand, a thin superficial tendinous strand appears, which inserts into the palmar aponeurosis at the level of the distal wrist crease (Figure 16–15).

The palmar aponeurosis is the superficial fascia and tendinous expansion that constrains the palm of the hand. Palpate for swelling or thickening along the course of the four fascial slips that run to the second to fifth fingers; this can be especially evident at the ulnar aspect. Deformity of the hand involving constant forced flexion of the fingers, such as a Dupuytren contracture, can be the result of

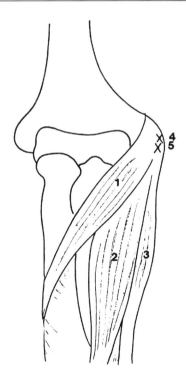

Figure 10–11 Right arm, volar view. **1**, Pronator teres muscle; **2**, flexor carpi radialis muscle; **3**, flexor carpi ulnaris muscle; **4**, site of the lesions of the origins of the above-mentioned muscles; **5**, site of the lesion of the musculotendinous junction.

pathological changes within the palmar apo-neurosis.

The median nerve is palpable deeply be-tween the tendons of the flexor carpi radialis and palmaris longus.

Flexor Carpi Ulnaris

Like the three muscles described above, the flexor carpi ulnaris also originates from the medial epicondyle (Figure 10–11).

Its tendon can be seen during simultaneous flexion and ulnar deviation of the hand. The muscle lies at the volar aspect of the posterior border of the ulna and is palpable along its entire length. At the wrist, the ulnar nerve and the palpable ulnar artery run just radial to the flexor carpi ulnaris tendon.

Lesions of the wrist flexor origins at the medial epicondyle, or at their musculotendi-nous junction, are called golfer's elbow (Fig-ures 10–5A and B and 10–11).

Palpation of the teno-osseous site is best performed with an extended elbow, whereas the musculotendinous junction is best pal-pated with a slightly flexed elbow.

To palpate the origin of the wrist flexors at the medial epicondyle, the examiner main-tains extension in the patient's elbow by ex-erting pressure against the dorsal aspect with the ipsilateral hand. The patient's hand and wrist are fixed between the examiner's arm and trunk. Now the examiner places the tip of the index finger at the volar aspect of the medial epicondyle; the thumb gives counterpressure dorsally. The palpation takes place in a lateral direction through a slight bending of the index finger. If this movement is repeated one-fourth inch more distally, the tendon can already be felt. How-ever, the tendon itself is rarely affected.

The musculotendinous junction of the wrist flexors can be felt by repeating the pal-pation just described, an additional one-fourth inch distally. A larger amplitude is re-quired during this palpation, and the patient's elbow is positioned in slight flexion.

Flexor Digitorum Superficialis

The flexor digitorum superficialis can be palpated at the distal two thirds of the fore-arm, between the flexor carpi ulnaris and flexor carpi radialis. Its tendons are palpable ulnar to the tendon of the palmaris longus at the wrist and run from there through the hand to the middle phalanxes of the fingers.

Flexor Digitorum Profundus

The tendons of the flexor digitorum pro-fundus run to the end phalanxes of the fin-gers. It is best palpated at its origin, directly volar to the posterior border of the ulna and dorsal to the flexor carpi ulnaris.

Flexor Pollicis Longus

The radial artery runs between the distal portions of the brachioradialis and the flexor carpi radialis. The flexor pollicis longus can be felt underneath this artery when the pa-tient flexes the thumb.

11

Examination of the Elbow

ELBOW JOINT (CUBITAL ARTICULATION)

Zero Position

Upper arm and supinated forearm are in the frontal plane.

Maximal Loose-Packed Position

Humeroulnar joint: The elbow is in approximately 70° flexion; the forearm is in approximately 10° supination.

Humeroradial joint: The elbow is in extension; the forearm is in maximal supination.

Maximal Close-Packed Position

Humeroulnar joint: The elbow is in maximal extension; the forearm is in maximal supination. For the part of the joint between the coronoid process and the humerus, the elbow is in maximal flexion.

Humeroradial joint: The elbow is in approximately 90° flexion; the forearm is in approximately 5° supination.

Capsular Pattern

For the humeroulnar joint, flexion is much more limited than extension (Figure 11–1).

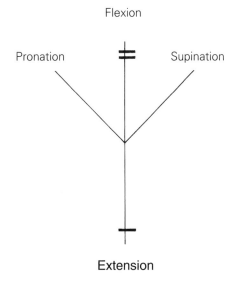

Figure 11–1 Capsular pattern of the humeroulnar joint.

FOREARM (ANTEBRACHII)

Zero Position

The arm is in the frontal plane; the elbow is in 90° flexion; the forearm is midway between pronation and supination.

221

Maximal Loose-Packed Position

Proximal radioulnar joint: The elbow is in approximately 70° flexion; the forearm is in approximately 35° supination.

Maximal Close-Packed Position

The forearm is in approximately 5° supination.

Capsular Pattern

There is minimal to no limitation of motion; pain is experienced at the end-range of each motion (pronation and supination).

OVERVIEW OF THE FUNCTIONAL EXAMINATION

General Inspection

The examining therapist can gain information immediately as the patient enters the room. The therapist observes the patient's general posture, facial expression, and the use of assistive devices. Attention is paid to how the patient holds the affected arm and to how the patient shakes hands. The use of a cast or brace can also be noted.

History

Age, Occupation, Hobbies, Sports

Some lesions are definitely age related. Dislocation of the radiohumeral and radioulnar joints is seen in children up to the age of about 8 years. Panner's disease is seen up to the age of about 10 years. In young throwers an avulsion fracture of the medial epicondyle can develop. From ages 15 to 20, osteochondrosis dissecans is found. Tennis elbow is seen particularly in the 35- to 60-year age group.

Some disorders, for instance tennis or golfer's elbow, can occur in both professional and recreational sports.

Chief Complaints

Depending on the type of elbow pathology, complaints can consist of one or more of the following:

- pain
- paresthesia
- loss of strength
- loss of sensation
- loss of range of motion
- locking of the joint

Pain in the region of the elbow often has a local cause. This may also be true of paresthesia at the elbow; however, it is usually the result of a cervical problem or occasionally a thoracic outlet syndrome. If a peripheral nerve is compressed at the level of the elbow, paresthesia is usually experienced further distally, particularly in the hand and fingers.

Generally, in instances of a loss of strength or sensation, a distinction has to be made between a cervical lesion and compression of a peripheral nerve.

Limitation of motion can have many causes. Often, the patient's age will point to the cause. For instance, a limitation of extension in a 15-year-old can be caused by osteochondrosis dissecans. In a 60-year-old, this limitation is usually part of a capsular pattern caused by arthrosis. Locking is often caused by loose bodies.

Sometimes pathology in the wrist area refers pain proximally. Therefore, when symptoms occur in the elbow region and the functional examination of the elbow is negative, a functional examination of the wrist should also be performed.

Onset

Several key points regarding onset can aid in establishing the diagnosis:

- Was there a trauma? The most often occurring traumatic lesion is traumatic arthritis, with or without accompanying instability and fractures.

- Did the complaints occur after overuse? Overuse usually results in the development of lesions of the contractile structures. Especially at the elbow joint, the origins of the tendons are involved. In such cases, the clinical stage of the tendinitis should be determined by conducting a thorough history.
- Is the cause unknown? Several types of arthritides or osteochondrosis dissecans develop in the elbow region without a known cause.

Localization of the Complaints

It is important to ask the patient whether the symptoms are local or radiating.

- The symptoms are local: The more local the symptoms, the greater the chance that the lesion is indeed localized at that site. Misleading pain and tenderness, however, always must be taken into account.
- The symptoms are radiating. Radiating pain occurs especially in tennis elbow (particularly in type 2) and in lesions of the biceps.

Factors That Influence the Symptoms

If possible, the patient should describe when the symptoms are experienced.

- Are they felt during movement (of the elbow, shoulder, head, or neck)? If the patient indicates that particular movements of the head cause the elbow pain, a cervical lesion should be suspected. If mainly shoulder movements cause the complaints, a shoulder problem should be considered.
- Are they felt at rest during the day? Knowing whether the pain occurs only during movement or also is present at rest helps determine the clinical stage of a tendinitis.

- Are they felt at rest during the night? If the patient complains chiefly about pain at night, the presence of a tumor should be ruled out

Involvement of Other Joints

If the patient has complaints about other joints, a systemic disease such as rheumatoid arthritis, psoriasis, ankylosing spondylitis, or gout should be considered.

Medication

Administering mechanical therapy such as mobilization, manipulation, or transverse friction is contraindicated if the patient is taking anticoagulants. When the patient is on antihypertensive medication, exercise programs should be closely monitored (to ensure that the patient maintains proper breathing).

Prior Treatment and Results

A tennis elbow that has been treated unsuccessfully with injections, without first having undergone physical therapy treatment, seldom reacts favorably when physical therapy is administered afterward.

Specific Inspection

Compare the position and contours of the affected elbow with those of the nonaffected side. Look for a valgus position or recurvation of the joint. Examine each side for color and condition of the skin. Look for local swelling. Always assess the patient's total posture. (See also Chapter 10.)

Palpation

Before starting the functional tests, the examiner palpates the elbow area for warmth. Palpation is also performed at the level of the radial head and at the ventral aspect of the medial epicondyle for possible swelling and synovial thickening (often the first sign of an arthritis). If there is visible swelling, consistency is assessed.

Functional Examination

Before the functional examination, note whether the patient is experiencing symptoms at that specific moment. With each test the examiner notes whether the symptoms change.

Procedurally, the affected side is always compared with the nonaffected side. The nonaffected side is tested first, to have an idea of what is "normal."

In the following description of the functional examination, the essential tests are indicated in **_boldface italic and underlined:_** these comprise the *basic functional examination*. The other tests are conditionally performed, depending on findings from the basic functional examination.

Tests—Active Motions

11.1.   Active extension of both elbows
11.2.   Active flexion of both elbows
11.3.   Active pronation of both forearms
11.4.   Active supination of both forearms

Tests—Passive Motions, Including Stability Tests

_11.5._   _Passive elbow extension_
_11.6._   _Passive elbow flexion_
_11.7._   _Passive forearm pronation_
_11.8._   _Passive forearm supination_
_11.9A._   _Passive valgus test_
_11.9B._   _Passive varus test_

Tests—Resisted Motions

_11.10._   _Resisted elbow flexion_
_11.11._   _Resisted elbow extension_
_11.12._   _Resisted forearm pronation_
_11.13._   _Resisted forearm supination_
_11.14._   _Resisted wrist extension_
11.15.   Resisted radial deviation of the wrist
11.16.   Resisted ulnar deviation of the wrist
11.17.   Resisted extension of fingers two to five

11.18.   Resisted extension of fingers two and three
_11.19._   _Resisted wrist flexion_

Palpation

After the functional examination, the elbow region is palpated again for warmth, swelling, tenderness, and synovial thickening.

Accessory Examinations in Limitations of Motion

If a limitation of motion in a noncapsular pattern has been found, the appropriate joint-specific translatory tests should be performed. These tests will help determine whether the limitation is indeed caused by the capsule.

Other Examinations

If necessary, other methods may be used to confirm a diagnosis or gain further information when a diagnosis cannot be based reliably on the functional examination. These methods include the following:

- imaging systems such as conventional radiographs, computed tomography (CT) scan, arthrography, arthro-CT, magnetic resonance imaging (MRI), and ultrasonography
- laboratory tests
- arthroscopy
- electromyography (EMG)

DESCRIPTION OF THE FUNCTIONAL EXAMINATION

Based on the patient's history, tests, and examinations, if it is still not clear whether pain in the elbow originates there, it may be necessary to look for possible causes at the cervical spine, thoracic outlet region, shoulder, or wrist.

Active Motions

Active motions are assessed to determine the amount of motion, course of movement, and provocation of pain.

In instances of limited movement, it should be determined whether this limitation is in a capsular pattern or noncapsular pattern. This can be assessed only on the basis of the passive movements.

11.1. Active Extension of Both Elbows

The patient extends both elbows actively.

This test allows for a quick assessment of the amount of motion (extension) in each elbow. The range of motion depends on the general mobility of the patient. More than 180° of extension indicates an increase of the valgus position.

An apparent limitation of motion can be correctly interpreted only after performing the passive extension test (Test 11.5).

11.2. Active Flexion of Both Elbows

The patient bends both elbows actively.

Compare left and right. The range of motion depends on the muscle mass at the anterior aspects of both arm and forearm. An apparent limitation of motion can be correctly interpreted only after performing the passive flexion test (Test 11.6).

If there is limitation of motion in a capsular pattern, the amount of flexion limitation is much greater than the extension limitation—for instance, a limitation of 60° in flexion compared with a limitation of 10° in extension.

11.3. Active Pronation of Both Forearms

The patient keeps the elbows 90° flexed and maximally pronates both forearms. The range of motion is generally approximately 90°.

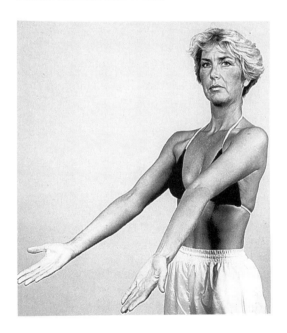

Test 11.1

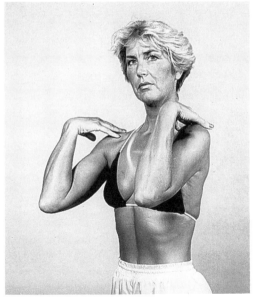

Test 11.2

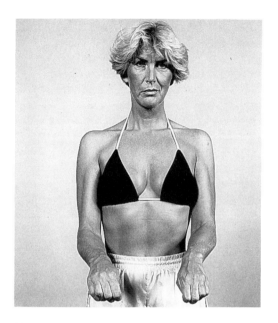

Test 11.3

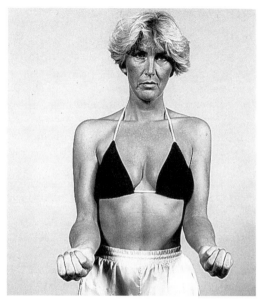

Test 11.4

Limitations of motion are seldom seen; they are usually the result of a fracture of the radial head or other parts of the radius.

Pain without a limitation of motion can be caused when the insertion of the biceps is compressed against the ulna.

11.4. Active Supination of Both Forearms

The patient keeps the elbows in 90° flexion and maximally supinates both forearms. The range of motion is generally 80° to 90°.

Limitations are seldom seen; they are usually the result of a fracture of the forearm.

Passive Motions

The amount of motion found during the passive evaluation is compared with results of the active evaluation. In limitations of motion, differentiation is made between capsular and noncapsular patterns. Limitations of motion in a capsular pattern indicate arthritis or arthrosis (osteoarthrosis). Determining and

correctly interpreting the end-feel is also of great importance in making a diagnosis and/ or a prognosis. As with the active motions, provocation of the patient's symptoms is also noted.

11.5. Passive Elbow Extension

With the ipsilateral hand, the examiner grasps the patient's forearm from the volar aspect, just proximal to the wrist. The other hand grasps the patient's elbow at the joint in such a way that the thumb is positioned anteriorly and the fingers posteriorly.

From a position of maximal extension and slight forearm pronation (the arthrokinematic coupling), the proximal hand flexes the elbow a few degrees and then performs an abrupt—but not forceful—extension. In so doing, the end-feel is assessed. The end-feel is normally hard. It is caused by the increase in tension in the anterior part of the capsule, which is reinforced by the anterior band of the ulnar collateral ligament.

If there is a loose body in the joint, the end-feel can be elastic or springy.

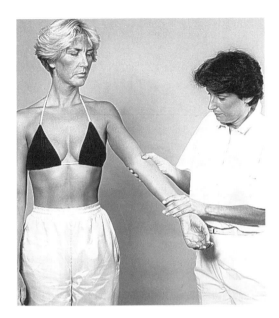

Test 11.5

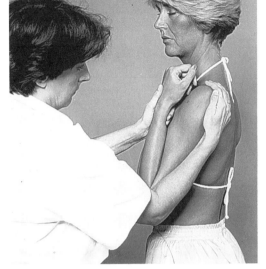

Test 11.6

Any limitations should be classified as occurring in a capsular or noncapsular pattern.

11.6. Passive Elbow Flexion

With the ipsilateral hand, the examiner grasps the patient's forearm just proximal to the wrist and flexes the elbow as far as possible. For stabilization, the other hand applies counterpressure at the posterior aspect of the patient's shoulder.

The end-feel is normally soft because of the interposition of soft tissue. However, in many people the end-feel is firm due to slight capsular changes caused by heavy labor or sports activities, such as boxing, volleyball, javelin throw, and others. In some cases, the firm end-feel exists without an apparent cause. For further interpretation, see Tests 11.2 and 11.5.

11.7. Passive Forearm Pronation

The patient's elbow is flexed to 90°. With the ipsilateral hand, the examiner pronates the patient's forearm: the thenar eminence is placed on the dorsal aspect of the patient's

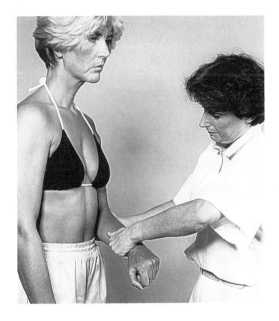

Test 11.7

radius, just proximal to the wrist. The examiner's contralateral hand stabilizes the elbow.

The end-feel is rather hard. This is caused mainly by the dorsal capsuloligamentous structures of the distal radioulnar joint.

Pain can be due to compression (impingement) of the insertion of the biceps against the ulna. In this case, there is no limitation of motion.

Limitation of motion is usually the result of a radial head fracture.

11.8. Passive Forearm Supination

With the thenar eminence of the ipsilateral hand, the examiner grasps the patient's forearm from the volar aspect just proximal to the wrist. The examiner supinates the patient's forearm while stabilizing the patient's elbow with the contralateral hand.

The end-feel is usually somewhat harder in supination than in pronation. The end-feel is caused by tension occurring at the volar capsuloligamentous structures of the distal radioulnar joint.

This test seldom provokes pain. When pain is induced, with or without a very slight limi-

tation of motion, there may be a distortion of the proximal radioulnar joint. A larger limitation, possibly accompanied by pain, is usually the result of a fracture of the radial head.

11.9A. Passive Valgus Test

With the ipsilateral hand, the examiner grasps the patient's forearm from ulnar, just proximal to the wrist. The patient's elbow is slightly flexed. The examiner's other hand grasps the patient's elbow from the radial side, placing the thenar eminence against the radius.

Both hands now work simultaneously to perform the passive valgus test. While the proximal hand exerts pressure ulnarly, the distal hand exerts pressure radially.

In the same manner, the test is performed with the arm in slightly more flexion, and in extension. In slight flexion, the entire ulnar collateral ligament is tested. In submaximal extension, the anterior band is emphasized, and in more flexion, particularly the posterior band of the ligament is tested. The examiner

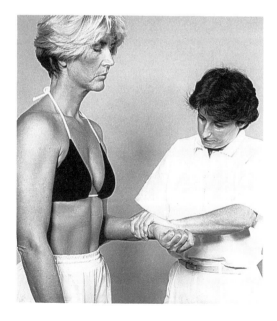

Test 11.8

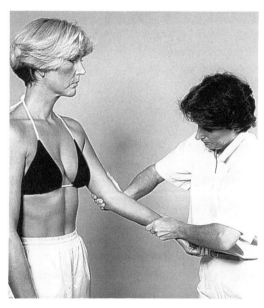

Test 11.9A

looks for provocation of pain or laxity of the ligament.

11.9B. Passive Varus Test

(not illustrated)

In the same way as described for the passive valgus test, the passive varus test is performed, but now from the medial aspect. This test is only performed particularly when a lesion of the radial collateral capsuloligamentous structures is suspected, which is seldom. Again, the examiner looks for provocation of pain or laxity.

Resisted Motions

By performing isometric resisted tests, contractile structures are evaluated. It is important to note weakness and pain provocation.

11.10. Resisted Elbow Flexion

The patient keeps the elbow in 90° flexion with the forearm supinated. The fingers remain relaxed.

The examiner places the ipsilateral hand just proximal to the patient's wrist at the volar aspect of the patient's forearm. The examiner's shoulder is positioned directly above the patient's wrist. The patient is now asked to bend the elbow while the examiner offers isometric resistance. The patient must keep the hand relaxed.

In this test, the elbow flexors are tested for strength and pain. The biceps is the most frequently affected muscle, the brachialis is seldom affected, and the brachioradialis is almost never affected.

11.11. Resisted Elbow Extension

There are several ways to perform this test. The initial positions of the examiner and the patient can be identical to the ones described for the resisted flexion (Test 11.10). There is an alternative method, however, that is especially useful when the examiner is shorter than the patient.

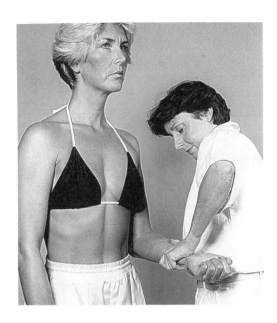

Test 11.10

With the patient's elbow in 90° flexion, the examiner grasps the patient's forearm from the dorsal aspect, just proximal to the wrist. In so doing, the examiner's elbow is positioned perpendicularly underneath the patient's wrist. The contralateral hand stabilizes the patient's elbow.

The patient is now asked to straighten the elbow while the examiner exerts isometric resistance. The patient's hand must remain relaxed.

With this test, the elbow extensors are tested for strength and pain. The most frequently affected muscle is the triceps. The anconeus is rarely affected.

11.12. Resisted Forearm Pronation

The patient holds the elbow in 90° flexion with the forearm in the zero position.

With the ipsilateral hand, the examiner grasps the patient's forearm from the volar aspect, just proximal to the wrist. In so doing the examiner's thenar eminence is placed

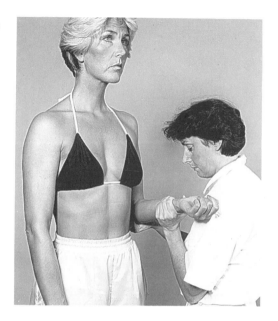

Test 11.11

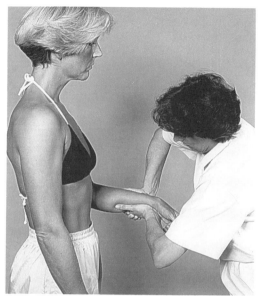

Test 11.12

against the patient's radius. The other hand reinforces the grasp from the dorsal aspect with the thenar eminence placed against the first hand's fingers, and the fingers resting at the dorsum of that hand. Both of the examiner's forearms are in line with each other. The patient is now asked to roll the forearm inward, without moving the upper arm, while the examiner exerts isometric resistance. The patient's hand must remain relaxed.

With this test, the pronators are tested for strength and pain.

The pronator teres is rarely affected. However, if the patient has a golfer's elbow, pronation against resistance is often painful. This is due to two factors. First, the pronator teres has part of its origin at the origin of the wrist flexors. Second, the flexor carpi radialis is also a pronator (against resistance).

If there is a compression neuropathy of the median nerve at the site where it runs in between or through one of the muscle bellies of the pronator teres, repeated pronation

against resistance can also be painful. The pronator quadratus is almost never affected.

11.13. Resisted Forearm Supination

This test is performed in manner similar to that described for Test 11.12. The only difference is that here the examiner grasps the patient's forearm from the dorsal aspect with the contralateral hand. In so doing, the examiner's thenar eminence is placed against the radius. The other hand reinforces the contralateral hand from the volar aspect.

The patient is now asked to roll the forearm outward, without moving the arm. The patient's hand should remain relaxed.

With this test, the supinators are tested for strength and pain.

The supinator muscle is rarely affected. A compression neuropathy of the posterior interosseus nerve can sometimes be painful during resisted supination because contraction of the supinator can compress the nerve.

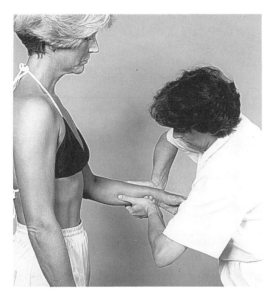

Test 11.13

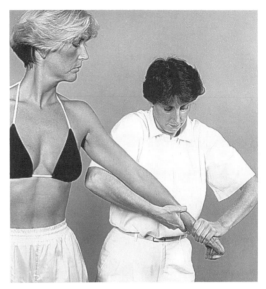

Test 11.14

In most cases, if the test produces pain, a lesion of the biceps (the most forceful supinator) or a tennis elbow can be suspected. In the latter instance, Tests 11.14, 11.15, and possibly 11.17 and 11.18 will also produce pain.

11.14. Resisted Wrist Extension

The examiner places the palm of the ipsilateral hand against the dorsal aspect of the patient's hand. In so doing, the examiner's forearm is positioned perpendicularly over the patient's forearm. The examiner's other arm supports the patient's extended arm, while the hand fixes the patient's forearm just proximal to the wrist.

The patient is now asked to extend the wrist with the fingers flexed and without moving the arm.

In this test, the wrist extensors are tested for strength and pain.

Pain is almost always due to a tennis elbow, a lesion of the extensor carpi radialis longus or brevis (sometimes the extensor digitorum is also affected).

11.15. Resisted Radial Deviation of the Wrist

The examiner's ipsilateral hand grasps the second metacarpal of the patient's hand from the radial aspect. The examiner's forearm is perpendicular to the patient's forearm. With the other hand, the examiner grasps the patient's forearm just proximal to the wrist. Both of the examiner's forearms are more or less in line with each other.

The patient is now asked to move the hand in the direction of the examiner's ipsilateral elbow.

In this test, the radial deviators of the wrist are tested for strength and pain. This test produces pain in a tennis elbow (see also Test 11.14).

11.16. Resisted Ulnar Deviation of the Wrist

The hand positioning for this test is similar to that described for Test 11.15. Here, however, the examiner places the contralateral

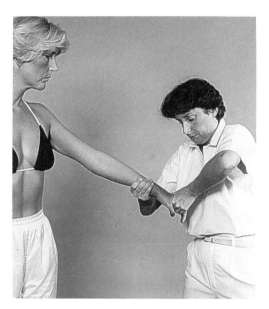

Test 11.15

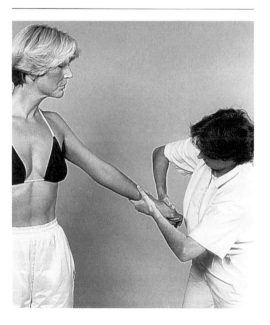

Test 11.16

hand against the ulnar aspect of the patient's fifth metacarpal, while the other hand grasps the patient's forearm from the radial aspect, just proximal to the wrist.

In this test, the ulnar deviators of the wrist are tested for strength and pain. In the elbow region, these are rarely affected.

11.17. Resisted Extension of Fingers Two to Five

The initial position is the same as that described for Test 11.14, except that the examiner now places the fingers against the dorsal aspect of the patient's extended fingers. The patient's elbow is extended, the wrist is in the zero position, and the metacarpophalangeal joints are in 90° flexion.

In this test, the extensor digitorum is tested. This test will often produce pain in a tennis elbow type 2 and will always be painful in a tennis elbow type 5. (In tennis elbow types 1, 3, and 4, this test should never be painful.)

11.18. Resisted Extension of Fingers Two and Three

The initial position for this test is the same as that described for Tests 11.14 and 11.17, but now the examiner offers resistance only to the second and third fingers.

This test is painful in a tennis elbow type 2, or in a combination of types 2 and 5.

The test can be repeated for extension of fingers four and five; if this test also produces pain, a type 5 tennis elbow condition exists. In a type 2, resisted extension of fingers four and five will not produce symptoms.

11.19. Resisted Wrist Flexion

The initial position is the same as that described for Test 11.14, except that here the

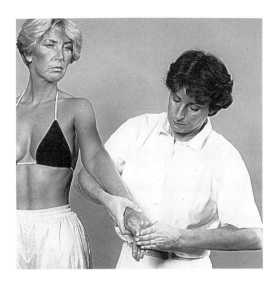

Test 11.17

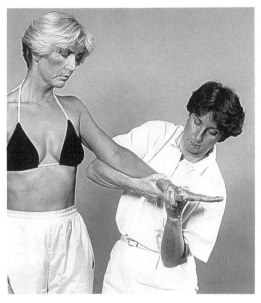

Test 11.19

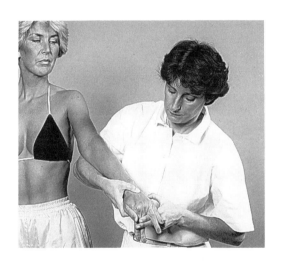

Test 11.18

examiner's ipsilateral hand offers resistance against the palmar aspect of the patient's hand. The patient's thumb should not be involved. The patient holds the fingers extended and is asked to move the hand in the direction of the examiner's ipsilateral elbow without moving the arm.

In this test, the wrist flexors are tested for strength and pain.

If this test produces pain, a golfer's elbow should be suspected. Golfer's elbow is a lesion of the palmar flexors of the wrist at the medial epicondyle of the elbow.

12

Pathology of the Elbow

12.1. ELBOW JOINT PATHOLOGY

PATHOLOGY WITH LIMITED MOTIONS IN A CAPSULAR PATTERN

Arthritis

In every form of arthritis, a capsular pattern of limitation occurs. Before initiating treatment, the cause of the arthritis must be determined. The patient history, functional examination, and laboratory tests generally provide enough information for the examiner to be able to make this diagnosis.

Traumatic Arthritis

Traumatic arthritis is an irritation of the synovial membrane as the result of a trauma. In the elbow joint, a hyperextension trauma is often seen, in which the anterior capsule and anterior part of the ulnar collateral ligament are sprained.

Clinical Findings.
- After a hyperextension trauma, the patient complains of diffuse elbow pain, especially at the medial aspect.
- Passive flexion is more limited than extension (capsular pattern), whereas pronation and supination have full range of motion and are not painful. If pronation and supination are painful, there is a significant chance of an accompanying fracture of the radial head.

- Stability always should be tested, and conventional radiographs should be taken.

Treatment. If there is an uncomplicated traumatic arthritis in adults, an intra-articular injection of a corticosteroid is generally very beneficial. If necessary, a second injection can be administered 1 week later. After each injection, the arm should be kept in a sling for 3 days.

In children, the arm first should be immobilized in a sling for 1 week, followed by gentle active and passive mobilization. An injection should not be given.

Distortion without Instability

Because of a trauma, one or more of the following parts of the capsuloligamentous structures can be injured: (1) ulnar collateral ligament (valgus trauma), (2) anterior capsule, mainly the ulnar part (hyperextension trauma), or (3) radial collateral ligament (varus trauma, rare).

Clinical Findings.
- Diffuse pain in the elbow develops as a result of the traumatic arthritis (see above).
- In the functional examination, a limitation in the capsular pattern is found, as well as pain during the passive valgus test (Test 11.9A), passive elbow exten-

234

sion (Test 11.5), and the passive varus test (Test 11.9B) (see Chapter 11).

Treatment. If there is an uncomplicated traumatic arthritis in adults, an intra-articular injection of a corticosteroid is generally very beneficial. If necessary, a second injection can be administered 1 week later. After each injection, the arm should be kept in a sling for 3 days. As soon as the arthritis symptoms disappear, the patient can carefully resume normal functions.

In children, the arm first should be immobilized in a sling for 1 week, followed by gradual return to normal use. An injection should not be given.

Nontraumatic Arthritis

Almost all existing arthritides can be located at the elbow joint.

Clinical Findings.
- The patient complains of local pain, swelling, and limitation of motion. The limitation is in a capsular pattern; flexion is much more limited than extension.

- Determining the cause of the arthritis is not always easy (Figure 12–1). Sometimes it involves a monarthritis with unknown cause; sometimes it is the manifestation of a systemic disease. In such cases laboratory testing is indicated.

Treatment. Treatment depends entirely on the cause and stage of arthritis. In most cases, the treatment is either medication or an intra-articular injection of a corticosteroid.

Arthrosis (Osteoarthrosis)

Arthrosis of the elbow is usually the result of a previously sustained trauma or severe arthritis. If the cause is traumatic, a badly healed intra-articular fracture or severe instability is often involved.

Repetitive, chronic microtrauma can lead to arthrotic changes. This is especially true in patients such as boxers or those who use jackhammers. In such cases, the disorder often

occurs bilaterally and is generally observed in individuals over age 45 years.

Clinical Findings.
- Except in severe cases, the patient does not usually complain of much pain. Sometimes there is pain after vigorous activities. Traumatic arthritis (activated arthrosis) causes the most complaints. The patient mainly complains of stiffness in the joint in the morning and pain at the end of the day.

- Crepitation and swelling develop in the later stages of this disorder.

- During the functional examination, a classical capsular pattern is found, sometimes with obvious crepitation. The end-feel is "bony" hard, both in extension and in flexion.

- Radiographs confirming the diagnosis will show narrowing of the joint space, sclerosis, osteophytes, and cysts.

- Sometimes loose bodies develop, which can cause sudden locking (internal derangement) and pain in the joint.

Treatment. In most cases, the disorder is not treated. If the symptoms are severe, it is likely the result of overuse.

In severe cases, loose bodies are removed surgically. Cleaning out the joint can be done either arthrotomically or arthroscopically.

PATHOLOGY WITH LIMITED MOTIONS IN A NONCAPSULAR PATTERN

Every limitation of motion that deviates from a limitation in a capsular pattern is called a noncapsular pattern. Disorders causing a limitation in the elbow in a noncapsular pattern occur fairly frequently.

Osteochondrosis Dissecans

Osteochondrosis dissecans is an aseptic necrosis of part of the subchondral bone. The disorder occurs mainly in young people be-

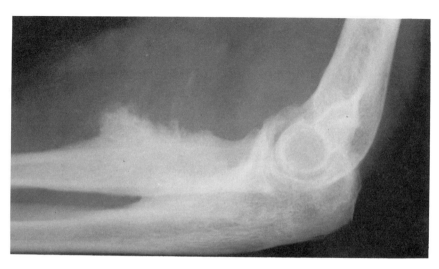

Figure 12–1 Conventional radiograph of the left elbow in a patient with severe limitation of motion in a capsular pattern. The patient is diagnosed with ankylosing spondylitis. On the radiograph, the proximal radius appears to demonstrate a malignant bone tumor. However, this could not be confirmed by pathological anatomical examination.

tween ages 15 and 20 years. It is seen approximately 90% more frequently in men than in women. It is almost always the dominant side that is affected. The most likely sites are the humeral capitulum, the humeral trochlea, and the radial head.

Often the disorder occurs in combination with foci of osteochondrosis dissecans in other joints. Because the disorder occurs more often in young patients engaged in sports featuring throwing motions, it is possible that radial hypercompression of the elbow could be an etiological factor.

Clinical Findings

Three different clinical stages can be discerned:

1. Early Stage.
- There is no pain, but there is recurrent mild joint effusion.
- There is usually a small limitation of motion in extension.

2. Middle Stage.
- The patient complains of activity-related pain and regular locking of the elbow.
- Both flexion and extension are limited.
- Often there is crepitation in the joint.

3. Late Stage.
- The pain is constant, and there are obvious impairments in activities of daily living (ADL).
- During the functional examination, pronation and supination are also limited.

Each clinical stage also reveals characteristic findings on radiography (Figure 12–2).

Treatment

The treatment of choice is usually surgery. In the early stage, the goal is to prevent the formation of a dissecate (a bony island). If a dissecate already exists, refixation (surgical reattachment) is used to prevent it from becoming loose in the joint. Refixation is mainly successful if performed prior to the middle

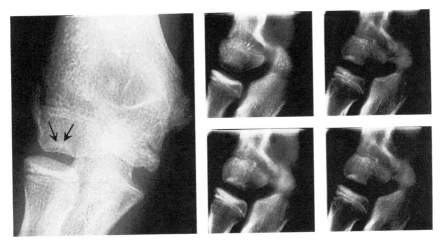

Figure 12–2 Radiograph and tomogram of an osteochondrosis dissecans at the level of the radial aspect of the elbow (***arrows***).

stage (or in the transition period of the early to middle stages). Subchondral retrograde bone drilling is performed to stimulate subchondral vascularization.

In the late stage, loose bodies as well as the accompanying arthrotic changes have to be removed (Figure 12–3).

Panner's Disease

Panner's disease is an aseptic necrosis of the epiphysis. It usually occurs around age 10 years, but can also be seen between ages 4 and 16 years. The disorder occurs almost exclusively in boys.

The etiology is unknown. However, many hypotheses are described in medical literature. They can be summarized as follows:

- constitutional disposition
- mechanical traumatic processes
- vascular disturbances

A combination of the above three factors is the most plausible cause. Although necrosis of the epiphysis can occur at many sites in the elbow, the most frequent site is the humeral capitulum.

Clinical Findings

- Clinical symptoms are usually minimal. In rare cases, activity-induced pain and minimal effusion can be found.
- The most frequent clinical sign is a painless limitation of extension, which leads to the medical consultation.
- The symptoms usually disappear after a period of 3 to 4 months, with functions returning to normal. In rare instances, a minimal limitation of elbow extension remains.
- Radiological examination confirms the diagnosis; the necrosis remains radiologically visible for up to 3 years.
- In some cases, the necrosis of the epiphysis is centered at the radial head or at the humeral trochlea. In these cases, there is generally less pain, less limitation, and less swelling. If the radial head is affected, pronation and supination are usually somewhat limited and slightly painful. At these sites, the healing process also takes only a few months. In rare cases, incongruence of the radiohumeral joint occurs, which later leads to the development of arthrosis.

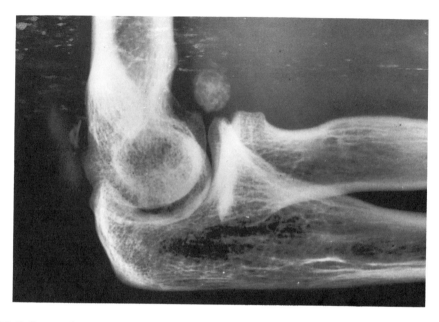

Figure 12–3 Conventional radiograph showing a loose body in the elbow joint, probably the result of an osteochondrosis dissecans.

Treatment

Because the disorder is self-limiting, treatment consists mainly of reassuring the parents and the child. It may be necessary to restrict or stop sports activities for a few months. Throwing activities (valgus stress) have to be avoided, especially when the radial head is involved.

In rare instances, surgical treatment is necessary (generally in older children) to prevent later arthrosis.

Loose Bodies in Adults

Even without the presence of one of the previously discussed disorders, a loose body can sometimes be diagnosed (with or without radiological confirmation). Although there may have been a trauma involved, the cause is usually unknown.

Clinical Findings

- The patient complains of sudden sharp pain in the elbow, mainly during movement. Often the pain is felt at the lateral aspect of the elbow. If this is the case, the examiner should test for a possible tennis elbow.
- Depending on the location of the loose body, extension and flexion can be painful and limited (Figures 12–4 and 12–5). The end-feel is often soft-springy in extension and too hard-springy in flexion.

Treatment

In most cases, manipulation is very effective, especially when extension is limited. If symptoms recur continually, arthroscopy or arthrotomy is indicated.

Synovial Osteochondromatosis

Synovial osteochondromatosis is a chondroid metaplasia of the synovial membrane where bone formation later occurs. As a result, numerous chondral or osteochondral loose bodies can develop (Figure 12–6). The disorder is twice as frequent in men as in

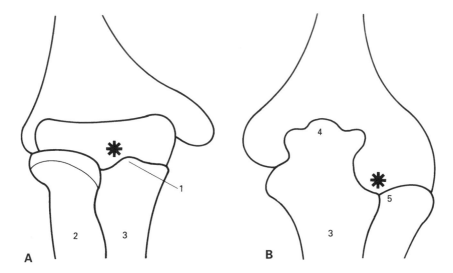

Figure 12–4 Two views of a right elbow. **A**, Anterior, site of a loose body in a flexion limitation; **B**, posterior, site of a loose body in an extension limitation. **1**, Coronoid process; **2**, radius; **3**, ulna; **4**, olecranon; **5**, head of the radius.

women, especially between ages 25 and 50 years.

Clinical Findings

- A painful swelling of the joint develops. Locking of the joint often occurs in either flexion or extension.
- Confirmation of the diagnosis is made through biopsy, computed tomography (CT) scan, or magnetic resonance imaging (MRI).

Treatment

The preferred treatment for synovial osteochondromatosis is surgical removal of the loose bodies or synovectomy.

PATHOLOGY OF THE CAPSULOLIGAMENTOUS COMPLEX

Instability

Of all joint dislocations, dislocations in the elbow have the second highest incidence, af-

ter shoulder dislocations. Despite their frequency, secondary instability is rarely observed in cases of elbow dislocations. When seen, secondary instability is characterized by chronic recurrent subluxation or dislocation of the humeroulnar or the proximal radioulnar joint. It is the result of irreversibly elongated capsuloligamentous structures or, in rare cases, arthropathies such as rheumatoid arthritis.

Analogous to those of the knee, stabilizers of the elbow joint are strongest at the medial aspect. The anterior band of the ulnar collateral ligament plays a particularly important role. This band serves as a stabilizer when hyperextension and valgus forces act on the joint.

The olecranon is not an important structure for maintaining stability. Stability remains intact even after the olecranon has been removed surgically. On the other hand, if the anterior band of the ulnar collateral ligament ruptures, severe instability develops.

The posterior band of the ulnar collateral ligament mainly restrains flexion of the el-

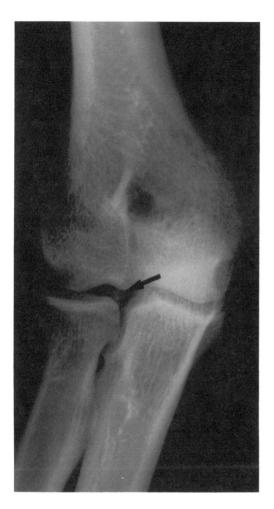

Figure 12–5 Conventional radiograph showing a loose body (**arrow**) in the elbow joint of a 28-year-old tennis instructor. The cause is unknown. In the functional examination, the only finding was a limitation of elbow extension.

bow. It is less important for stability of the joint.

Rupture of the anterior part of the capsuloligamentous structures occurs mainly during movements in which valgus forces act on a relatively extended elbow. Some examples of such movements are throwing (especially javelin throwing), falling on an outstretched hand, or using a sledge hammer.

The first defense against these valgus forces is contraction of the wrist flexors. It is interesting to note, however, that ruptures of the flexors at the level of the medial epicondyle are rarely observed. In adolescents, avulsion fractures of the apophysis of the epicondyles can occur. Sprains of the tendinous insertion of the wrist flexors occur more frequently in adults.

Fractures of the medial humeral epicondyle usually happen in combination with a posterior or posterolateral instability of the elbow. Complications that can develop from this are impingement of the medial epicondyle in the joint and, sometimes, compression of the ulnar nerve.

At the lateral aspect of the elbow, compression fractures can occur as the result of a valgus trauma. This is analogous to the medial compression fractures in the foot as the result of an inversion trauma.

Four main forms of instability are seen: (1) medial, (2) lateral, (3) anterior, and (4) posterior.

Clinical Findings

Medial Instability.

- Medial instabilities have a characteristic patient history. After a trauma, the patient complains of pain at the anterior and medial aspects of the elbow. Sometimes there is also lateral pain as a result of compression.

- Usually a moderate to severe flexion limitation is present, due to the hemarthrosis, along with an obvious extension limitation. If the condition of the patient will tolerate it, the valgus stress test (with minimal force) in 20° flexion demonstrates an abnormal amount of mobility.

- In chronic secondary instability, the patient complains of the sudden onset of fatigue in the arm. Sometimes the patient also has the feeling that something is "shifting" in the joint, or that there is a "snapping" in the joint.

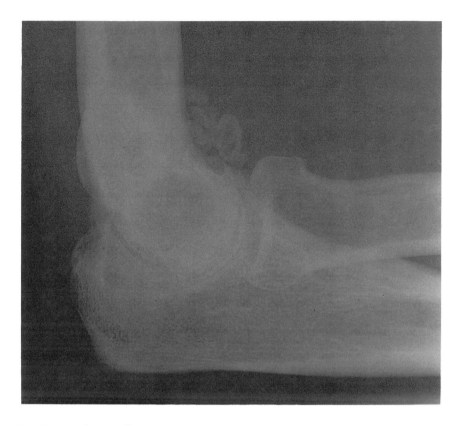

Figure 12–6 Conventional radiograph showing osteochondromatosis of the right elbow in a 54-year-old man. In the functional examination, both flexion and extension were limited by approximately 30°.

- The valgus stress test provokes pain and demonstrates laxity. The excess motion can be confirmed through radiographs.
- If the dislocation still exists, the functional examination is impossible to perform because of pain; however, the abnormal position and form of the joint are obvious.

Lateral Instability.

- Lateral instability occurs as the result of an insufficient lateral collateral ligament and is a rare disorder. In adults, subluxations as well as dislocations of the proximal radioulnar joint can occur. This can result in a tendency to subluxate or dislocate anterolaterally as well as pos-

teriorly. Remarkably, the clinical symptoms are usually minimal. In a subluxation of the radial head, sometimes a snapping is noticed during alternating pronation and supination. If the radial head is dislocated, a severe limitation of flexion of the elbow is observed, and the radial head is palpable within the cubital fossa.

- Dislocation of the radial head in children is a form of lateral instability. Subluxation and dislocation of the radial head in children are usually caused by traction on the forearm. This can occur when a parent swings a child around or pulls on the child's arm, particularly when the motion is unexpected and the arm is relaxed. This generally occurs in children who are younger than 8 years of age. Pain is localized at the radial side of the elbow and often is also felt in the hand (distal radioulnar joint). The child holds the elbow in approximately 90° flexion, the extension is approximately 20° limited, and the end-feel is "rubbery."

Anterior Instability. In very rare instances, a subluxation or dislocation of the radius or ulna occurs in an anterior direction.

Posterior Instability. There are three kinds of posterior instability: posterior, posteromedial, and posterolateral subluxation or dislocation. A chronic instability develops in only 2% of all cases. In over 80% of all cases, posterior dislocations in children and adolescents are the result of a trauma. Most frequently, the posterolateral instability occurs.

The patient with a chronic instability usually avoids maximal elbow extension because of fear of subluxation or dislocation. During the functional examination, the varus stress test in approximately 20° elbow flexion produces symptoms. A medial instability often will be present as well.

Treatment

Surgery almost always has to be performed. However, in cases of a dislocated joint, after radiological examination, an attempt is usually made to reposition the joint first.

Generally, in younger patients with only a posterior instability, immobilization in a cast for 4 to 6 weeks leads to full recovery.

If the instability is minor and the complaints are minimal, specific muscle-strengthening exercises can be performed.

In subluxation or dislocation of the radial head in children, manipulative reduction is usually fairly simple. The physician flexes the patient's elbow to 90°, supporting it with one hand at its posterior aspect. The other hand pushes the radius, via the wrist, in the direction of the elbow while performing a fast, alternating pronation and supination of the forearm. Reduction takes place during maximal supination and is accompanied by a click.

12.2 PATHOLOGY OF THE BURSAE

SUBCUTANEOUS OLECRANON BURSITIS

Inflammation of the subcutaneous olecranon bursitis can be caused by chronic irritation, such as in leaning on the elbows ("student's elbow"), or by rheumatoid arthritis. Also, a blow to the elbow or a fall on the elbow can cause bleeding into the bursa which will, in many cases, result in inflammation of the bursa (Figure 12–7).

Differential Diagnosis

Subcutaneous nodules in rheumatoid arthritis or urate tophi in gout can also be located at the level of the olecranon. Instead of the expected soft palpation of the bursa, hard bumps are felt.

Clinical Findings

After a trauma or when leaning on the elbow, the patient complains of pain at the posterior aspect. Often, there is a palpable thickening. Especially after a trauma, swelling can be apparent at the olecranon.

Treatment

Posttraumatically, the bursa should be aspirated. Usually, the bursa contains hemorrhagic fluid. If the bursa is inflamed as a result

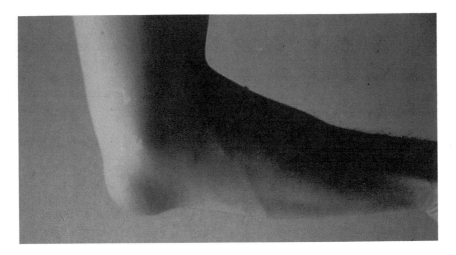

Figure 12–7 Clinical picture of a subcutaneous olecranon bursitis. The patient is a soccer goalie who developed the bursitis from a direct blow to the elbow caused by a fall.

of microtrauma, the aspiration usually shows a clear fluid. After the aspiration, a corticosteroid is injected. Usually, this treatment has to be repeated one or two times.

A rheumatoid bursitis is also aspirated first, and then a corticosteroid is injected. If there is recurrence, the bursa may have to be removed surgically.

12.3   PATHOLOGY OF THE MUSCLE-TENDON UNIT

STRAINS OR OVERUSE OF THE BRACHIALIS

Sprains of the brachialis muscle are rare. Overuse usually occurs from activities such as weight lifting or long distance running when the elbows are held in 90° or more of flexion.

Clinical Findings

- As in lesions of the biceps, the pain is felt at the anterior aspect of the distal part of the arm.
- Unlike lesions of the biceps, resisted supination is not painful.
- Resisted elbow flexion is painful.

Treatment

Through palpation, the exact localization of the lesion is determined; it is usually in the muscle belly of the brachialis, at the level of the musculotendinous junction of the biceps. If possible, the treatment is causal.

In addition, local treatment is administered. In our experience, transverse friction is very beneficial. Usually, after four to six treatments the symptoms have completely disappeared.

It is advisable to restrict the pain-provoking activities as much as possible; however, it is seldom necessary to stop these activities completely.

MYOSITIS OSSIFICANS

In the elbow region, myositis ossificans almost always occurs in the brachialis and is usually the result of a trauma. Bone formation develops in the muscle. In some instances of severe neurological disorders, which are accompanied by paresis or paralysis of the arm, bone formation (ectopic calcification) occurs in the brachialis muscle within a few weeks.

Clinical Findings

- After a trauma the patient experiences pain in the middle third of the arm, at its anterior aspect. A few weeks to 1 month later, a limitation of motion can develop in both flexion and extension.
- In a massive myositis ossificans (visible on a radiograph), the patient can move the elbow only a few degrees in either direction from a position of 90° flexion.
- Flexion against resistance is often weak and painful.

Treatment

There are no therapeutic measures known to be effective in treating myositis ossificans. Sometimes, with varying degrees of success, the calcification is removed surgically. Usually the disorder resolves within approximately 2 years.

LESIONS OF THE BICEPS

Lesions of the tendon of the long head of the biceps are described in Part I, The Shoulder. The muscle can be affected at three sites in the region of the elbow.

Site 1: Muscle Belly. The lesion is a sprain or partial tear, usually at the posterior aspect of the muscle belly.

Site 2: Musculotendinous Junction. The lesion is usually a sprain. This is a rare disorder.

Site 3: Teno-osseus Insertion. Of all of the lesions of the biceps that can manifest themselves at the level of the elbow, the insertion tendopathy has the highest incidence.

Clinical Findings

Regarding Sites 1, 2, and 3.

- Usually the pain is localized at the site of the lesion. However, it is possible for the pain to radiate proximally as well as distally.
- Resisted elbow flexion and resisted forearm supination are painful.

Regarding Site 3.

- If the teno-osseus insertion is affected, the pain is usually severe and there is a fair amount of radiating pain. The diagnosis should differentiate between a biceps lesion and a possible irritation of the bursa (not always present) between the tendon and the radius.
- Resisted elbow flexion and resisted forearm supination are painful. Passive pronation is painful at end-range (with the elbow in 90° flexion). This is because in pronation, the swollen insertion of the tendon at the radial tuberosity is compressed against the ulna. Sometimes passive extension of the elbow is painful because of the stretch on the muscle.

Treatment

Regarding Site 1. In acute cases, injection of a local anesthetic is helpful. If the lesion is more chronic, transverse friction is usually quite effective.

It is wise to restrict the load on the muscle during the treatment period. Without treatment, the lesion can remain for several years.

Regarding Site 2. Transverse friction massage usually provides quick relief of pain.

Regarding Site 3. Injection of a corticosteroid is usually quite effective. This injection is given with the forearm in maximal pronation and the elbow extended. The needle is inserted at the posterior aspect of the elbow (not at the anterior aspect) to avoid puncturing the brachial artery.

After the injection, the patient should keep the arm relatively immobilized in a sling for 3 days. As soon as the functional examination is negative, muscle-strengthening exercises should be initiated.

LESIONS OF THE TRICEPS

Triceps lesions are rare and are usually the result of either a direct trauma or overuse. An often-occurring trauma results from a fall on the hand with the elbow bent. In this situation, fracture of the olecranon (the insertion of the triceps) can occur. Overuse is mainly observed in patients who engage in throwing and racket sports, often as the result of a poor throwing or swinging technique.

Clinical Findings

- The patient complains of pain at the posterior aspect of the elbow, either at or just proximal to the olecranon. There is usually minimal or no referred pain.
- Resisted elbow extension is painful. Passive flexion is sometimes slightly painful.
- If a fracture of the olecranon is involved, resisted extension is markedly weak, and there is a severe limitation of both flexion and extension.

Treatment

In all cases—except of course with a fracture—transverse friction and stretching are very effective forms of treatment. The patient needs to perform the stretching exercises at home on a daily basis. In cases of poor technique in athletes, improving the technique is important. Strengthening exercises should be initiated as soon as the functional examination is negative.

GOLFER'S ELBOW (MEDIAL HUMERAL EPICONDYLITIS)

Golfer's elbow is a tendinitis of the common tendon of the wrist flexors (flexor carpi radialis, flexor carpi ulnaris, and, if present, the palmaris longus) at the medial humeral epicondyle. The pronator teres also has its origin in this area.

This lesion occurs chiefly among athletes who participate in sports requiring throwing activities; however, it is also incurred by individuals whose occupations demand repetitive use of their wrist flexors (such as gardeners, painters, and toolmakers). The lesion also afflicts golfers (very rarely) and racket athletes who use poor techniques.

Golfer's elbow is most frequently located at the teno-osseous insertion or, less often, at the musculotendinous junction of the wrist flexors. The tendon found in between is rarely affected.

Differential Diagnosis

- Traumatic arthritis: Usually pain from a traumatic arthritis of the elbow is initially experienced only at the medial epicondyle.
- Compression neuropathy: At the posterior aspect of the epicondyle, the ulnar nerve can become irritated due to several causes. In a pronator teres syndrome (compression neuropathy of the median nerve), pain is also experienced on resisted forearm pronation.
- There is referred pain from the cervical spine.
- If acute pain occurs in young athletes (15 to 20 years of age) during and after a throw, an avulsion fracture of the medial epicondyle of the humerus is usually present.

Clinical Findings

- The patient complains of pain at the medial aspect of the elbow with almost no referred pain.

- With an extended elbow, resisted flexion of the wrist is painful. Sometimes resisted finger flexion is also painful.
- Resisted pronation can be painful because one head of the pronator teres originates just proximal to the medial epicondyle, and some of its fibers are interwoven with fibers from the common flexor tendon. In addition, against resistance, the flexor carpi radialis assists in pronation.

Treatment

If possible, treatment should be causal. Local treatment also should be administered.

Both the teno-osseous and musculotendinous sites react very well to transverse friction and stretching. Healing of the teno-osseous lesion usually takes longer than healing at the musculotendinous site.

Transverse friction massage should be administered on a daily basis in athletes, and at least three times a week for others. Stretching is performed by the patient, preferably once an hour during the first week of treatment. In the second week, the patient is instructed to stretch every other hour, and from the third week on, four or five times per day.

If transverse friction and stretching are unsuccessful, an injection with a local anesthetic can be administered (at weekly intervals). If results are unsatisfactory after three injections, a corticosteroid can be injected very locally, but only if the teno-osseous site is involved. The arm should be partially immobilized in a sling for 3 or 4 days after the injection of corticosteroid.

TENNIS ELBOW (LATERAL HUMERAL EPICONDYLITIS)

A tennis elbow is a lesion of the wrist extensors at or near their origin, in the region of the lateral epicondyle (Figure 12–8). Numerous suggestions have been made as to the etiology of a "tennis elbow"; however, they remain only postulations. Some researchers attribute the cause to overuse, others to degenerative changes (Figure 12–9). Allander[3] examined 15,000 individuals between ages 34 and 74 years. He found a lower incidence of tennis elbow after age 42 years, leading to the assumption that degenerative changes are not involved.

In the clinic, diverse activities appear to be the cause of this frequently encountered lesion (wringing, screwing, playing tennis, and similar movements). Upon closer analysis, however, all of these activities seem to have something in common: the hand does not have a supportive function during activities; instead it is functioning predominantly to grasp some sort of object.

With this in mind, Snijders[4] analyzed the forces and moments that affect the wrist. He concluded that the force generated in the finger flexors during the grasping of objects forms a moment in relation to the axis of rotation of the wrist, causing the hand to move in a palmar direction around this axis. To prevent this, a moment in an extension direction is necessary. This moment could be supplied by the extensor digitorum, but contraction of the extensor digitorum would interfere with the grasping function of the flexors. Thus, the required extension moment is best generated by the extensors carpi radialis longus and brevis, which attach to the metacarpals.

It is possible that this mechanism plays a role in patients with tennis elbow who also have a limitation of motion at the wrist. Empirically we have found that patients with therapy-resistant tennis elbow respond very well to mobilization of the carpus when limitations in this region have also been found.

In almost every case, the lesion in a tennis elbow is localized at the anterior aspect of the lateral epicondyle, which is the origin of the extensor carpi radialis brevis. The disorder is observed chiefly in homemakers, tennis players, and individuals who frequently extend the wrist during their daily activities. In order to prescribe effective causal treatment, it is

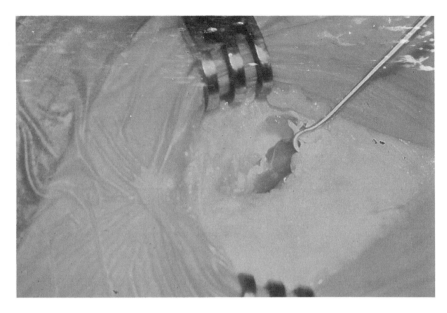

Figure 12–8 This preoperative picture shows a tear of the tendon of the extensor carpi radialis brevis. The patient had tennis elbow complaints that were not alleviated by conservative therapy.

very important to analyze specifically the motion patterns of the patient when engaged in professional or sport activities.

Clinically, tennis elbow is defined by five types (Figure 12–10).

Type 1. Tennis elbow type 1 is a lesion of the muscular origin of the extensor carpi radialis longus, just proximal to the lateral epicondyle. These lesions are rare.

Type 2. Either alone or in combination with type 5, tennis elbow type 2 is the most often occurring type of tennis elbow. It is an insertion tendopathy of the extensor carpi radialis brevis (Figures 12–8 and 12–9).

In a study concerning the effect of phonophoresis and transverse friction massage, only 9 of the 40 patients (23%) had a tennis elbow type 2. Through experience with thousands of course participants, however, we have concluded that the exact location of this lesion is not easy to determine. The affected site of type 2 can be missed completely if the palpation is performed too medially.

The tendon, type 3, and musculotendinous junction, type 4, are tender areas on everyone. These observations make some of the findings questionable.

On histological examination of the affected sites in a tennis elbow, old and new scar tissue is found. The old scar tissue develops as a result of microruptures at the teno-osseous insertion. With repetitive forceful extension of the wrist, small tears of the tendon fibers occur, causing the formation of new scar tissue. Eventually, a large tear can develop.

Type 3. Like type 1, type 3 is a rare type of tennis elbow. Type 3 is a tendinitis of the extensor carpi radialis brevis tendon at the level of the radial head.

Type 4. A sprain of the musculotendinous junction or proximal part of the muscle belly of the extensor carpi radialis brevis is a type 4 tennis elbow. This condition is found only occasionally.

Type 5. Type 5 tennis elbow occurs frequently, but seldom in isolation. It is almost

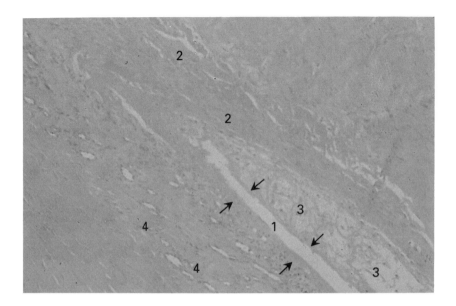

Figure 12–9 Histological view of the tendinous tissue of the extensor carpi radialis brevis at its origin showing significant degenerative changes in a patient with complaints and clinical signs of a tennis elbow type 2. Histologically, there is a tear (***arrows***) in a zone of mucoid degeneration. In addition, a fibrinoid necrosis (**2**) and a mucoid degeneration of the tendon tissue (**3**) can be seen. An inflammatory reaction with proliferation of capillary vessels (**4**) is also present. From a histological point of view there is not only a degeneration but also an inflammation.

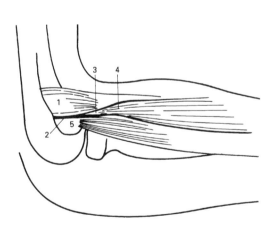

Figure 12–10 The five types of tennis elbow. **1**, Origin of the extensor carpi radialis longus; **2**, origin of the extensor carpi radialis brevis; **3**, tendon of the extensor carpi radialis brevis; **4**, muscle belly/musculotendinous junction of the extensor carpi radialis brevis; **5**, origin of the extensor digitorum.

always seen in conjunction with type 2. In type 5, the origin of the extensor digitorum at the laterodistal aspect of the lateral epicondyle is affected.

Combinations of lesions often occur. The combination of type 2 with type 4 or type 5 is seen frequently.

A tennis elbow, of any type, is mainly seen in patients who are between ages 40 and 60 years. Seldom is a patient younger than 20 years. The incidence of tennis elbow decreases after the age of 42.[3]

Differential Diagnosis

- Contusion of the proximal radioulnar joint, in which mainly passive supination is painful
- Status post distortion of the elbow
- Compression neuropathy of the posterior interosseous nerve
- Loose body

- Referred pain from the cervical spine
- Sprain of the supinator muscle

Clinical Findings

The patient usually complains of pain at the lateral aspect of the elbow in which most of the pain is localized at the lateral epicondyle. The pain can radiate down the dorsal aspect of the forearm to the wrist or the dorsum of the hand. Often, the middle and ring fingers are also painful. In some cases, the pain also radiates up the arm, sometimes even reaching the shoulder. As in other tendopathies, the onset of pain usually has to do with exertion that is characterized by repetitive or forced extension of the wrist combined with squeezing or grasping.

Functional Examination

- Passive extension of the elbow can be painful at end-range because of stretch. Sometimes resisted supination is painful.
- The most painful test is resisted wrist extension, performed with the elbow in extension. (In this position, the extensor tendons are somewhat stretched.) Resisted radial deviation of the wrist is also painful.
- In a type 2 tennis elbow, resisted extension of the second and third fingers is painful. If resisted extension of the fourth and fifth fingers is painful, a type 5 tennis elbow is involved as well.

Treatment

Cause and duration of the lesion determine the appropriate therapy. The most often occurring tennis elbow (type 2) is self-limiting; it recovers without treatment within a period of 8 to 13 months. The rarer types (1, 3, and 4) can remain painful for a much longer period of time—sometimes years—if not treated. Thus intensive treatment should not be administered to a patient whose type 2 tennis elbow has been present for 1 year. The self-limiting

nature of the problem offers recovery soon enough. Reassuring the patient, giving a tennis elbow strap, and teaching stretching exercises are usually sufficient treatments. Of course, for all types of tennis elbow, the sooner the patient is seen for the appropriate treatment, the sooner the patient will recover.

One example of causal therapy is elimination of a carpal limitation of motion. Sometimes the equipment of a person who participates in tennis or other racket sports must be adjusted. For instance, a racket grip that is too large or too small can be the primary cause of the problem; the athlete has to grasp too hard, resulting in not only an overuse of the finger flexors but of the wrist extensors as well.

The tension and the conduction of vibration of the racket can also be significant. If the pain occurs mainly during the backhand stroke in a tennis player, it is wise to switch to a double-handed backhand in order to decrease the load on the wrist extensors.

The eye-to-ball contact also plays a very important role. If the ball is not hit precisely in the middle of the racket, vibrations occur that are conducted to the elbow via the forearm. In this instance, causal therapy could consist of improving the eye-to-ball contact by teaching the tennis player to follow the ball with the eye as long as possible in order to position the racket effectively throughout execution of the stroke.

Type 1. This infrequent type of tennis elbow is curable within a short period of time with the proper exercise program and only a few treatments of transverse friction massage. Of course, to prevent recurrence, steps must be taken to eliminate the causes.

Type 2.

- In addition to eliminating causes, the preferred local treatment is to counteract the pain of scar tissue by stretching. Relief from painful scar tissue can also be obtained using the Mills manipulation, preceded by transverse friction massage for its analgesic effect.

- Stretching exercises are the most effective conservative treatment. Transverse friction massage, as a sole treatment, does not appear to offer permanent results. The patient should perform the stretching exercises each hour throughout the day during the first week. The stretches should last 10 to 60 seconds, depending on pain and muscle splinting. In the second week, the stretching exercise should be performed every other hour, and from the third week on, four or five times per day. Tennis players and other athletes involved in racket sports should perform these exercises before and after playing.

- When the functional examination no longer provokes pain, muscle strengthening is initiated.

- Unfortunately, too often, patients with a tennis elbow have the joint immobilized in a cast. This increases the adaptation of the muscles into a shortened position and causes muscle atrophy—the exact opposite of the goals set in therapy (elongation and hypertrophy of the muscle).

- If stretching and transverse friction massage do not provide sufficient relief (within 3 months), the preferred treatment is injection of a corticosteroid. If an injection also is unsuccessful, surgical tenotomy may be indicated. In this instance, however, careful differential diagnosis should be performed preoperatively to rule out a compression neuropathy of one of the branches of the radial nerve.

Type 3. Regardless of the duration of the symptoms, this lesion reacts very well to transverse friction massage and stretching. Usually four to eight treatments suffice.

Causal therapy to prevent recurrence is important.

Type 4. In the last few years, we have had excellent results in treating type 4 tennis elbow with transverse friction and stretching. In 1978, Cyriax[5] indicated that transverse friction massage was not effective for this type of tennis elbow. We think we understand the reason for his statement: as a result of the palpation technique proposed by Cyriax for this type of tennis elbow (the site of the lesion is compressed between thumb and index finger), the superficial ramus of the radial nerve is compressed. If transverse friction massage is administered in the same way as the palpation, the pain does not resolve. We have developed a transverse friction technique that avoids putting pressure on the radial nerve.

Regardless of the duration of the complaints, results of treatment employing transverse friction massage and stretching are very good. Four to six treatments are sufficient in providing complete relief of the symptoms. Of course, causal treatment is also necessary to prevent recurrence.

Injection of a local anesthetic is always a possible treatment alternative.

Type 5. The treatment for type 5 tennis elbow is the same as that for type 2. In most cases, along with the causal treatment, transverse friction massage and stretching are very effective.

In all types of tennis elbow, a tennis elbow strap can be an effective adjunct to the primary therapy.

Neurological disorders are discussed in Chapter 14, Peripheral Compression Neuropathies in the Elbow Region.

For an overview of the common pathologies of the elbow, refer to Appendix B, Algorithms for the Diagnosis and Treatment of Upper Extremities.

13

Treatment Techniques in Lesions of the Elbow

CUBITAL JOINT ARTHRITIS

Functional Examination

- There is painful limitation of flexion and extension in a capsular pattern; passive flexion is more limited than passive extension, in a ratio of 4:1 or 5:1.

Intra-articular Injection

Intra-articular injection is indicated for traumatic arthritis in adults and for arthritides that are rheumatic in nature (ie, rheumatoid arthritis, ankylosing spondylitis, Reiter's disease, gout, and the like).

Position of the Patient

The patient lies prone with the arm placed alongside the body. The elbow is supported in maximal extension with a small pillow or towel roll. Maximal extension and positioning take into account the capsular pattern of limitation.

Position of the Physician

The physician stands next to the patient's affected side.

Performance

A solution of 1 to 2 mL of triamcinolone acetonide, 10 mg/mL (for a traumatic arthri-

tis), or 1 mL of triamcinolone acetonide, 40 mg/mL (for rheumatic arthritis), and a thin, 2-cm long needle are used for the injection.

The physician palpates the joint space between the radial head and the humerus and follows this until reaching the radial edge of the ulna. The needle is inserted vertically just lateral to this radial edge of the ulna. After the needle passes through the anconeus muscle and the joint capsule, the solution is injected (Figures 13–1A and 13–1B).

Follow-Up

The patient is instructed to immobilize the affected arm partially in a sling for 3 days.

After 1 week, the patient returns for reassessment. Another injection is sometimes necessary at this time. More than two injections are seldom needed to achieve complete relief of pain.

If effective, the injection can be repeated at 4-month (or longer) intervals for patients who cannot obtain relief from medication. In our opinion, there is no danger of steroid arthropathy when this injection is repeated at these intervals over a number of years.

LOOSE BODIES

Functional Examination

- There is flexion and/or extension limitation of motion in a noncapsular pattern.

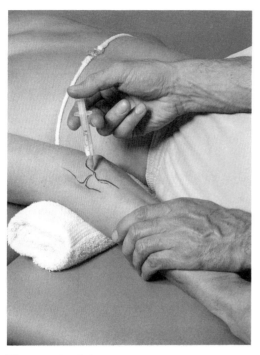

Figure 13–1A Intra-articular injection of the elbow joint.

Manipulation

An extension limitation in the elbow due to the presence of one or more loose bodies can generally be treated with a manipulation (Figure 13–2). This is true regardless of the cause (idiopathic, traumatic, osteochondrosis dissecans, or arthrosis). The benefits of manipulation vary. If the loose body is the result of osteochondrosis dissecans or there are several loose bodies such as found in synovial osteochondromatosis, the benefits of this treatment technique will be only temporary. On the other hand, if the loose body is due to unknown (idiopathic) causes, trauma, or osteoarthritis, the manipulation can give lasting relief. A limitation of motion in extension generally responds very well to the manipulation. Flexion limitations are much more difficult to treat. In these instances, manipulations are seldom successful.

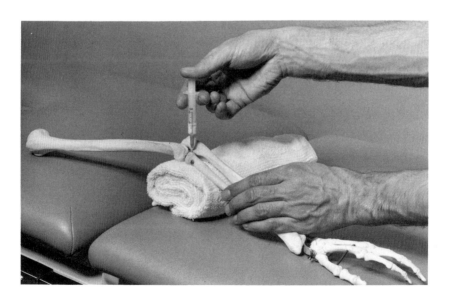

Figure 13–1B Intra-articular injection of the elbow joint in a skeletal model.

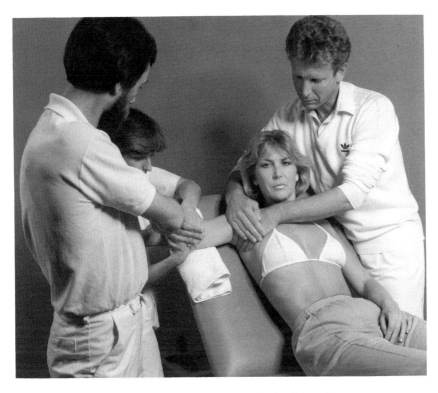

Figure 13–2 Manipulation of an extension-limiting loose body of the elbow.

Position of the Patient

The patient sits against the inclined head of the treatment table with the upper arm in a horizontal position and the elbow over the edge of the table. The elbow is flexed to approximately 80°.

A small hand towel or pillow is placed behind the arm, just proximal to the elbow.

Position of the Therapist

The therapist stands on the patient's affected side. If the right elbow is to be treated, the therapist grasps the distal end of the patient's radius with the right hand (Figures 13–3A and 13–3B). With the other hand, the therapist first checks to make sure that the ulna moves freely in relation to the radius, after which this hand reinforces the grasp of the right hand from the ulnar aspect (Figures 13–3C and 13–3D).

The therapist places the left foot on the floor perpendicularly under the patient's elbow, or slightly forward. This foot is braced against the right foot of the assistant, who is fixing the patient's upper arm (Figure 13–4).

Position of the Assistant

The manipulation is best performed with two assistants. (If there are no assistants available, the patient can also be fixed with belts.) One assistant stands behind the patient, fixes the patient's upper arm against the table, and places the right foot forward to brace the therapist's left foot.

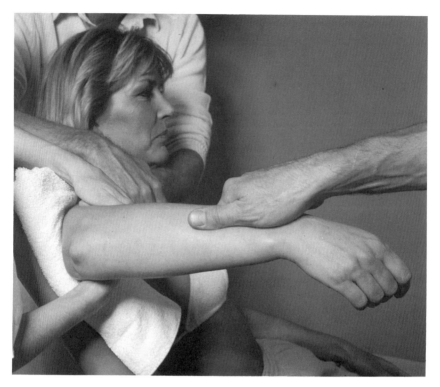

Figure 13–3A Beginning hand positions.

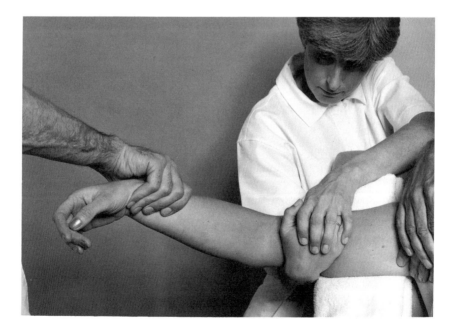

Figure 13–3B One hand grasps the radius.

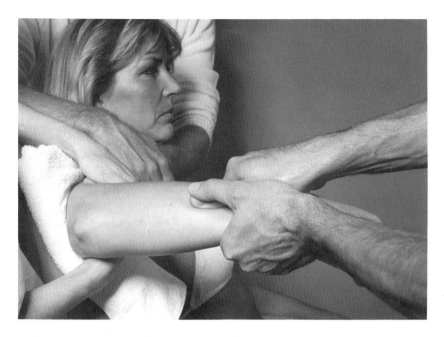

Figure 13–3C The other hand reinforces the grip of the first hand.

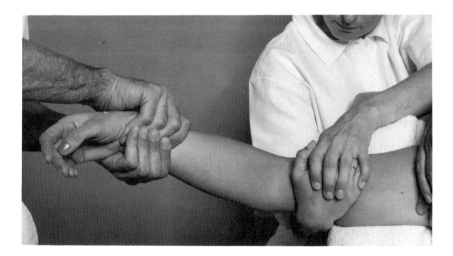

Figure 13–3D Now the forearm is supinated.

The other assistant stands on the patient's nonaffected side and fixes the patient's thorax and shoulder at the affected side.

Performance

The therapist stands on the left leg and lifts the right leg. By slightly shifting the body weight to the right, the therapist exerts traction on the radius.

The traction should not be too forceful, otherwise muscle splinting results. From maximal forearm supination, the therapist (1) *quickly* brings the forearm into maximal pronation (Figure 13–5A), and (2) shifts the

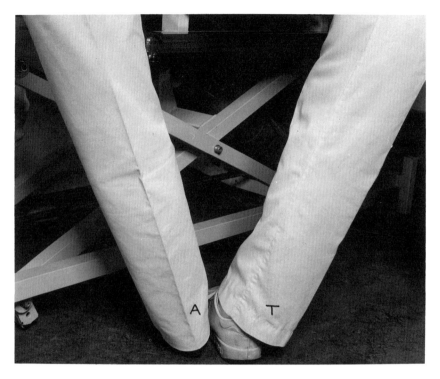

Figure 13–4 The therapist's foot (**T**) braces against the assistant's foot (**A**).

right foot backward in order to (3) bring the elbow further into extension; (4) then, the forearm is *slowly* supinated (Figure 13–5B). This quick pronation and slow supination maneuver is repeated three or four times while moving from the starting position of 80° flexion into extension (always stopping short of the limitation).

At the end of the last pronation movement, the therapist sidebends the trunk away from the patient, exerting an extra traction on the radius (Figure 13–5C).

It is very important to stop before reaching maximal extension (before reaching the patient's limitation of motion). If the elbow is brought into forced extension, traumatic arthritis can occur.

After the manipulation, the elbow is reassessed. If there is improvement in the amount of extension, the manipulation can be re-peated. If there is no improvement in extension, a supination manipulation is performed; starting with the forearm in pronation, a manipulative movement is made into supination. In so doing, the therapist's left hand grasps the patient's radius from the radial aspect while the right hand reinforces the grip from the ulnar aspect (Figure 13–6).

Usually significant improvement is achieved in two to four manipulations. In cases of idiopathic loose bodies, the chance of permanent relief is the greatest.

If there is a loose fragment in an osteochondrosis dissecans, the preferred treatment is surgery. Usually, in synovial osteochondromatosis, the manipulation has only a temporary effect, and surgery is also the treatment of choice. Loose bodies in an arthrotic joint may need to be removed surgically in severe cases.

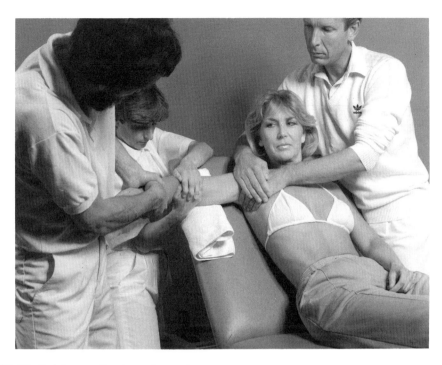

Figure 13–5A Quick pronation is performed.

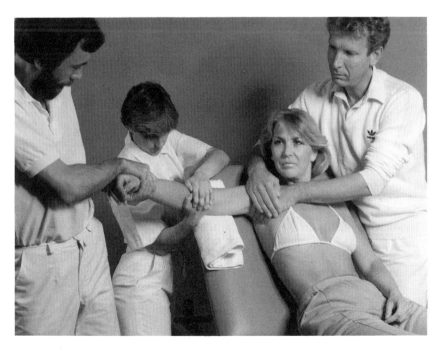

Figure 13–5B The forearm is brought slowly back into supination, and then the forearm is further extended.

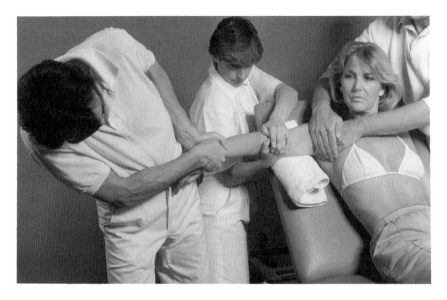

Figure 13–5C The therapist sidebends the trunk, increasing traction on the radius.

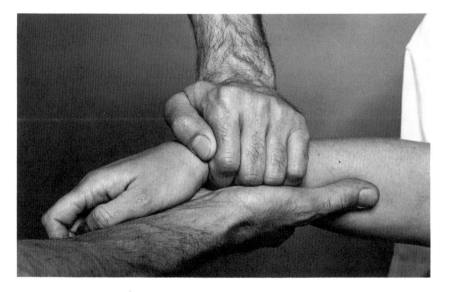

Figure 13–6 Therapist's grip in supination manipulation.

Follow-Up

After approximately 1 week, the patient should be reassessed and manipulated again if necessary.

In many cases, full extension is achieved after the first treatment, but the end-feel remains slightly altered. Usually, the latter improves spontaneously after 1 week.

SUBLUXATION/DISLOCATION OF THE RADIAL HEAD (SUNDAY AFTERNOON ARM)

Reposition

In young children (to about age 8 years), the undeveloped radial head can subluxate or dislocate from its ligamentous sleeve after sudden traction on the forearm or as the result of a trauma.

Position of the Patient

The child sits on the treatment table. Automatically, the child holds the elbow in approximately 90° flexion.

Position of the Physician

The physician stands next to the treatment table at the patient's affected side. With one hand, the physician grasps the 90° flexed elbow and fixes it against the inclined end of the table. The other hand grasps the child's forearm and wrist.

Performance

The hand that grasps the forearm exerts slight pressure in the direction of the elbow and induces quick, but cautious, alternating pronation and supination motions. During this maneuver, the physician can also bring the elbow into slightly more extension.

When a slight click is heard—usually during supination—the radial head is repositioned (Figure 13–7). The function is restored immediately. If the child continues to have complaints several days later, radiographs should be taken in order to rule out or confirm a radial fracture.

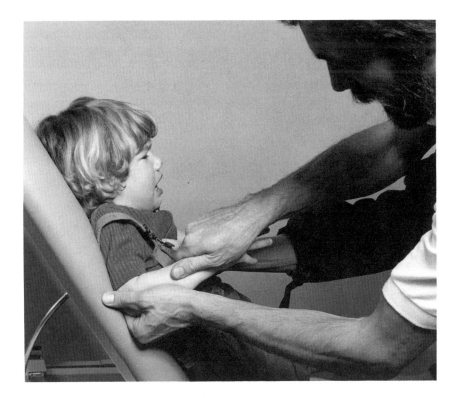

Figure 13–7 Reposition of the radial head.

STRAIN/OVERUSE OF THE BRACHIALIS MUSCLE BELLY

Functional Examination

- Passive elbow extension is sometimes painful (due to stretch of the muscle).
- Resisted elbow flexion is painful.
- Resisted forearm supination is painful.

Transverse Friction

Lesions of the brachialis muscle belly are rare. They are most often seen in long-distance runners and cross-country skiers who have trained inadequately for the long distances.

Position of the Patient

The patient sits next to the short side of the treatment table. The elbow is positioned in 90° flexion and the forearm rests on the table in maximal supination.

Position of the Therapist

The therapist sits next to the long side of the treatment table diagonally facing the patient.

The site of the lesion is localized by palpation. In most cases, the affected site is directly in the middle (between medial and lateral) of the muscle belly, at the level of the biceps musculotendinous junction.

If the right brachialis muscle is being treated, the therapist places the left thumb just lateral to the musculotendinous junction of the biceps. The other hand holds the patient's forearm in maximal supination.

Performance

To reach the site of the lesion, the therapist first pushes the biceps musculotendinous junction as far as possible medially with the thumb (Figure 13–8A). After exerting pressure posteriorly, the therapist performs the transverse friction in a lateral direction by deviating the wrist radially (Figure 13–8B).

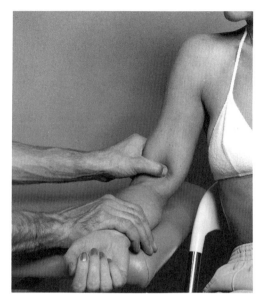

Figure 13–8A Transverse friction of the brachialis muscle, initial position.

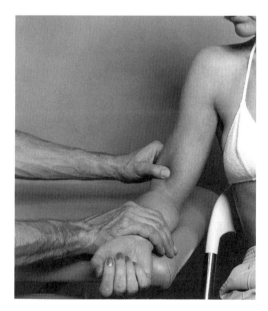

Figure 13–8B End position of the transverse friction of the brachialis muscle.

Duration of Treatment

The transverse friction should be performed for 10 to 15 minutes two to three times per week. Generally, only four to eight treatments of transverse friction are necessary to reach full recovery.

STRAIN/OVERUSE OF THE MUSCLE BELLY/MUSCULOTENDINOUS JUNCTION OF THE BICEPS

Functional Examination

- Passive extension of the elbow can be painful (due to stretch of the muscle).
- Resisted elbow flexion is painful.
- Resisted forearm supination is painful.

Transverse Friction

Lesions of the biceps muscle belly or musculotendinous junction can occur as a result of carrying a heavy object or forceful throwing or smashing activities.

Position of the Patient

The patient sits next to the short side of the treatment table. The elbow is positioned in 90° flexion with the forearm resting in supination on the treatment table.

Position of the Therapist

The therapist sits next to the long side of the treatment table, diagonally facing the patient.

If the right side is to be treated, the therapist localizes the site of the lesion with the right hand. This is done by means of a "pinch grip"; the posterior aspect of the muscle belly is "pinched" between the therapist's thumb and index finger (Figure 13–9).

The other hand fixes the patient's forearm in supination.

Performance

The "active" phase of the transverse friction occurs through a "flat" pinching together of the thumb and index finger with simultaneous extension of the wrist. This pulls the

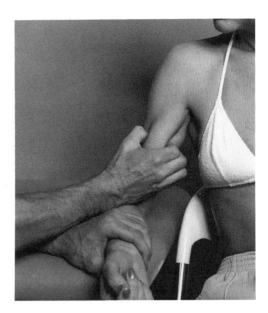

Figure 13–9 Transverse friction of the biceps muscle belly.

muscle belly fibers transversely through the fingers.

Musculotendinous Junction. In principle, transverse friction is performed in the same manner as described above. However, in this instance it may be easier to use the other hand for the transverse friction because of limited space distal to the lesion (Figure 13–10).

Duration of Treatment

Usually only a few sessions of 10 to 15 minutes of transverse friction, performed two or three times a week, are necessary to achieve complete relief of pain. In extremely acute cases, 2 mL of local anesthetic can be injected.

INSERTION TENDOPATHY OF THE BICEPS

Functional Examination

- Passive extension of the elbow can be painful (due to stretch of the muscle).

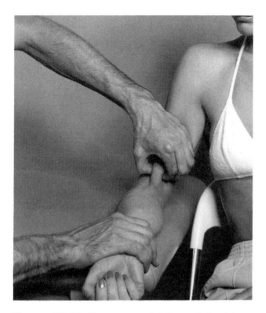

Figure 13–10 Transverse friction of the biceps musculotendinous junction.

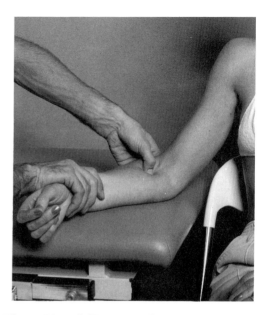

Figure 13–11A Transverse friction of the biceps insertion, initial position.

- Resisted elbow flexion is painful.
- Resisted forearm supination is painful.
- Passive pronation is usually painful (due to compression of the insertion against the ulna).

Transverse Friction

Insertion tendopathies of the biceps are seen relatively often. They are usually caused by chronic overuse.

Position of the Patient

The patient sits next to the short side of the treatment table. The elbow is positioned in 90° flexion with the forearm resting in supination on the treatment table.

Position of the Therapist

The therapist sits next to the long side of the treatment table, diagonally facing the patient.

To localize the biceps insertion at the radial tuberosity, the therapist follows the lateral

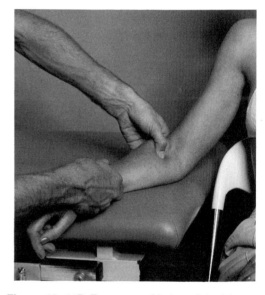

Figure 13–11B Transverse friction of the biceps insertion, end position.

tendon of the biceps distally until it is no longer palpable. If the right side is being treated, the therapist places the tip of the left thumb on the radial tuberosity. The other hand grasps the patient's supinated forearm, just proximal to the wrist (Figure 13–11A).

Performance

With the left thumb, pressure is exerted directly medial to the biceps insertion at the radial tuberosity. While maintaining pressure with the thumb, the other hand pronates the patient's forearm to a point just beyond the middle position (Figure 13–11B). Pressure is then released and the forearm is brought back into supination.

In the treatment of biceps tendopathies, transverse friction can be combined with stretching exercises.

Duration of Treatment

The patient should be seen three to five times per week for 10 to 15 minutes of transverse friction per session. Generally 3 to 6 weeks of treatment are required to gain complete pain relief.

If there is no improvement after six treatments of transverse friction, an injection may be indicated. In elderly patients, the treatment of choice is often an injection. In these cases, the friction can be too much load on the brachial artery, which is difficult to avoid.

If there is no reduction in pain during the transverse friction, the bursa (which lies between the tendon and the radial tuberosity) may be affected. In this case, the preferred treatment is injection. The technique is the same as that described for the tendon insertion.

Stretch

Static stretching of the biceps is combined with transverse friction in the treatment of a biceps insertion tendopathy.

Position of the Patient

The patient sits against the inclined head of the treatment table with the affected side as close as possible to the edge. The shoulder is positioned over the edge of the table.

Position of the Therapist

The therapist stands behind the patient. If the right side is being treated, the therapist grasps the patient's distal forearm with the right hand. The other hand fixes the patient's shoulder against the table.

Performance

With the right hand, the therapist brings the patient's shoulder slowly into extension, in a plane parallel to a line connecting the corocoid with the posterior corner of the acromion, being careful to avoid internally rotating the shoulder. The patient's forearm is then pronated and subsequently the elbow is extended, taking care to avoid pain and muscle splinting (Figure 13–12). By placing a firm object behind the back, the patient can perform this exercise several times per day at home.

Injection

For older patients for whom the transverse friction may be too uncomfortable (due to load on the brachial artery), as well as for patients who had minimal or no improvement with transverse friction, an injection into the biceps insertion is indicated.

Position of the Patient

The patient lies prone with the arm alongside the body. The elbow is positioned in maximal extension with the forearm in maximal pronation.

Position of the Physician

The physician stands next to the patient's affected side. The joint space between the radial head and the humerus is palpated. Approximately 2 to 3 cm distal from the humeroradial joint space, the radius is palpated in an ulnar direction until the edge of the ulna is reached.

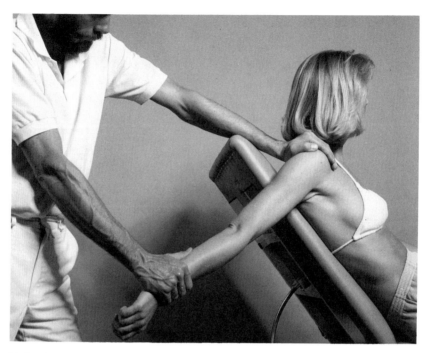

Figure 13–12 Static stretch of the biceps.

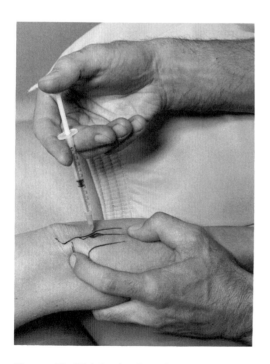

Figure 13–13 Injection into the insertion of the biceps.

Performance

A syringe filled with 0.5 mL of triamcinolone acetonide, 10 mg/mL, and a 3-cm long needle are used for the injection. The needle is inserted vertically until a "tough" moderate resistance is felt and the patient's pain is provoked (Figures 13–13 and 13–14). At that point, one drop of solution is injected. The needle is then withdrawn slightly and redirected to a slightly different spot; a drop of solution is again injected when the patient's pain is provoked. This step is repeated several times until the lesion has been injected in a dropwise fashion, corresponding to the patient's pain.

The advantage to this injection technique with its dorsal approach is that there is no danger of puncturing the brachial, radial, or ulnar arteries.

Follow-Up

The patient is instructed to wear a sling for 3 or 4 days and to limit activities for another 4

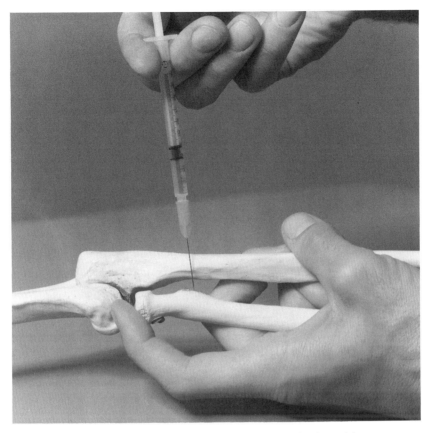

Figure 13–14 Injection into the insertion of the biceps brachii, skeletal model.

days. Activities are slowly increased after 1 week.

In 2 weeks the patient is seen for reassessment. Depending on the functional examination, a second injection may be necessary. The follow-up is the same as that after the first injection. More than three injections are seldom necessary.

SUBTENDINOUS BURSITIS OF THE BICEPS

Functional Examination

- The symptomatology and findings from the functional examination are essentially the same as those seen in an insertion tendopathy of the biceps.

- Resisted elbow flexion with the forearm in a neutral position is painful both in a biceps insertion tendopathy and in a biceps subtendinous bursitis. A bursitis can often be differentiated from an insertion tendopathy in the following manner: The resisted elbow flexion test is repeated two more times, first with the forearm in maximal pronation and then with the forearm in maximal supination.

- If the patient has a *tendinitis*, *both* pronation and supination tests will be painful; if the patient has a *bursitis*, the resisted flexion test with the forearm in pronation will be very painful, but the resisted flexion test with the forearm in supination will provoke minimal symptoms or not be painful at all. (The bursa is no longer compressed between the biceps tendon and the radius when the test is performed in forearm supination.)

Injection

Position of the Patient

See Insertion Tendopathy of the Biceps, Injection.

Position of the Physician

See Insertion Tendopathy of the Biceps, Injection.

Performance

An injection of the bursa is given at almost the same location as for the biceps insertion (see Insertion Tendopathy of the Biceps, Injection). However, usually the needle has to be directed somewhat more proximally.

A localizing sign for the bursa is that the patient experiences pain before any resistance is felt with the needle.

Because of the obstinate character of this bursitis, a solution of cortisone should be administered as a first injection. In cases of doubt, a local anesthetic can be injected first, to confirm the diagnosis.

INSERTION TENDOPATHY OF THE TRICEPS

Functional Examination

- Resisted elbow extension is painful.

Transverse Friction

Transverse friction is indicated for lesions in the musculotendinous junction (rare), the tendon, or the teno-osseous insertion of the triceps.

Position of the Patient

The patient lies prone on the treatment table with the upper arm resting on the table and the forearm hanging over the edge of the table (Figure 13–15).

Position of the Therapist

The therapist sits next to the patient at the patient's affected side.

After the functional examination, the exact site of the lesion is confirmed by palpation. With one hand, the therapist holds the patient's elbow in slightly more than 90° flexion. The thumb of the other hand is placed at the site of the lesion, while the fingers of this hand grasp the patient's forearm (Figure 13–16A).

Performance

The transverse friction is performed by adducting the thumb and simultaneously slightly extending the wrist (Figure 13–16B).

Transverse friction combined with stretching is almost always successful in relieving the patient's pain.

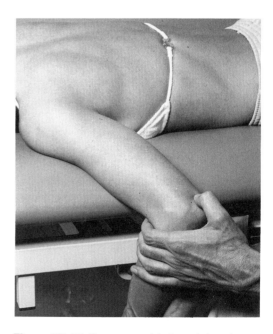

Figure 13–15 Transverse friction of the triceps.

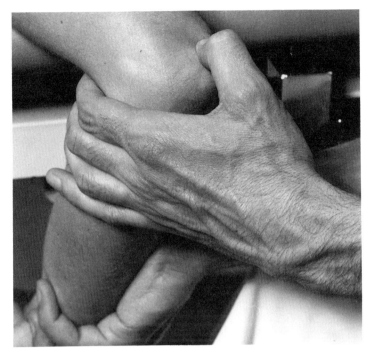

Figure 13–16A Transverse friction of the insertion of the triceps, initial position.

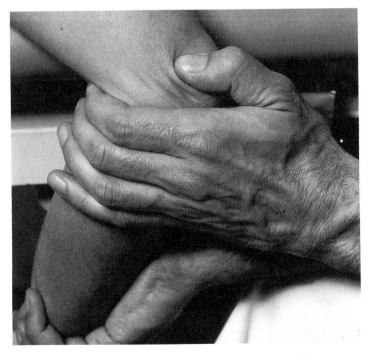

Figure 13–16B Transverse friction of the insertion of the triceps, end position.

Duration of Treatment

Transverse friction should be administered for approximately 15 minutes per treatment. Treatment is given daily for athletes and not less than three times per week for others. Generally, the treatment period lasts 2 to 4 weeks. During this period, pain provoking activities should be avoided.

An injection is indicated only in rare cases, when the transverse friction does not offer satisfactory results.

Stretch

Static stretching of the triceps is combined with the treatment of transverse friction.

Position of the Patient

The patient sits on a chair or stool with the arm in maximal elevation. The elbow is flexed and the forearm is supinated.

Position of the Therapist

The therapist stands at the nonaffected side of the patient.

If the left side is being treated, the therapist uses the left hand to grasp the patient's forearm just proximal to the wrist. The therapist places the right forearm as cranial as possible against the ventral aspect of the patient's thorax; the fingers grasp the spine of the scapula and acromion, and the thumb can be placed against the inside of the upper arm.

Performance

With the right hand, the therapist fixes the patient's scapula as far as possible ventrally. Simultaneously, the thumb pushes the upper arm slightly dorsally. With the left hand, the therapist cautiously and very slowly (taking care to avoid pain and muscle splinting) pulls the patient's entire arm backward and downward and at the same time flexes the elbow (Figure 13–17).

By firmly placing the scapula against a solid surface, such as a wall, the patient can per-

form the exercise at home; this should be done several times per day.

Injection

Injection of the teno-osseous insertion of the triceps is indicated only in the rare instances when transverse friction offers minimal to no results.

Position of the Patient

The patient lies in a prone position. The arm is supported on the table and the forearm hangs over the edge of the table.

Position of the Physician

The physician sits next to the affected side of the patient. The most tender spot on the olecranon is localized through palpation.

Performance

A 2-cm long needle and 0.5 mL of triamcinolone acetonide, 10 mg/mL (local anesthesia is not effective here), is used for the injection. The needle is inserted vertically, and the lesion is infiltrated in a dropwise fashion corresponding to the patient's pain (Figure 13–18).

Follow-Up

The patient is instructed to wear a sling for 3 or 4 days and limit activities as much as possible for the next 4 days. After this, activities can be increased gradually.

Two weeks later the patient is seen for reassessment. A second injection is given if the functional examination still produces pain. Follow-up is the same as that after the first injection. More than two injections are seldom necessary.

GOLFER'S ELBOW (TENDOPATHY OF THE WRIST FLEXORS)

Functional Examination

- Passive elbow extension is sometimes painful (due to stretch of the muscle).

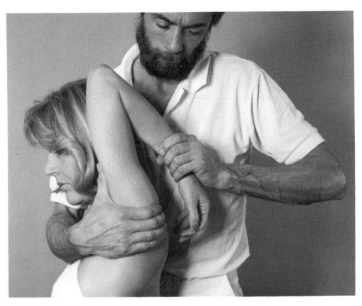

Figure 13–17 Static stretch of the triceps.

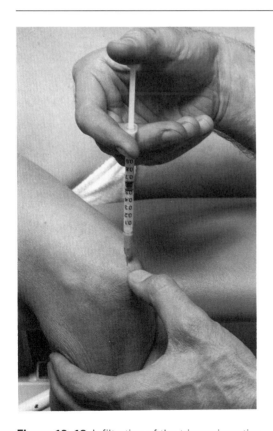

Figure 13–18 Infiltration of the triceps insertion.

- Resisted forearm pronation can be painful.
- Resisted wrist flexion must be painful.

Overuse of the wrist flexors can lead to either an insertion tendopathy at the medial humeral epicondyle or a lesion of the musculotendinous junction.

Transverse Friction Type 1: Insertion Tendopathy at the Medial Humeral Epicondyle

Position of the Patient

The patient sits against the inclined head of the table with the affected arm elevated sideways to just below the horizontal. The elbow is extended and the forearm is supinated.

Position of the Therapist

The therapist sits on a chair or stool next to the patient.

If the right elbow is to be treated, the therapist positions the patient's hand between the upper arm and thorax. The right hand grasps the patient's forearm just distal to the elbow and holds the elbow in extension (Figures 13–19A and 13–19B). To determine the most painful site of the lesion, the tip of the left index finger carefully palpates the anterior plateau of the medial humeral epicondyle.

Performance

The tip of the index finger is reinforced by the tip of the middle finger. In both fingers, all the joints are positioned in slight flexion (Figure 13–20A). During the active phase of the friction, the joint position of the fingers does not change. The friction motion consists of minimal wrist extension and an even smaller amount of adduction of the arm (Figure 13–20B).

Duration of Treatment

Athletes should be seen daily. Other patients should be treated up to three times a week. Each session of transverse friction should last approximately 15 minutes. The treatment of transverse friction is combined with stretching. These stretching exercises also should be performed by the patient several times per day.

Usually 3 to 6 weeks of treatment are required to achieve complete relief of pain. If the results are unsatisfactory after the first six treatments, an injection of a local anesthetic can be performed.

During the treatment period, activities that load the affected muscle group and provoke pain should be avoided.

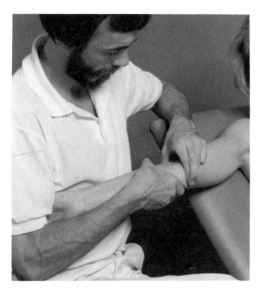

Figure 13–19A Transverse friction of the origin of the wrist flexors.

Transverse Friction Type 2: Lesion of the Musculotendinous Junction

If the musculotendinous junction is being treated, the therapist holds the arm of the patient in slight elbow and wrist flexion. Otherwise the fibers in this region are too taut (Figure 13–21).

Performance

The site of the lesion is found approximately 1 cm distal to the insertion (Figure 13–22A). The musculotendinous junction is 1.5 to 2 cm wide; thus the transverse friction

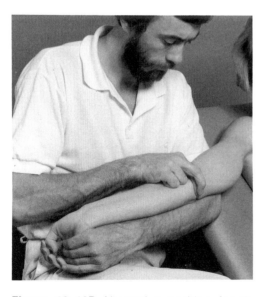

Figure 13–19B Alternative position for the therapist.

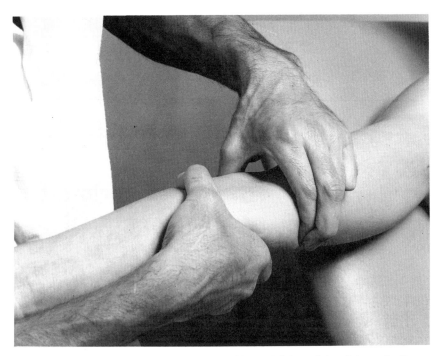

Figure 13–20A The initial position of the transverse friction of the origin of the wrist flexors.

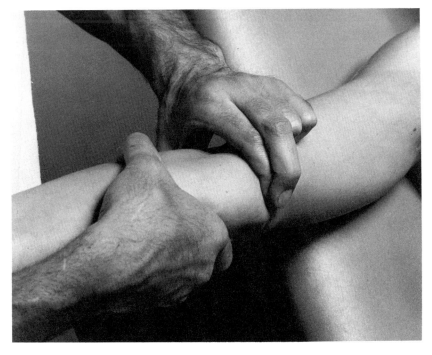

Figure 13–20B The end position of the transverse friction.

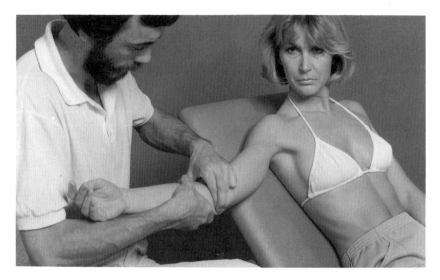

Figure 13–21 Transverse friction of the musculotendinous junction of the wrist flexors.

here has a much longer area of coverage than at the origin. During the active phase, the therapist's wrist makes a larger extension motion. In addition, the arm adduction is greater (Figure 13–22B).

Duration of Treatment

Generally, the musculotendinous junction heals faster than the origin. Usually four to ten treatments are sufficient to resolve the problem.

Here, too, the treatment of transverse friction is combined with stretching exercises.

Stretch

The function of the wrist flexors is flexion of the elbow, pronation of the forearm, and flexion of the wrist. Stretching treatments are effective for both the insertion tendopathy and a lesion of the musculotendinous junction. These treatments are always combined with transverse friction.

Position of the Patient

The patient sits on a chair with the affected arm elevated approximately 80° sideways.

The elbow is slightly flexed, the forearm supinated, and the wrist extended.

Position of the Therapist

The therapist stands behind the patient.

If the right arm is being treated, the therapist uses the right hand to bring the patient's wrist and fingers into as much extension as possible.

With the other hand, the therapist supports the patient's elbow from ulnar. The forearm fixes the patient's shoulder at the anterior aspect, preventing the patient from making compensatory motions (Figure 13–23).

Performance

While holding the wrist in maximal extension, the therapist very slowly extends the patient's elbow. As soon as pain or muscle splinting occurs, the motion is stopped and the elbow is brought slightly back into more flexion. If the pain disappears after a few seconds, the elbow can be brought further into extension.

Self-Stretch

Frequent self-stretching is very important for the patient. The more often the stretch is

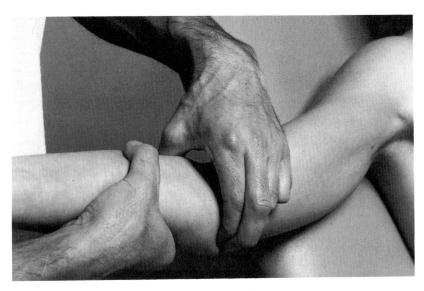

Figure 13–22A Initial position for transverse friction of the musculotendinous junction of the wrist flexors.

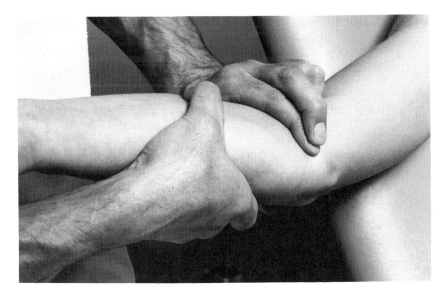

Figure 13–22B The end position for transverse friction.

performed, the better (and faster) the results. The patient should perform the stretching exercise two or three times daily at home, particularly first thing in the morning and before and after sports or other vigorous activities. Athletes should perform a more intensive stretching exercise program with stretching hourly recommended during the first week of treatment, then every 2 hours in the second week of treatment. In the third

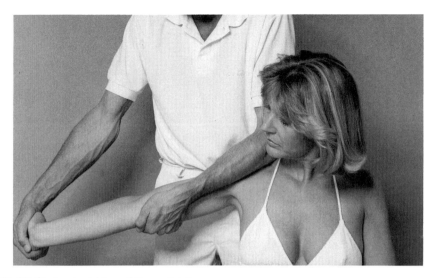

Figure 13–23 Static stretching of the wrist flexors.

week, the athlete should stretch two or three times per day.

Sometimes, patients with a tennis elbow develop a golfer's elbow (and vice versa), generally—but not always—on the same side. Therefore, in cases of golfer's elbow or tennis elbow, the patient must additionally stretch the wrist extensors or flexors on both sides as a preventive measure.

Performance. The patient grasps the fingers of the hand on the side to be stretched. The forearm is supinated and the elbow is flexed (Figure 13–24A). With care to avoid pain and muscle splinting, the elbow is now slowly extended (Figure 13–24B).

Injection

If transverse friction and stretching of the origin of the wrist flexors offer minimal to no improvement, an injection of a local anesthetic is indicated.

Position of the Patient

The patient sits next to the short end of the treatment table. The elbow is positioned in maximal extension with the forearm in maximal supination.

Position of the Physician

The physician sits next to the long side of the treatment table at the ulnar side of the patient's forearm.

With the tip of the thumb, the physician locates the most tender spot of the insertion of the wrist flexors. The tender area should be very small, 4 × 4 mm at most, at the anterior aspect of the medial humeral epicondyle.

Performance

A syringe is filled with 0.5 to 1 mL of local anesthetic. A 2-cm long, thin needle is inserted almost vertically, and the site of the lesion receives the injection in a dropwise fashion (Figure 13–25). As in all injections, a drop of solution is injected only when specific pain is provoked.

Follow-Up

The patient is instructed to limit activities for a few days after the injection.

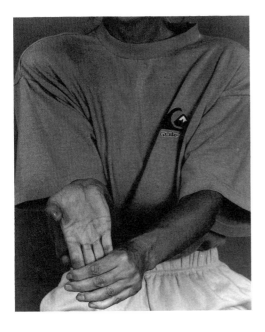

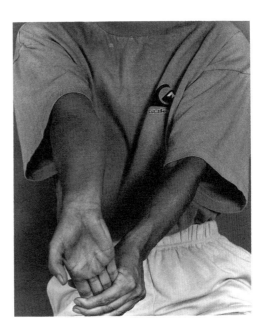

Figure 13–24A Initial position in self-stretching of the wrist flexors.

Figure 13–24B Self-stretching the wrist flexors, end position.

After 1 week, the patient's condition is re-assessed. If there has been improvement, but the patient still has pain, the injection can be repeated. Following these procedures, up to four injections may be given in conjunction with weekly reassessments.

If there is no change in the symptoms, a solution of corticosteroid can be injected. The follow-up after an injection of a corticosteroid consists of wearing a sling for 3 or 4 days and restricting all load on the wrist flexors for the following 4 days. After 1 week, activities can be increased gradually.

Two weeks later the patient is seen again for reassessment. A second injection is given if the functional examination still provokes pain. The follow-up is the same as that after the first injection. More than two injections are seldom necessary to achieve complete relief of pain.

TENNIS ELBOW TYPE 1 (INSERTION TENDOPATHY OF THE EXTENSOR CARPI RADIALIS LONGUS)

Functional Examination

- Passive elbow extension can be painful (due to stretch of the muscle).
- Resisted forearm supination is some-times painful.
- Resisted radial deviation of the hand is painful.
- Resisted wrist extension is the most painful.

Transverse Friction

The insertion of the extensor carpi radialis longus is rarely affected.

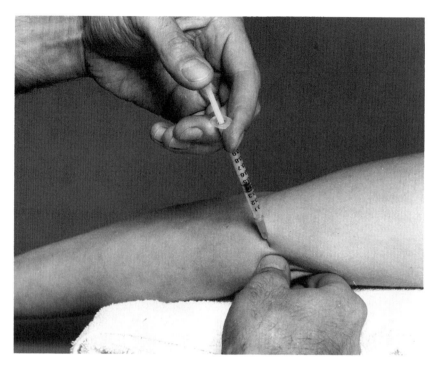

Figure 13–25 Injection of the insertion of the wrist flexors at the medial humeral epicondyle.

Position of the Patient

The patient should sit next to the short end of the treatment table. The arm is positioned in 45° abduction and 90° elbow flexion, with the forearm in supination.

Position of the Therapist

The therapist sits diagonally across from the patient, at the long side of the treatment table.

If the right elbow is being treated, the therapist grasps the patient's forearm just above the wrist with the right hand, fixing the forearm in supination. The tip of the thumb of the other hand is placed against the anterior aspect of the humerus, just proximal to the lateral humeral epicondyle (Figure 13–26A). The therapist's left forearm is in line with the patient's forearm.

Performance

During the active phase of the transverse friction, pressure is exerted posteriorly against the humerus. The transverse friction is performed from distal to proximal by simultaneously adducting the thumb, extending the wrist, slightly supinating the forearm, and slightly adducting the shoulder (Figure 13–26B).

Duration of Treatment

Usually only four to eight treatment sessions, two or three times per week, are necessary to achieve complete recovery. The transverse friction should be applied for 15 minutes each session.

The treatment is always combined with stretching exercises. (Refer to Tennis Elbow Type 2 for a description of the stretching exercise.) Injections are almost never indicated.

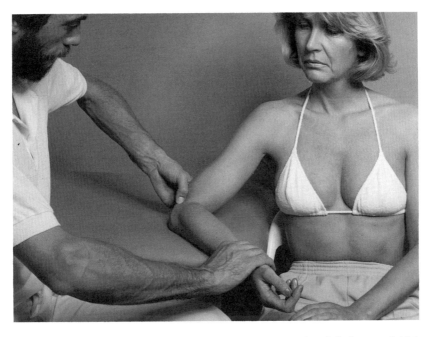

Figure 13–26A Transverse friction of the origin of the extensor carpi radialis longus, initial position.

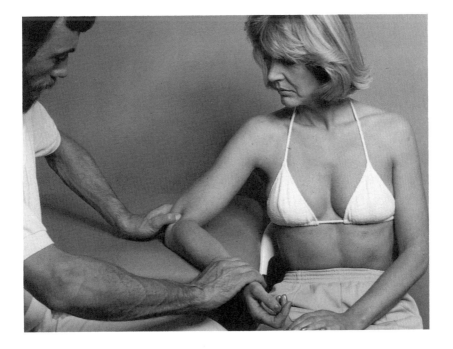

Figure 13–26B Transverse friction, end position.

TENNIS ELBOW TYPE 2 (INSERTION TENDOPATHY OF THE EXTENSOR CARPI RADIALIS BREVIS)

Functional Examination

- Passive elbow extension can be painful (due to stretch of the muscle).
- Resisted forearm supination is sometimes painful.
- Resisted radial deviation of the hand is painful.
- Resisted extension of the second and third fingers can be painful.
- Resisted wrist extension is the most painful test.

Transverse Friction

Type 2 tennis elbow is the most-often occurring type of tennis elbow. Initial approaches to treatment should be directed toward discovering and eliminating causes. For example, tennis players can develop tennis elbow as a result of a poor hitting technique or insufficient eye-to-ball contact (in which the ball does not hit the "sweet spot" of the racket). In these instances, the player has to squeeze the grip of the racket too hard in order to keep the racket from tipping. A grip that is too thick or too thin, or string tension of the racket that is too soft or too hard, can also be a causal factor. Elimination of causes such as these should be the first step in a therapy that may require therapeutic techniques as well.

Transverse friction is a fast-working analgesic therapy. This treatment is indicated in the acute and subacute stages and during the first months of the chronic stage of a tennis elbow. Sometimes, however, relief is only temporary.

Many patients with a tennis elbow have shortened wrist extensors. In this instance, the most important therapeutic measure, besides the causal treatment, is to stretch the wrist and finger extensors.

If the lesion had a *sudden* onset, the arm was immobilized in a cast or a splint for a period of time, or an injection of a corticosteroid was administered previously, transverse friction—as well as any other physical therapeutic treatment and injections—will not be effective.[6]

In most instances, however, this is a self-limited lesion. Therefore, if the lesion has not been injected and the symptoms have been present for longer than 6 months, the patient should be told that, with precautions, the condition should gradually disappear. The patient should be given detailed information about this particular condition along with instruction in a home self-stretching exercise program. During pain-provoking activities, the patient should wear a tennis elbow strap.

Position of the Patient

The patient sits next to the short end of the treatment table. The upper arm is positioned in 45° abduction with the elbow in 90° flexion and the forearm supinated.

Position of the Therapist

The therapist sits diagonally facing the patient, next to the long side of the treatment table.

If the right side is being treated, the therapist uses the tip of the left thumb to palpate the horizontal (in this position) plateau of the lateral humeral epicondyle and locate the most tender site of the lesion. The therapist's forearm is in line with the patient's upper arm.

The other hand fixes the patient's supinated forearm, just proximal to the wrist.

Performance

By flexing the shoulder, the therapist brings the tip of the thumb (as well as the whole hand) approximately 5 mm in a medial direction. If the thumb is moved too far medially, fibers of the extensor carpi radialis longus are reached (Figure 13–27).

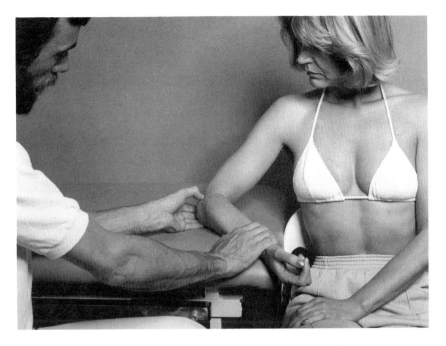

Figure 13–27 Transverse friction of the origin of the extensor carpi radialis brevis.

Note: If even the slightest pressure from the thumb is severely painful, ice first can be applied locally and cautious stretching can be performed.

Duration of Treatment

The patient should be seen three to five times per week for transverse friction and stretching. Transverse friction is performed for 10 to 15 minutes per treatment session. The total number of treatments required to achieve complete relief of pain can vary from only 3 to up to 20.

After the transverse friction, stretching always should be performed, either statically or manipulatively. In addition to the treatment of transverse friction and stretching, classic massage of the entire extensor muscle group is recommended. The treatment can be reinforced by taping or wearing a specific tennis elbow strap.

The patient also should perform stretching exercises two to three times daily at home, particularly first thing in the morning and before and after sports or other vigorous activities. Athletes should perform a more intensive stretching exercise program: stretching hourly is recommended during the first week of treatment, then every 2 hours in the second week of treatment. In the third week, the athlete should stretch two or three times per day.

Significant improvement should be noted after six treatments. If this does not occur, an injection may be indicated.

Stretch

Stretching of the extensor carpi radialis brevis (Figure 13–28) is always combined with stretching of the extensor carpi radialis longus and extensor digitorum, and is indicated in all types of tennis and golfer's elbow. The function of the extensor brevis carpi radialis muscle is flexion of the elbow, supination of the forearm, and extension and radial deviation of the wrist.

Position of the Patient

The patient sits on a stool or chair. The upper arm is held horizontally, with the elbow 90° flexed, the forearm pronated, and the wrist flexed.

Position of the Therapist

The therapist stands behind, or sits next to, the patient.

If the right side is being stretched, the therapist uses the right hand to grasp the patient's right hand. In so doing, the wrist is positioned in maximal flexion and ulnar deviation, with the forearm in maximal pronation (Figure 13–28A). The other hand grasps the upper arm of the patient just proximal to the elbow (Figure 13–28B).

Performance

Without changing the position of the patient's hand and forearm, the elbow is brought very slowly into extension while monitoring the patient's pain or muscle splinting (Figures 13–28C and 13–28D).

Manipulative Stretch

Instead of slowly stretching to maximal extension, the last few degrees to maximal elbow extension can be achieved through a manipulation (Mills' manipulation). This manipulation is indicated only in patients with type 2 tennis elbow. There are two prerequisites for the manipulation: (1) during the functional examination, the elbow joint has full extension with a normal end-feel, and (2) during the stretch, the elbow demonstrates only a slight limitation of motion (which, in this instance, is due to soft tissue adhesions). Transverse friction generally is given before Mills' manipulation is performed.

Performance

When the elbow is almost straight, the therapist bends in the direction of the patient's hand until the therapist's shoulder is directly over the hand at the patient's elbow. By means of an abrupt, short extension movement of the elbow, the therapist maximally extends the patient's elbow (Figure 13–29).

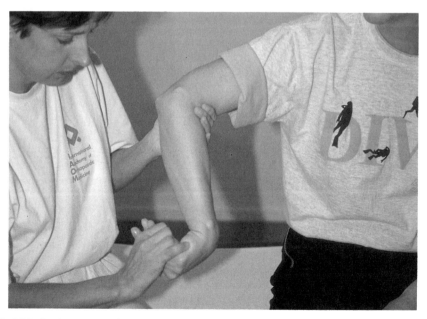

Figure 13–28A Static stretch of the extensor carpi radialis brevis.

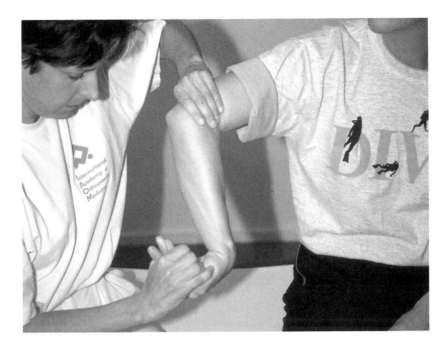

Figure 13–28B Hand positioning in the initial position for stretching of the extensor carpi radialis brevis.

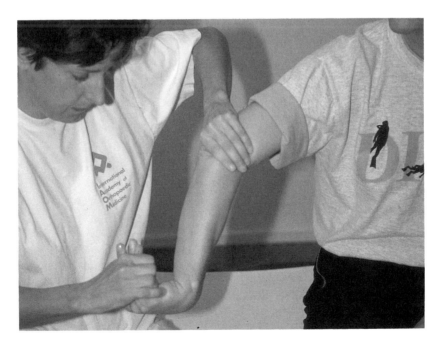

Figure 13–28C Stretching of the extensor carpi radialis brevis; while the position of the patient's hand and forearm remains unchanged, the elbow is slowly extended.

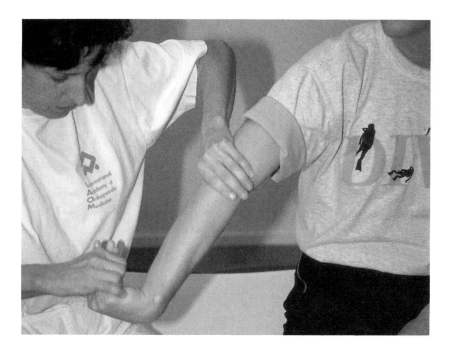

Figure 13–28D Stretching of the extensor carpi radialis brevis. The end position has almost been reached.

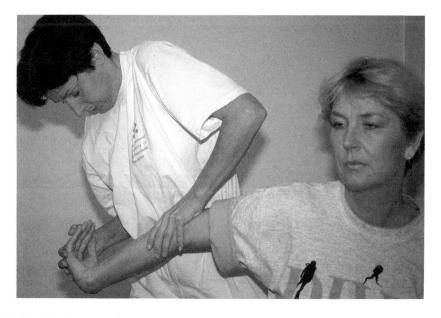

Figure 13–29 Mills' manipulation.

Sometimes a sound like the tearing of cloth is heard. This manipulation is performed only one time per treatment.

Note: If the manipulation is not performed correctly, a traumatic arthritis of the elbow can occur.

Self-Stretch

Stretching exercises for the wrist and finger extensors are always performed bilaterally. This is an important preventive measure, because patients with a tennis elbow often eventually develop a tennis elbow on the nonaffected side. In addition, the wrist flexors also should be stretched: a golfer's elbow is a frequent complication of the tennis elbow.

Performance

Phase 1. With the elbow flexed, the patient brings the arm being stretched into a horizontal position in which the hand is more or less at the level of the sternum. The wrist is flexed, with the little finger and other fingers in the horizontal plane (Figure 13–30A).

Phase 2. With the other hand, the patient grasps the fingers so that the fingertips are just visible (Figure 13–30B).

Phase 3. The patient tries to make the distance between the fingertips and the patient's head as small as possible, without allowing the elbow to bend further. In this way, the wrist is brought into maximal ulnar deviation and flexion, and the forearm is brought into maximal pronation (Figure 13–30C).

Phase 4. Being careful to avoid pain and muscle splinting, the patient slowly straightens the elbow (Figure 13–30D). The stretch should be held for approximately 40 seconds.

Phase 5. Against very slight resistance (performed by the other hand), the arm is then brought back to the original position. Finally, the wrist is extended. This stretching procedure is repeated six times.

After stretching the affected side, the entire procedure is repeated on the nonaffected side.

Injection

If the desired results are not achieved after six treatments of transverse friction and intensive stretching, an injection of corticosteroid is indicated.

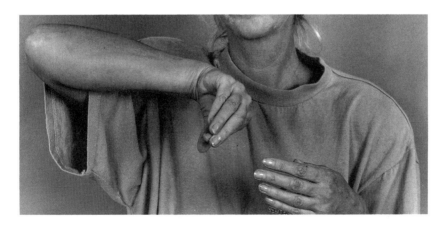

Figure 13–30A The first phase of the stretch.

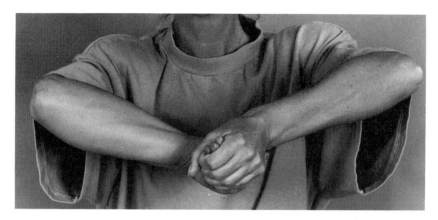

Figure 13–30B The second phase of the stretch.

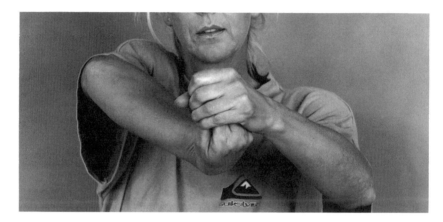

Figure 13–30C The third phase of the stretch.

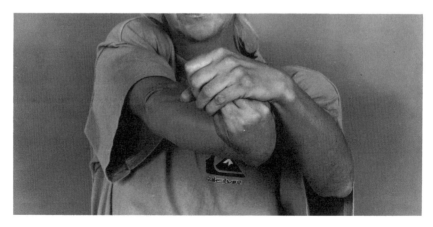

Figure 13–30D The fourth phase of stretching.

This treatment is particularly effective when there is no actual shortening of the wrist and finger flexors. This would apply to patients with a tennis elbow who can hyperextend their arms during the stretching exercise.

Position of the Patient

The patient sits next to the short end of the treatment table.

The upper arm is abducted 45°, the elbow is flexed 90°, and the forearm is positioned in maximal supination. To maintain the position of maximal supination, the patient grasps the forearm of the side being treated with the nonaffected hand.

Position of the Physician

The physician sits diagonally facing the patient, next to the long side of the treatment table.

With the thumb, the horizontal plateau of the lateral humeral epicondyle is palpated and the most tender spot is localized.

Performance

A 2-cm long needle and syringe with 0.5 to 1 mL of triamcinolone acetonide, 10 mg/mL, is used for this injection.

An injection of a local anesthetic provides no therapeutic benefit.

The needle is inserted at an angle of 45° to the horizontal, just over the physician's thumb (Figure 13–31). As soon as the needle is through the subcutaneous tissue, it is brought into a vertical position and the area of the lesion is infiltrated in a dropwise fashion corresponding to the patient's pain.

Follow-Up

As in all injections of a corticosteroid in tendon insertions of the upper extremity, the arm is immobilized in a sling for 3 or 4 days. For the following 3 or 4 days, the arm should be used as little as possible. After 1 week, activities can be increased gradually, and the patient should resume the stretching exercises. The tennis elbow strap is again applied.

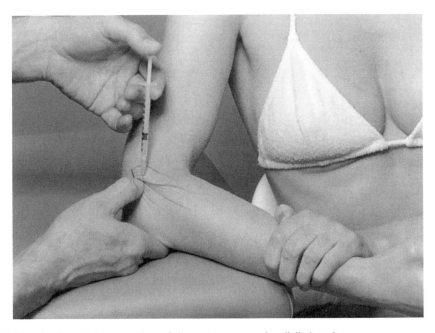

Figure 13–31 Injection of the insertion of the extensor carpi radialis brevis.

After 2 weeks the patient is reassessed. Depending on the functional examination, a second injection may be necessary. The follow-up is the same as that after the first injection. Usually, two to four injections are needed to achieve complete relief of pain during the functional examination.

TENNIS ELBOW TYPE 3 (TENDINITIS OF THE EXTENSOR CARPI RADIALIS BREVIS)

Functional Examination

- Passive elbow extension can be painful (due to stretch of the muscle).
- Resisted forearm supination is sometimes painful.
- Resisted radial deviation of the hand is painful.
- Resisted extension of the second and third fingers can also be painful.
- Resisted wrist extension is the most painful test.

Transverse Friction

Overuse of the tendon of the extensor carpi radialis brevis is seldom seen. In most cases, the origin of this muscle is affected.

Position of the Patient

The patient sits next to the short end of the treatment table. The upper arm is positioned in 45° abduction, with the elbow in approximately 20° flexion and the forearm in pronation.

Position of the Therapist

The therapist sits next to the long side of the treatment table, diagonally facing the patient.

If the right side is being treated, the therapist uses the right hand to grasp the patient's pronated forearm from above, just proximal to the wrist. With the left thumb, the therapist localizes the tendon of the extensor carpi radialis brevis (Figure 13–32A). In the pronated forearm, the extensor carpi radialis brevis tendon runs over the radial head. In most cases, one tendon is felt, which is the common tendon of the extensor carpi radialis brevis and the extensor digitorum. If the thumb is moved quickly over this tendon, slight extension occurs in the metacarpophalangeal joint of the middle or index finger. Sometimes two tendons are palpated; the medial one is the extensor carpi radialis brevis.

Performance

The active phase of the transverse friction massage is performed by moving the thumb from medial to lateral over the tendon. This is achieved by performing radial deviation of the wrist (Figure 13–32B).

Duration of Treatment

The patient should be seen two or three times per week, and the transverse friction treatment should last for approximately 15 minutes each session. Three to four weeks of treatment generally are required to achieve complete relief of pain.

As in the other types of tennis elbow, the patient also should perform stretching exercises several times per day, as described for type 2 tennis elbow.

The use of a tennis elbow strap can help to reinforce the treatment.

TENNIS ELBOW TYPE 4 (STRAIN OF THE MUSCULOTENDINOUS JUNCTION AND/OR PROXIMAL MUSCLE BELLY OF THE EXTENSOR CARPI RADIALIS BREVIS)

Functional Examination

- Passive elbow extension can be painful (due to stretch of the muscle).
- Resisted forearm supination is sometimes painful.

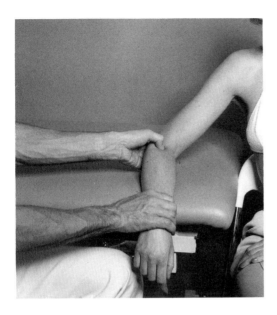

Figure 13–32A Initial position of transverse friction of the tendon of the extensor carpi radialis brevis.

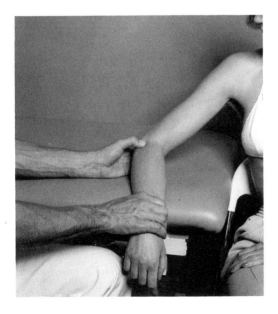

Figure 13–32B End position of the transverse friction.

- Resisted radial deviation of the hand is painful.
- Resisted wrist extension is the most painful test.

Transverse Friction

Type 4 tennis elbow is seen most frequently after types 2 and 5. Sometimes it occurs solitarily; however, most of the time it is seen in combination with either type 2 or type 5.

Position of the Patient

The patient sits next to the short side of the treatment table. The upper arm is abducted 45°, the elbow is flexed 90°, and the forearm is slightly supinated.

Position of the Therapist

The therapist sits next to the long side of the treatment table, diagonally facing the patient. By palpation, the therapist locates the most painful site of the musculotendinous junction or proximal muscle belly. The palpation is performed as follows:

The therapist supports the patient's forearm in supination and holds the elbow in more than 90° flexion. The amount of flexion depends on relaxation of the extensor muscle group as well as the amount of room available for the fingers. The therapist grasps the musculotendinous junction of the extensor carpi radialis brevis from the dorsal aspect by placing the thumb on soft tissue at the level of the neck of the radius and from the ventral aspect by placing the index and middle fingers in the cubital fossa just radial to the biceps tendon.

The therapist then squeezes the thumb and fingers together. By performing radial deviation of the wrist, the musculotendinous junction is pulled transversely between the thumb and fingers. The same procedure is repeated over a distance of approximately 1.5 to 2 cm distally until the most tender site of the musculotendinous junction or proximal muscle belly is localized.

Performance

Because the palpation technique can cause irritation of the radial nerve if performed over a long period of time, a different technique is used in administering the transverse friction massage.

The therapist places the volar aspect of the distal phalanx of either one or both thumbs just radial to the site of the lesion. If one thumb is used, it is reinforced by the other thumb (Figure 13–33). If both thumbs are used, they are placed end to end.

Before performing the actual transverse friction massage, the muscle is first moved ventrally, away from the radial nerve. The therapist then applies pressure toward the radius, and performs the active part of the transverse friction by moving the thumbs from radial to ulnar over the site of the lesion. When performing the transverse friction in this way, there is no danger of irritating the radial nerve.

Duration of Treatment

The transverse friction massage should last for 10 to 15 minutes per session, and treatments should be administered three to five times per week. Generally 1 to 2 weeks of treatment are required to attain complete relief of symptoms. Of course, if this lesion is seen in conjunction with type 2 or type 5, these lesions have to be treated as well.

As in the other types of tennis elbow, the patient should perform stretching exercises several times per day (described under Tennis Elbow Type 2).

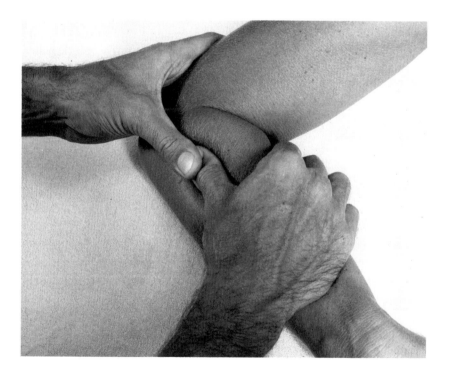

Figure 13–33 Transverse friction of the musculotendinous junction and/or the muscle belly of the extensor carpi radialis brevis.

The use of a tennis elbow strap can help to reinforce the treatment.

Injection

Injection of the musculotendinous junction or proximal muscle belly of the extensor carpi radialis brevis is indicated in the rare instances when transverse friction massage and stretching do not result in pain relief.

Position of the Patient

The patient sits at the short end of the treatment table with the arm abducted 45°, the elbow flexed 90°, and the forearm in maximal supination. The patient maintains the position of maximal supination with the other hand.

Position of the Physician

The physician sits next to the long side of the treatment table, diagonally facing the patient. If the right side is being treated, the physician palpates the musculotendinous junction and proximal part of the muscle belly between the thumb and index finger. The most tender site is located.

Performance

A 5-cm long needle and 2 to 5 mL of local anesthetic are used for this injection. The needle is inserted vertically, and the lesion is infiltrated in a dropwise fashion corresponding to the patient's pain (Figure 13–34).

Immediately after the injection, resisted wrist extension should no longer be painful. If it is still painful, either the injection was not performed in the right spot or the diagnosis was incorrect.

Follow-Up

Activities should be limited for several days, and the patient should be reassessed after 1 week.

Depending on the functional examination, a second injection can be given, again with a local anesthetic. The follow-up is the same as

that described above. Relief of pain and a negative functional examination are usually achieved with two to four injections. The patient should continue wearing a tennis elbow strap. Daily stretching exercises should be performed at home, as described under Tennis Elbow Type 2.

TENNIS ELBOW TYPE 5 (INSERTION TENDOPATHY OF THE EXTENSOR DIGITORUM)

Functional Examination

- Passive elbow extension can be painful (due to stretch of the muscle).
- Resisted forearm supination is sometimes painful.
- Resisted extension of the second and third fingers is painful.
- Resisted extension of the fourth and fifth fingers is also painful.
- Resisted wrist extension is the most painful test.

Transverse Friction

Type 5 tennis elbow is seen most frequently after type 2, usually in combination with types 2 and 4. It is rarely seen as a solitary lesion.

Position of the Patient

The patient sits next to the treatment table. The elbow is almost fully extended, with the forearm in the zero position.

Position of the Therapist

With one hand, the therapist grasps the patient's forearm. The tip of the thumb of the other hand is placed against the distal aspect of the lateral humeral epicondyle (Figure 13–35).

Performance

Pressure is exerted in a proximal direction, maintaining firm contact with the underside

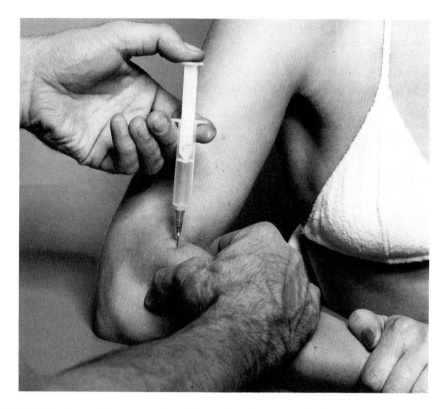

Figure 13–34 Injection of the musculotendinous junction or proximal muscle belly of the extensor carpi radialis brevis.

of the lateral epicondyle. The active phase of the transverse friction massage is performed by moving the thumb from medial to lateral over the insertion.

Duration of Treatment

The transverse friction massage should last for 10 to 15 minutes per session, and treatments should be administered three to five times per week. Generally, 2 to 3 weeks of treatment are required to attain complete relief of symptoms.

Of course, if other types of tennis elbow are present in combination with type 5, they should be treated as well.

As in the other types of tennis elbow, the patient should perform stretching exercises several times per day (described under Tennis Elbow Type 2). The use of a tennis elbow strap can help reinforce the treatment.

If the lesion does not react satisfactorily to the conservative treatment, an injection of corticosteroid, administered very locally and in a dropwise fashion, might be indicated.

TENNIS ELBOW, ALL TYPES

Taping

The easy-to-apply bandage-tape construction procedure can supplement the previously described treatments for the various types of tennis elbow. Taping can be used instead of a prefabricated tennis elbow strap.

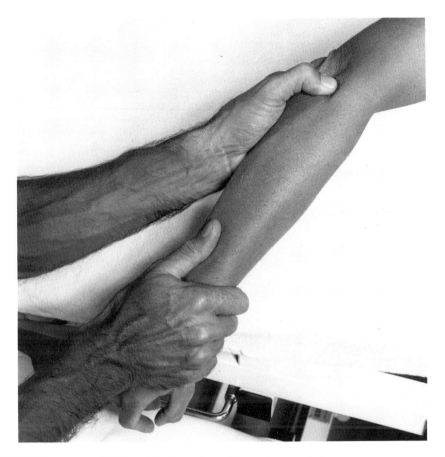

Figure 13–35 Transverse friction of the insertion of the extensor digitorum.

Position of the Patient

The patient either sits or stands and holds the elbow in approximately 100° flexion.

Position of the Therapist

The therapist sits or stands next to the patient.

Performance

If necessary, shave the hair in the area to be taped. Apply a 6- to 8-cm wide adhesive elastic tape to the thickest part of the forearm (Figure 13–36A). Proximally, the tape touches the upper arm. If desired, a small pad for applying additional pressure can be placed between the skin and the tape at the

level of the tendon of the extensor carpi radialis brevis. Finally, a 2- to 3-cm wide adhesive nonelastic tape is wrapped in a circular fashion around the forearm, approximately 1 cm from the proximal edge of the elastic tape (Figure 13–36B).

SUBCUTANEOUS OLECRANON BURSITIS

Functional Examination

- Sometimes both active and passive flexion are painful at the end-range of motion.

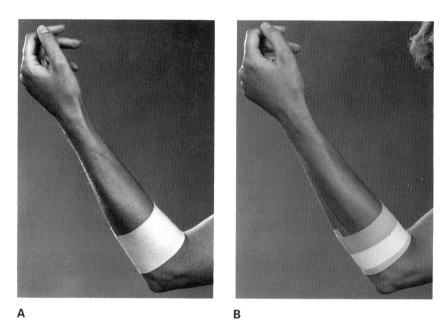

A   **B**

Figure 13–36 Taping for all types of tennis elbow.

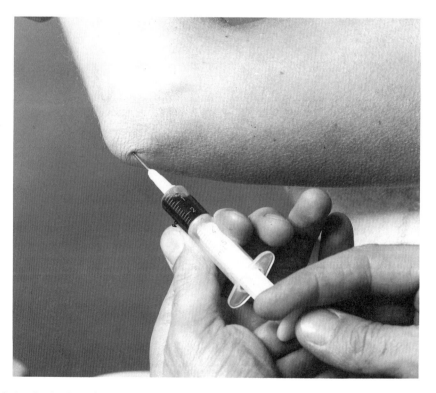

Figure 13–37 Aspiration of a hemorrhagic subcutaneous olecranon bursitis.

Injection

As the result of trauma, an acute hemorrhagic bursitis can occur. Because of repeated irritation (from friction with increased compression), a chronic bursitis can develop (eg, "student's elbow"). In both cases, aspiration followed by injection is indicated.

Position of the Patient

The patient sits with the upper arm positioned in such a way that the proximal part rests on the treatment table and the elbow (with the swollen bursa) lies over the edge of the table. The arm can also be held up by an assistant, whereby the elbow is held in slight flexion.

Position of the Physician

The physician stands or sits next to the affected side of the patient.

Performance

An aspiration needle, as thick as possible, with a 5-mL syringe is used to aspirate the bursa (Figure 13–37). After the aspiration, the same needle can be used to inject 2 mL of corticosteroid. A compression wrap is then placed around the elbow for 1 week.

Follow-Up

During the first week, any possible irritation of the bursa must be avoided. Generally, the desired results can be achieved in two or three injections. Should the bursitis recur, surgery to remove the bursa may be indicated.

14

Peripheral Compression Neuropathies in the Elbow Region

FUNCTIONAL ANATOMY

Although motor deficits do not occur in every compression syndrome of the upper extremity, an overview of the normal innervation of the muscles should be kept on hand. Of course, these innervations are subject to significant variance, particularly distal in the extremity. In various anatomy books, descriptions of branching patterns and topography differ. Even the distribution of the segments is subject to interindividual differences. Therefore, the overview presented in Table 14–1 should be used only as a rough guide.

Regarding sensory innervation, there is even greater variance among individuals. Therefore, the examiner who is making a diagnosis should not hold rigidly to one diagram. Regarding innervation of the hand, however, the following rules generally apply:

- The fifth finger and the ulnar aspect of the fourth finger are supplied entirely by the ulnar nerve.
- The other parts of the fingers are supplied dorsally by the radial nerve and palmarly by the median nerve.

RADIAL NERVE

The radial nerve (C5 to T1) arises from the posterior cord of the brachial plexus. The nerve curves behind the humerus, initially running between the long head and medial head of the triceps and later in a groove covered by the lateral head of the triceps.

On reaching the lateral side of the humerus, it pierces the lateral intermuscular septum from posterior to anterior. After that, the nerve runs at the anterior aspect of the elbow, between the brachialis (medial) and brachioradialis (lateral). At the level of the anterior aspect of the lateral epicondyle, the nerve splits into a deep branch and a superficial branch (Figure 14–1).

Generally, the deep branch (posterior interosseous nerve) first gives motoric branches to the extensor carpi radialis brevis and supinator muscles, and a sensory branch to the region of the lateral epicondyle, before running posteriorly between the fibers of the supinator. The superficial branch usually runs distally, superficial to the extensor carpi radialis brevis and supinator muscles.

Compression of the superficial branch can occur if it runs through the extensor carpi radialis brevis, instead of over it. The most likely site of compression of the deep branch is along the trajectory of the small ramus (recurrent nerve), which innervates the region of the lateral epicondyle. The deep branch as a whole (posterior interosseous nerve) can be compressed as it enters the supinator muscle. Symptoms are based on the innervation patterns.

Just proximal to its bifurcation, the radial nerve is responsible for innervation of the brachioradialis, extensor carpi radialis longus, and the lateral part of the brachialis muscle.

Table 14–1 Normal Innervation of the Muscles

Muscle	Nerve	Neurological Segments
Biceps	Musculocutaneous	C5, C6
Brachialis	Musculocutaneous	C5, C6
	Radial (only lateral)	C7
Triceps	Radial	C6 to C8
Pronator teres	Median	C6, C7
Flexor carpi radialis	Median	C6, C7
Palmaris longus	Median (sometimes ulnar)	C6, C7 (C8)
Flexor carpi ulnaris	Ulnar	C7, C8
Flexor digitorum superficialis	Median	C7 to T1
Flexor digitorum profundus	Ulnar (ulnar part)	C8, T1
	Median (radial part)	C8, T1
Flexor pollicis longus	Median	C8, T1
Pronator quadratus	Median	C8, T1
Brachioradialis	Radial	C5 to C7
Extensor carpi radialis longus	Radial	C6, C7
Extensor carpi radialis brevis	Radial	C7, C8
Extensor digitorum	Radial	C7, C8
Extensor carpi ulnaris	Radial	C7, C8
Anconeus	Radial	C7, C8
Supinator	Radial	C5, C6

Distal to the bifurcation, the deep branch provides sensory innervation to the region of the lateral epicondyle. It provides motoric innervation to the extensor carpi radialis brevis, supinator, extensor digitorum, extensor digiti minimi, extensor carpi ulnaris, extensors pollicis longus and brevis, abductor pollicis longus, and extensor indicis.

The extensor carpi radialis brevis muscle can also be innervated by the superficial branch of the radial nerve. In addition, the superficial branch is mainly responsible for afferent innervation of the back of the hand (ie, the dorsal aspect of the thumb, second and third fingers, and the radial part of the fourth finger).

Compression of the Radial Nerve

Superficial Branch (Sensory)

Functional Anatomy. Compression of the superficial branch of the radial nerve is usually the result of an abnormal trajectory, particularly when it runs through, instead of over, the extensor carpi radialis brevis muscle. Compression may be caused by a fracture with dislocation of the radial head or neck or a subluxation of the radial head (primarily in children). Often, however, compression is caused by overuse or hypertrophy of the wrist extensors.

Differential Diagnosis.
- Tennis elbow (lateral epicondylitis) (In therapy-resistant cases of lateral tennis elbow, always suspect a radial nerve compression syndrome.)
- de Quervain's disease (tenosynovitis of the tendons running through the first extensor tunnel of the wrist, the abductor pollicis longus and extensor pollicis brevis)

Clinical Findings. The patient complains of pain and sensory disturbances (hy-

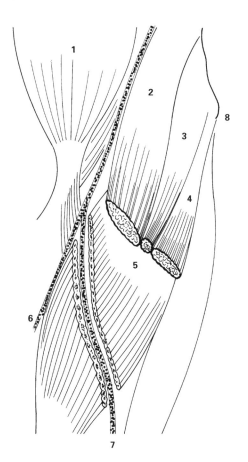

Figure 14–1 Anteroradial aspect of the left elbow. **1**, Biceps brachii muscle; **2**, brachioradialis muscle; **3**, extensor carpi radialis longus muscle; **4**, extensor carpi radialis brevis muscle; **5**, supinator muscle; **6**, radial nerve, superficial branch; **7**, radial nerve, deep branch (posterior interosseous nerve); **8**, lateral humeral epicondyle.

peresthesia, hypoesthesia, anesthesia) at the dorsal aspect of the thumb and the second and third fingers and the radial half of the fourth finger.

Treatment. The patient should be advised to refrain from activities that provoke the symptoms. If necessary, an injection of a corticosteroid can be administered at the site of the compression. The injection must be performed perineurally, and *not* intraneurally. In severe cases, surgery may be indicated.

Deep Branch (Mainly Motoric)

Functional Anatomy. Compression of the posterior interosseous nerve can occur at the site where the nerve runs under the extensor carpi radialis brevis and through the supinator muscle further distally. Sudden resisted supination in combination with extension or radial deviation of the wrist can lead to nerve compression at this site. For example, an incorrectly executed backhand stroke in tennis with maximal contraction of the extensor carpi radialis brevis and supinator muscles may produce this condition.

Differential Diagnosis.
- Tennis elbow (lateral epicondylitis) (In therapy-resistant cases of lateral tennis elbow, always suspect a radial nerve compression syndrome.)

Clinical Findings. The patient usually complains of sharp, localized pain at the lateral humeral epicondyle. This is often the result of compression of a small branch that has split from the deep branch and runs to the lateral epicondyle (recurrent nerve).

Treatment. The patient should be advised to refrain from activities that provoke the symptoms. If necessary, an injection of a corticosteroid can be administered at the site of the compression. The injection must be performed perineurally, and *not* intraneurally. In severe cases, surgery may be indicated.

ULNAR NERVE

The ulnar nerve (C8, T1) arises from the medial cord of the brachial plexus. Often a branch from the seventh cervical root also runs with the ulnar nerve. Initially, the nerve runs distally between the brachial artery and vein. Halfway down the arm, the nerve pierces the intermuscular septum from anterior to posterior, and then runs anterior to the medial head of the triceps toward the cubital tunnel.

At the cubital tunnel, the nerve runs in the epicondylar groove (located at the posterior elbow region) between the medial epicondyle and the olecranon (Figure 14–2). In the area of the cubital tunnel, branches are given off to the elbow joint. Traumatic compression can occur, particularly in the cubital tunnel (cubital tunnel syndrome).

Distal to the site of possible compression, the ulnar nerve supplies sensory innervation to the fifth finger and ulnar half of the fourth finger (palmar aspect as well as dorsal aspect). The ulnar nerve provides motoric branches to the flexor carpi ulnaris muscle, ulnar part of the flexor digitorum profundus muscle, muscles of the hypothenar eminence,

palmaris brevis and (sometimes) longus muscles, interosseous muscles, lumbrical muscles III and IV, flexor pollicis brevis muscle (see also Median Nerve), and adductor pollicis muscle.

The ulnar nerve enters the forearm region from between the two heads of the flexor carpi ulnaris. Distal to the elbow, the ulnar nerve runs on the medial side of the forearm, anterior to the flexor digitorum profundus. In the proximal half of the forearm, the nerve is covered by the flexor carpi ulnaris; in the distal half of the forearm, it lies radial to this muscle. In the forearm, the ulnar nerve gives off a number of branches that are responsible for sensory innervation of the ulnar aspect of the midhand region and particularly the dorsal aspect of the fifth finger and the ulnar half of the fourth finger.

In the carpal region, the ulnar nerve runs through a space called Guyon's tunnel (Figure 14–3). The tunnel is bordered by the pisiform at its proximoulnar edge and by the hook of the hamate bone at its distoradial edge. The floor and roof of the tunnel are formed by the deep ulnar and superficial ulnar layers of the flexor retinaculum (see also Median Nerve).

Note: The ulnar nerve does *not* run through the carpal tunnel, where the roof is formed by the flexor retinaculum proper. The ulnar nerve *is* covered by the superficial layer of the flexor retinaculum, however.

At the level of the carpus, the ulnar nerve splits into a deep motor ramus and a (mainly) superficial sensory ramus. The superficial ramus runs distally, radial to the pisiform; it sends motor branches to the palmaris brevis and sensory branches to the palmar aspect of the entire little finger and the ulnar aspect of the fourth finger.

The deep motor ramus of the ulnar nerve runs further distally between the abductor and flexor digiti minimi muscles, before piercing the opponens digiti minimi. It is this branch that is mainly responsible for the motoric innervation of the hypothenar eminence

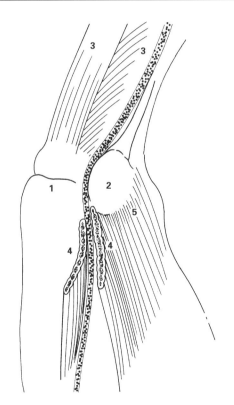

Figure 14–2 Cubital tunnel of the left elbow. **1**, Olecranon **2**, medial humeral epicondyle **3**, triceps brachii muscle; **4**, flexor carpi ulnaris muscle; **5**, flexor carpi radialis and palmaris longus muscles.

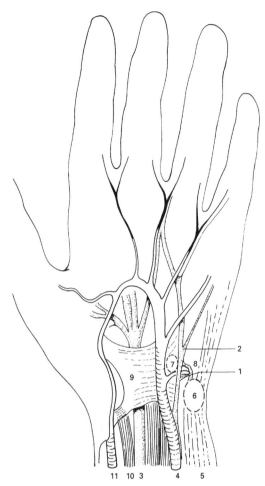

Figure 14–3 Volar aspect of the left hand. **1**, Ulnar nerve, deep ramus; **2**, ulnar nerve, superficial ramus; **3**, median nerve; **4**, ulnar artery; **5**, flexor carpi ulnaris muscle; **6**, pisiform; **7**, hook of the hamate; **8**, Guyon's tunnel; **9**, flexor retinaculum; **10**, tendon of the flexor carpi radialis muscle; **11**, radial artery.

muscles, the interossei, lumbricals III and IV, adductor pollicis, and flexor pollicis brevis.

Compression of the ulnar nerve in the wrist region (distal compression of the ulnar nerve) can occur at three sites: (1) proximally against the pisiform, (2) distally against the pisiform, or (3) against the hook of the hamate bone. In principle, compression in Guyon's tunnel is also possible; precise diagnostic differentiation is difficult to determine and is of little clinical importance.

Compression can occur as the result of a trauma or a teno-osseous tendinitis of the flexor carpi ulnaris. This is particularly true when the site of compression is proximally against the pisiform.

The sensory terminal branches of the superficial ulnar nerve, which innervate the palmar aspect of the little finger and the ulnar part of the fourth finger, run in the area of the fingers through so-called metacarpal tunnels (Figure 14–4). The metacarpal tunnels are passages between the deep and superficial transverse metacarpal ligaments, located between the heads of the metacarpal bones. The sensory terminal branches of the median nerve, which innervate the palmar aspects of the rest of the fingers, also run through these tunnels. The distribution of branches from the ulnar and median nerves is subject to variation. Usually these branches are called the common palmar digital nerves. Each common palmar digital nerve can become compressed in a metacarpal tunnel as a result of trauma or a space-occupying lesion.

Cubital Tunnel Syndrome

Functional Anatomy

In the cubital tunnel syndrome, compression of the ulnar nerve (C7-T1) occurs directly posterior to the medial humeral epicondyle in the epicondylar groove. The cause can be a direct trauma or repeated microtrauma. Such would be the case in an individual with cubitus valgus (sometimes even years after a fracture); the nerve is stretched again and again every time the elbow is extended.

Subluxation of the nerve from the groove can also lead to a neuropathy. In this instance, there is no compression. Each time the elbow flexes, the nerve subluxes. During elbow extension the nerve reduces again.

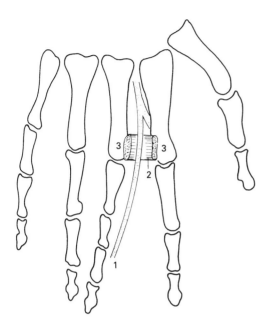

Figure 14–4 Metacarpal tunnel. **1**, Common palmar digital nerve; **2**, deep transverse metacarpal ligament; **3**, superficial transverse metacarpal ligament (cut).

Clinical Findings

- The patient often complains of burning pain in the fifth finger and the ulnar half of the fourth finger. First there is hyperesthesia, which then progresses to anesthesia.

- Initially, motor deficit of the interossei, the flexor pollicis brevis, and the adductor pollicis is evident, along with atrophy. Later, motor deficit is also noted in the ulnar part of the flexor digitorum profundus and the entire flexor carpi radialis.

Treatment

Conservative therapy generally provides minimal to no improvement. Surgical transfer of the nerve, anteriorly, is the recommended treatment.

MEDIAN NERVE

The median nerve (C5 to T1) arises from the lateral and medial cords of the brachial plexus. Initially, the nerve runs distally, lateral to the brachial artery. At the level of the insertion of the coracobrachialis the nerve crosses over the brachial artery and continues running medially along the brachial artery further distally to the cubital fossa. In the cubital fossa, the median nerve lies posterior to the bicipital aponeurosis and anterior to the brachial artery (Figure 14–5).

Particularly in hypertrophy of the pronator teres, compression of the median nerve can occur (pronator teres syndrome).

Proximal to the site of possible compression, the median nerve innervates the brachial artery (vasomotor). From the region of the cubital fossa, the nerve sends one branch to the pronator teres. At the level of the elbow joint, branches innervate the cubital articulation, including the proximal radioulnar joint.

Distal to the site of possible nerve compression, motor branches from the median nerve innervate the flexor carpi radialis, palmaris longus (see also Ulnar Nerve), flexor digitorum superficialis, flexor digitorum profundus (the radial part), flexor pollicis longus, pronator quadratus, abductor pollicis brevis, opponens pollicis, flexor pollicis brevis (see also Ulnar Nerve), and lumbricals I and II.

Sensory branches supply the joints of the carpus, and particularly the palmar skin of the thumb to the radial side of the fourth finger.

After the median nerve enters the forearm through the two heads of the pronator teres, it runs distally under the collagenous bridge between both heads of the flexor digitorum superficialis. The nerve then lies superficial to the flexor digitorum profundus. Approximately 5 cm proximal to the wrist, the nerve comes out from under the flexor digitorum superficialis and continues on into the palm through the carpal tunnel.

The carpal tunnel is formed by the flexor retinaculum proper, which spans the concave

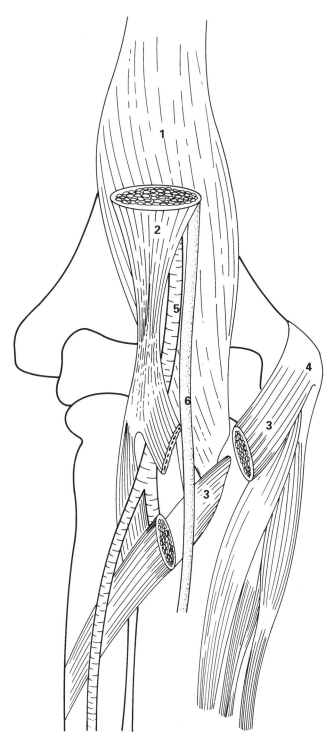

Figure 14–5 Anterior aspect of the elbow. **1**, Brachialis muscle; **2**, biceps brachii muscle; **3**, pronator teres muscle; **4**, origin of the wrist flexors; **5**, brachial artery; **6**, median nerve.

carpus. The tendons of the flexor pollicis longus and flexors digitorum superficialis and profundus run together with the median nerve through the carpal tunnel. At the level of the tunnel, the median nerve lies between the tendons of the flexor digitorum superficialis and the tendon of the flexor pollicis longus.

There are several causes of compression in the carpal tunnel. It can occur as a result of a trauma, such as after a Colles fracture, fracture of the scaphoid, or dislocation of the lunate. It may also be caused by a space-occupying lesion, such as a tumor, ganglion, tophi occurring in gout, tenosynovitis of the flexor digitorum profundus, or rheumatoid arthritis. In all of these instances, the symptoms are primarily caused by compression of the median nerve.

Distal to the carpal tunnel, the median nerve innervates the abductor pollicis brevis, opponens pollicis, flexor pollicis brevis (see also Ulnar Nerve), and lumbricals I and II. In addition, the distal branches of the median nerve play an important vasomotor role in the hand. The distal median nerve also contains afferent fibers from the palmar skin of the thumb and the second and third fingers as well as the radial aspect of the fourth finger.

Pronator Teres Syndrome

Functional Anatomy

The median nerve can become compressed between the two heads of the pronator teres muscle. Possible causes are as follows:

- structural hypertrophy or sudden forceful or repeated contraction of the pronator teres
- tendonlike bands in the pronator teres
- direct trauma (rare)
- tumors (extremely rare)

Clinical Findings

- The patient complains of pain along the trajectory of the median nerve distal to the elbow. There is tenderness to palpation at the biceps aponeurosis. Sometimes the palmar aspects of the thumb and index finger feel numb.
- Often, the pain can be provoked by repeated pronation against resistance.

Treatment

The patient should be advised to refrain from activities that provoke the symptoms. If necessary, an injection of a corticosteroid can be administered at the site of the compression. In cases of recurrence, surgery may be indicated.

PART II—ELBOW REVIEW QUESTIONS

1. Which structure stops extension of the elbow?

2. Name the predilection sites for a golfer's elbow.

3. During which age span does osteochondrosis dissecans present itself and during which age span does Panner's disease present itself?

4. What is the main difference in treatment between osteochondrosis dissecans and Panner's disease?

5. Name the two most common forms of elbow instability.

6. Name three complications of a medial instability.

7. Name three lesions of the elbow whereby a loose body can occur.

8. Describe the maximal loose-packed position of the humeroulnar joint and the humeroradial joint.

9. Describe the maximal close-packed position of the humeroulnar joint and the humeroradial joint.

10. Describe the function of the extensor carpi radialis brevis muscle.

11. With golfer's elbow, why is resisted pronation of the forearm painful?

12. Name the five predilection sites of a tennis elbow.

13. Name the nerve and the site of compression in a pronator teres syndrome and in a cubital tunnel syndrome.

14. Why is painful passive pronation of the forearm a localizing sign for a lesion of the biceps brachii muscle insertion?

15. Which lesion at the medial side of the elbow can occur in young throwers?

16. What is the treatment of choice for a traumatic arthritis of the elbow (when there are no associated injuries)?

17. In the elbow region, which muscle is usually affected with myositis ossificans?

18. Which bursitis is most commonly seen in the elbow area?

19. In which position is the interosseous membrane most taut?

20. Which type of tennis elbow is most common?

21. Where are the sites of predilection for osteochondrosis dissecans in the elbow?

22. What treatment is indicated for a radial head dislocation in children?

23. In which sports is overuse of the brachialis muscle most frequently seen?

24. Which muscles pronate the forearm?

25. Which muscles supinate the forearm?

26. What kind of joint is the proximal radioulnar joint?

27. What kind of trauma can result in a lesion of the triceps brachii muscle? Name a possible complication.

28. List some important differential diagnosis possibilities for a tennis elbow.

29. What kind of joint is the humeroulnar joint?

30. Describe the maximal loose-packed position and the maximal close-packed position of the proximal radioulnar joint.

PART II—ELBOW REVIEW ANSWERS

1. The capsular ulnar (medial) collateral ligament, anterior part.

2. The musculotendinous junction and the insertion of the wrist flexors at the medial humeral epicondyle.

3. Osteochondrosis dissecans: 15 to 20 years of age; Panner's disease: average, 10 years of age.

4. Osteochondrosis dissecans: surgery; Panner's disease: reassuring the patient and family, advising to decrease or stop participation in sports temporarily.

5. Medial instability and lateral instability.

6. In adolescents: apophyseal avulsion fracture of the humeral medial epicondyle; in adults: ulnar nerve entrapment, compression fracture laterally.

7. Arthrosis; osteochondrosis dissecans; synovial osteochondromatosis.

8. Humeroulnar joint: approximately 70° elbow flexion and 10° forearm supination; humeroradial joint: maximal elbow extension and forearm supination.

9. Humeroulnar joint: maximal elbow extension and forearm supination; humeroradial joint: approximately 90° elbow flexion and 5° forearm supination.

10. Extension and radial deviation of the wrist, supination of the forearm, and flexion of the elbow.

11. —The pronator teres muscle attaches via the insertion of the wrist flexors to the medial humeral epicondyle.

    —Against resistance, the flexor carpi radialis also pronates.

12. —Insertion of the extensor carpi radialis longus.

    —Insertion, tendon, and musculotendinous junction/proximal muscle belly of the extensor carpi radialis brevis.

    —Insertion of the extensor digitorum communis.

13. Pronator teres syndrome: median nerve, between the muscle bellies of the pronator teres; cubital tunnel syndrome: ulnar nerve, in the groove on the posterior side of the medial humeral epicondyle.

14. The tendon insertion is compressed against the ulna.

15. An avulsion fracture of the medial humeral epicondyle.

16. Intra-articular injection of a corticosteroid.

17. Brachialis muscle.

18. Olecranon bursitis.

19. The zero position of the forearm.

20. Type 2, insertion tendopathy of the extensor carpi radialis brevis.

21. Humeral capitulum, humeral trochlea, and head of the radius.

22. Manual reduction.

23. Long-distance running, weight lifting.

24. Pronator quadratus, pronator teres, and flexor carpi radialis.

25. Supinator, biceps brachii, extensors carpi radialis longus and brevis.

26. A single-axis rotating joint, trochoid articulation.

27. Fall on the hand with a bent elbow; avulsion fracture of the olecranon.

28. —Compression neuropathy of the recurrent branch of the radial nerve.
    —Compression neuropathy of the deep branch of the radial nerve (posterior interosseous).
    —Loose body in the elbow joint.
    —Lesion of the supinator muscle.

29. "Pivot joint," trochlear joint.
30. Proximal radioulnar joint, maximal loose-packed position: approximately 70° elbow flexion and 35° forearm supination; maximal close-packed position: approximately 5° forearm supination.

Part II—References

1. Kopell HP, Thompson WAL. *Peripheral Entrapment Neuropathies*. New York: RE Krieger; 1976:113–144.
2. Frankel VH, Nordin M, Snijders CJ, eds. *Biomechanica van het Skeletsysteem: Grondslagen en Toepassingen*. Lochem: De Tijdstroom; 1984.
3. Allander E. Prevalence, incidence, and remission rates of some common rheumatic diseases and syndromes. *Scand J Rheumatol*. 1974;3:145–153.
4. Snijders CJ. Grip van de handen. In: Frankel VH, Nordin M, Snijders CJ, eds. *Biomechanica van het Skeletsysteem: Grondslagen en Toepassingen*. Lochem: De Tijdstroom; 1984:373.
5. Cyriax J. *Textbook of Orthopaedic Medicine*, Vol 1: *Diagnosis of Soft Tissue Lesions*. 7th ed. London: Baillière Tindall; 1978.
6. Winkel D, Martens M, Wyffels P. *Orthopedische Casuïstiek*. Zaventem: Bohn Stafleu Van Loghum; 1992.

PART II—SUGGESTED READING

Albright JA, Jokl P, Shaw R, Albright JP. Clinical study of baseball pitchers: correlation of injury to the throwing and with method of delivery. *Am J Sports Med*. 1978;6:15–21.

Andrews JR, Wilson F. Valgus extension overload in the pitching elbow. In: Zarins B, Andrews JR, Carson WG, eds. *Injuries to the Throwing Arm*. Philadelphia: Saunders; 1985:250–257.

Ansink BJJ, van Meerwijk GM, et al. *Neurologie voor Paramedische Beroepen*. Utrecht: Bunge; 1982.

Babhulkar SS. Triceps contracture caused by injections. *J Bone Joint Surg [Br]*. 1985;67:94–96.

Bachum A van, Elkhuizen JW, Tilstra S. Epicondylalgia lateralis. *Tijdschr Man Ther*. 1983;2:2–19.

Baker BE, Bierwagen D. Rupture of the distal tendon of the biceps brachii: operative versus non-operative treatment. *J Bone Joint Surg [Am]*. 1985;67:414–417.

Banniza U, Bazan V, Jani L. Kongenitale Veränderungen am Ellbogengelenk. *Orthopaedie*. 1988;17:347–352.

Basset FJ, Nunley JA. Compression of the musculocutaneous nerve at the elbow. *J Bone Joint Surg [Am]*. 1982;64:1050–1052.

Baumann JU. Neuro-orthopädische Probleme im Ellbogengelenksbereich. *Orthopaedie*. 1988;17:382–389.

Bell MJ, Hill RJ, McMurtry RY. Ulnar impingement syndrome. *J Bone Joint Surg [Br]*. 1985;67:126–129.

Boyd HB, Mcleod AC. Tennis elbow. *J Bone Joint Surg [Am]*. 1973;55:1183–1187.

Brok AGMF. De epicondylitis medialis humeri bij sportmensen. *Geneeskd Sport*. 1982;15:144.

Burton AK, Edwards VA. Electromyography and tennis elbow straps. *Br Osteopath J*. 1982;14:83–86.

Clain A, ed. *Hamilton Bailey's Demonstrations of Physical Signs in Clinical Surgery*. Bristol: John Wright & Sons; 1965.

Cleary JE, Omer GE. Congenital proximal radio-ulnar synostosis: natural history and functional assessment. *J Bone Joint Surg [Am]*. 1985;67:539–545.

Coonrad RW, Hooper WR. Tennis elbow: its course, natural history, conservative and surgical management. *J Bone Joint Surg [Am]*. 1973;55:1177–1183.

Crawford Adams J. *Outline of Orthopaedics*. 6th ed. London: Churchill Livingstone; 1967.

Cyriax JH. The pathology and treatment of tennis elbow. *J Bone Joint Surg*. 1936;18:921–940.

De Haven KE, Evarts CM. Throwing injuries of the elbow in athletes. *Orthop Clin North Am*. 1973;4:301.

Dias JJ, Wray CC, Jones JM, Gregg PJ. The value of early mobilization in the treatment of Colles' fractures. *J Bone Joint Surg [Br.]*. 1987;69:463–467.

Eichenauer M, Wödlinger R. Aseptishe Nekrosen und Osteochondrosis dissecans des Ellbogengelenks. *Orthopaedie.* 1988;17:374–381.

Elias N. *Über den Prozeß der Zivilisation.* Two Vol. 5th ed. Baden-Baden: Suhrkamp; 1978.

Feindel W, Stratford J. The role of the cubital tunnel in tardy ulnar palsy. *Can J Surg.* 1985;1:287–300.

Fowles JV, Kassab MT, Douik M. Untreated posterior dislocation of the elbow in children. *J Bone Joint Surg [Am].* 1984;66:921–926.

Fowles JV, Kassab MT, Moula T. Untreated intra-articular entrapment of the medial humeral epicondyle. *J Bone Joint Surg [Br].* 1984;66:562–565.

Fowles JV, Sliman N, Kassab MT. The Monteggia lesion in children: fracture of the ulna and dislocation of the radial head. *J Bone Joint Surg [Am].* 1983;65:1276–1282.

Gainor BJ, Jeffries JT. Pronator syndrome associated with a persistent median artery: a case report. *J Bone Joint Surg [Am].* 1987;69:303–304.

Gardner E, Gray DJ, O'Rahilly R. *Anatomy.* Philadelphia: Saunders; 1975.

Geary N. Late surgical decompression for compartment syndrome of the forearm. *J Bone Joint Surg [Br].* 1984;66:745–748.

Gelberman RH, Pfeffer GB, Galbraith RT, Szabo RM, Rydevik B, Dimick M. Results of treatment of severe carpal tunnel syndrome without internal neurolysis of the median nerve. *J Bone Joint Surg [Am].* 1987;69:896–903.

Geukens C. Medial stress-syndrome osteochondritis en gewrichtsmuizen. Presented at the Elbow Congress, organized by the V.V.S.S. 1983; Diepenbeek, Belgium.

Goldie I. Epicondylitis lateralis humeri (epicondylalgia or tennis elbow): a pathological study. *Acta Chir Scand.* 1964;339 .

Good AB. Examination and manipulative management of tennis elbow. *Br Osteopath J.* 1983;15:83–86.

Gray H, Williams PL, Warwick R. *Gray's Anatomy.* 36th ed. London: Churchill Livingstone; 1980.

Greene CP. The curve ball and the elbow. In: Zarins B, Andrews JR, Carson WG, eds. *Injuries to the Throwing Arm.* Philadelphia: Saunders; 1985.

Haak A, Steendijk R, de Wijn IF. *De samenstelling van het menselijk lichaam.* Assen: Van Gorcum; 1968.

Hafferl A. *Lehrbuch der topographischen Anatomie des Menschen.* Berlin: Springer Verlag; 1957.

Halpern AA, Nagel DA. Compartment syndromes of the forearm: early recognition using tissue pressure measurements. *J Hand Surg.* 1979;4:258–263.

Hamilton WJ, Simon G, Hamilton SGI. *Surface and Radiological Anatomy.* 5th ed. London: Macmillan Press Ltd; 1976.

Hartz CR, et al. The pronator teres syndrome: compression neuropathy of the median nerve. J Bone Joint Surg [Am]. 1981;63:6.

Haymaker W, Woodhall B. *Peripheral Nerve Injuries.* 2nd ed. Philadelphia: Saunders; 1956.

Healy EJ, Seybold WD. *A Synopsis of Clinical Anatomy.* Philadelphia: Saunders; 1969.

Heerkens YF, Meijer OG. *Tractus-anatomie.* Interfaculty Physical Education. Amsterdam; 1980.

Hirayama T, Takemitsu Y. Isolated paralysis of the descending branch of the posterior interosseous nerve: report of a case. *J Bone Joint Surg [Am].* 1988;70:1402–1403.

Hirayama T, Takemitsu Y, Yagihara K, Mikita A. Operation for chronic dislocation of the radial head in children: reduction by osteotomy of the ulna. *J Bone Joint Surg [Br].* 1987;69:639–642.

Hirschfeld P, Winkel D. *Video-Seminar Orthopädische Medizin.* Pt 4: *Der Ellbogen.* Erlangen: Perimed Verlag; 1985.

Hoppenfeld S. *Physical Examination of the Spine and Extremities.* New York: Appleton-Century-Crofts; 1976.

Hunter SC. Little leaguer's elbow. In: Zarins B, Andrews JR, Carson WG, eds. *Injuries to the Throwing Arm.* Philadelphia: Saunders; 1985:228–234.

Huskisson EC, Hart FD. *Joint Disease: All the Arthropathies.* 3rd ed. Bristol: John Wright; 1978.

Janis JL, Mahl GF, Kagan J, Holt RR. *Personality, Dynamics, Development, and Assessment.* New York: Harcourt, Brace and World, Inc; 1969.

Johnson RK. Median nerve entrapment syndrome in the proximal forearm. *J Hand Surg.* 1979;4:48–51.

Josefsson PO, Gentz CF, Johnell O, Wendeberg B. Long-term sequelae of simple dislocation of the elbow. *J Bone Joint Surg [Am].* 1984;66:927–929.

Josefsson PO, Gentz CF, Johnell O, Wendeberg B. Surgical versus non-surgical treatment of ligamentous injuries following dislocation of the elbow joint: a prospective randomized study. *J Bone Joint Surg [Am].* 1987;69:605–608.

Karanjia ND, Stiles PJ. Cubital bursitis. *J Bone Joint Surg [Br].* 1988;70:832–833.

King JW, Breslford HJ, Tullos HS. Analysis of the pitching arm of the professional baseball pitcher. *Clin Orthop.* 1969;67:116.

Kingma MJ. *Nederlands Leerboek der Orthopedie.* Utrecht: Bohn, Scheltema & Holkema; 1982.

Klein Rensink GJ, Smits M. Entrapment neuropathieën. *Tijdschr Ned Belg Vereniging Orthop Geneeskd.* 1983;3:33–48.

Kuschner S, Reid DC. Manipulation in the treatment of tennis elbow. *J Orthop Sports Phys Ther.* 1986;7:264–272.

La Frenière JG. Tennis elbow: evaluation, treatment, and prevention. *Phys Ther.* 1979;59:742–746.

Lohman AGM. *Vorm en beweging. Leerboek van het bewegingsapparaat van de mens.* 4th ed. Utrecht: Bohn, Scheltema & Holkema; 1977.

London JT, Kinematics of the elbow. *J Bone Joint Surg [Am].* 1981;63:529–535.

McAuliffe TB, Hilliar KM, Coates CJ, Grange WJ. Early mobilization of Colles' fractures: a prospective trial. *J Bone Joint Surg [Br].* 1987;69:727–729.

McMinn RMH, Hutching RT. *A Color Atlas of Human Anatomy.* London: Wolfe Medical Publications Ltd; 1977.

Meerwijk GM van. *Syllabus Onderzoeken en Behandelen.* Amsterdam: Stichting Akademie voor Fysiotherapie Amsterdam; 1979; chap 16.

Mehlhoff TL, Noble PC, Bennett JB, Tullos HS. Simple dislocation of the elbow in the adult: results after closed treatment. *J Bone Joint Surg [Am].* 1988;70:244–249.

Mitchell JD, Reid DM. Reversible neurological causes of tennis elbow. *Br Med J.* 1983;286:1703–1704.

Morrey BF. A biomechanical study of normal functional elbow motion. *J Bone Joint Surg [Am].* 1981;63:872–876.

Morrey BF, Askew LJ, An KN, Dobyns JH. Rupture of the distal tendon of the biceps brachii: a biomechanical study. *J Bone Joint Surg [Am].* 1985;67:418–421.

Morrison DL. Berust de hardnekkige tenniselleboog echt op inklemming van de N. radialis? *Mod Med.* September 1982:1409–1410.

Mumenthaler M. *Der Schulter-Arm-Schmerz.* Bern: Hans Huber; 1982.

Mumenthaler M, Schliack H. *Läsionen peripherer Nerven.* Stuttgart: Georg Thieme Verlag; 1977.

Nause E. Rationelle Epikondylitisbehandlung. *Man Med.* 1987;25:82–85.

Nirschl RP. The etiology and treatment of tennis elbow. *J Sports Med.* 1974;2:308.

Ogilvie-Harris DJ, Fornasier VL. Pseudomalignant myositis ossificans: heterotopic new bone formation without a history of trauma. *J Bone Joint Surg [Am].* 1980;62:1274–1283.

Petherick M, Rheault W, Kimble S, Lechner C, Senear V. Concurrent validity and intertester reliability of universal and fluidbased goniometers for active elbow range of motion. *Phys Ther.* 1988;68:966–969.

Pluymers RJ. De tenniselleboog also sportletsel. *Geneeskd Sport.* 1978;2:123–127.

Priest JD, Braden V, Gerberich SG. The elbow and tennis, part 1: an analysis of players with and without pain. *Phys Sports Med.* 1980;8:81–91.

Putz R, Müller-Gerbl M. Funktionelle Anatomie des Ellbogengelenkes. *Orthopaedie.* 1988;17:338–346.

Quinton DN, Finlay D, Butterworth R. The elbow fat pad sign: brief report. *J Bone Joint Surg [Br].* 1987; 69:844–845.

Russe O, Gerhardt JJ, King PS. *An Atlas of Examination, Standard Measurements and Diagnosis in Orthopaedics and Traumatology.* Bern: Hans Huber Verlag; 1972.

Schwab GH, Bennett JB, Woods GW, Tullos HS. Biomechanics of the elbow instability: the role of the medial collateral ligament. *Clin Orthop.* 1980;146:42–52.

Seth MK, Khurana JK. Bony ankylosis of the elbow after burns. *J Bone Joint Surg [Br].* 1985;67:747–749.

Seyffarth H. Primary myosis in m. pronator teres as cause of lesion of n. medianus (pronator syndrome). *Acta Psychol Neurol Suppl.* 1951;74:251–254.

Snijders CJ, Volkers ACW, Mechelse K, Vleeming A. Provocation of epicondylalgia lateralis (tennis elbow) by power grip or pinching. *Med Sci Sports Exerc.* 1987;19:518–523.

Sobotta J, Becher PH. *Atlas of Human Anatomy.* Vol 1, 2 and 3. 9th English ed. Berlin: Urban & Schwarzenberg; 1975.

Steininger K, Stöferle B, Wörsdörfer O. Nachbehandlung bei Operationen am Ellbogengelenk: dargestellt am Beispiel der Osteochondrosis dissecans eines jugendlichen Kunstturners. *Physikal Ther.* 1984;5(suppl):611–617.

Stewart HD, Innes AR, Burke FD. Functional cast-bracing for Colles' fractures: a comparison between cast-bracing and conventional plaster casts. *J Bone Joint Surg [Br].* 1984;66:749–753.

Tanabu S, Yamauchi Y, Fukushima M. Hypoplasia of the trochlea of the humerus as a cause of ulnar-nerve palsy: report of two cases. *J Bone Joint Surg [Am].* 1985;67:151–154.

Tarr RR, Garfinkel AI, Sarmiento A. The effects of angular and rotational deformities of both bones of the forearm: an in vitro study. *J Bone Joint Surg [Am].* 1984;66:65–70.

Thomas W, Tillmann B. Engpaßsyndrome des Nervus radialis im Ellenbogenbereich im Rahmen der Epicondylosis humeri radialis: klinisch-anatomische Untersuchung. *Zeitschr Orthop.* 1980;118,1:41–46.

Thompson WAL, Kopell HP. Peripheral entrapment neuropathies of the upper extremity. *N Engl J Med.* 1959;260:1261–1265.

Tullos HS, Bryan WJ. Examination of the throwing elbow. In: Zarins B, Andrews JR, Carson WG, eds. *Injuries to the Throwing Arm.* Philadelphia: Saunders; 1985: 191–199.

Tullos HS, Bryan WJ. Functional anatomy of the elbow. In: Zarins B, Andrews JR, Carson WG, eds. *Injuries to the Throwing Arm.* Philadelphia: Saunders; 1985: 201–209.

Villar RN, Marsh D, Rushton N, Greatorex RA. Three years after Colles' fracture: a prospective review. *J Bone Joint Surg [Br].* 1987;69:635–638.

Wadsworth TG. Tennis elbow: conservative, surgical and manipulative treatment. *Br Med J.* 1987;294:621–624.

White SH, Goodfellow JW, Mowat A. Posterior interosseous nerve palsy in rheumatoid arthritis. *J Bone Joint Surg [Br].* 1988;70:468–471.

Wiley JJ, Galey JP. Monteggia injuries in children. *J Bone Joint Surg [Br].* 1985;67:728–731.

Wilhelm A. Unklare Schmerzzustände an der oberen Extremität. *Orthopaedie.* 1987;16:458–464.

Williams JGP. *A Color Atlas of Injury in Sport.* London: Wolfe Medical Publications; 1980.

Williams PL, Warwick R, eds. *Gray's Anatomy.* 36th ed. Edinburgh: Longman; 1980.

Wilson FD, Andrews JR, Blackburn TA, McCluskey G. Valgus extension overload in the pitching elbow. *Am J Sports Med.* 1983;2:83.

Winkel D. *Elleboog en Pols.* Rijswijk: Squibb; 1982.

Winkel D. Onderzoek, diagnostiek en behandeling van de tenniselleboog. *Geneeskd Sport.* 1987;2:79–81.

Winkel D, Fisher S. *Schematisch handboek voor onderzoek en behandeling van weke delen Aandoeningen van het Bewegingsapparaat.* 6th ed. Delft: Nederlandse Akademie voor Orthopedische Geneeskunde; 1982.

Wirth CJ. Sekundäre Bandinstabilitäten im Ellbogengelenksbereich. *Orthopaedie.* 1988;17:353–358.

Zenker H, Bruns H. Epicondylitis humeri: Behandlungsrichtlinien und Ergebnisse nach der Operation von Hohmann, G. *Muench Med Wochenschr.* 1978;120:1159–1162.

Part III

The Wrist and Hand

Functional Anatomy of the Wrist and Hand

15.1 FUNCTIONAL ANATOMY OF THE WRIST

If considered in isolation, the term *wrist* is misleading. Considered anatomically, the wrist is a structure that has numerous connections with very intricate, interrelated motions. Although it may be possible to differentiate among the various *anatomical* connections, in a functional context, isolated movements of wrist joints are impossible. Movement in one joint implies movement in the other joints.

Motions such as pronation and supination of the entire hand take place in the proximal and distal radioulnar joints, at the same time influencing the motions of the carpal and metacarpal connections. Thus, there is even a relationship between movements in the wrist and movements in the elbow.

JOINT MORPHOLOGY

Radiocarpal Joint (Articulatio Radiocarpea)

The radiocarpal joint forms the actual wrist joint. Considered anatomically, it is a two-axis, ellipsoid joint.

The proximal joint partner consists of the distal end of the radius along with the distal surface of the articular disc (which lies between the ulna and the carpus, and is one of the structures making up the so-called triangular fibrocartilaginous [TFC] complex). The distal joint partner consists of the scaphoid, lunate, and triquetrum. The pisiform does not articulate with the forearm.

Together, the distal bones of the radiocarpal joint form an almost uniform convexity that fits quite well into the concave joint surface formed by the radius and disc.

The joint cavity is isolated from the distal radioulnar joint as well as from the intercarpal (or midcarpal) joint. The capsule is reinforced by several ligaments (Figure 15–1).

Intercarpal (Midcarpal) Joints (Articulationes Intercarpeae)

Anatomically, it is useful to describe the intercarpal joints as proximal and distal rows of carpal bones. The first row is formed (from radial to ulnar) by the scaphoid, lunate, and triquetrum with the volar lying pisiform. The distal row consists of the trapezium, trapezoid, capitate, and hamate. Movement of these two rows in relation to each other takes place in the so-called midcarpal joints. It is not yet clear, however, whether the bones of the proximal row move in directions and degrees of motion similar to those of the distal row.

Joints between the bones of the carpus are strengthened by ligaments.

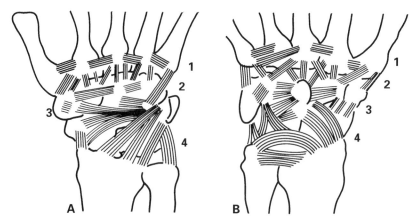

Figure 15–1 Collagenous reinforcement of the capsule. **A**, Dorsal view; **B**, ventral view; **1**, ligaments between the metacarpal bones; **2**, ligaments from the carpus to the metacarpus; **3**, ligaments between the carpal bones; **4**, ligaments between the forearm and carpus.

Except for the synovial cavity between the triquetrum and pisiform, the synovial cavities between the various carpal bones are connected to each other.

Carpometacarpal Joints (Articulationes Carpometacarpeae)

The first carpometacarpal joint is unlike the other four. It is a saddle joint (between the trapezium and metacarpal I). There is an ample joint capsule, and its synovial cavity is separate from the other four joints. On its palmar, dorsal, and lateral sides, the capsule is reinforced by ligaments.

The forms of the second, third, fourth, and fifth carpometacarpal joints are more intricate than is generally imagined. Sometimes the joint surfaces have curves that appear to be similar to that of a saddle joint. Joint surfaces on the metacarpal bones of the intermetacarpal connections are often continuous with the joint surfaces of the carpometacarpal joints. Ligaments are present at the dorsal, palmar, and interosseous aspects of the joints. The synovial cavities are often continuous with those of the intercarpal joints.

MUSCULATURE

The same forearm muscles guide the active motions of the radiocarpal and midcarpal joints. These include motions such as flexion, extension, radial deviation, ulnar deviation, and combinations of these (such as circumduction).

Palmar muscles involved in movements of these joints are the wrist flexors. These also have a function in finger motions (except for the flexors carpi radialis and ulnaris). The extensors are extrinsic hand muscles as well, with the exception of the extensors carpi radialis longus and brevis and the extensor carpi ulnaris. The latter three muscles function exclusively at the level of the carpus.

The muscles mentioned above as exceptions (the flexors carpi radialis and ulnaris, extensors carpi radialis longus and brevis, and extensor carpi ulnaris) are particularly involved in radial and ulnar deviation.

OTHER STRUCTURES

Median Nerve and Carpal Tunnel

The bones of the carpus do not lie flat. Actually, they form a gutter with a dorsal convexity. This gutter is spanned by the transverse carpal ligament (flexor retinaculum).

On the radial side, the transverse carpal ligament is attached to the scaphoid and trapezium. On the ulnar side, it has attachments to the pisiform and hook of the hamate bone. The carpal tunnel has a distinctive form, that of a flattened cone with the tip pointed distally. The smallest part of the carpal tunnel is approximately 2.5 cm distal to the entrance located at the level of the proximal border of the flexor retinaculum.

The most significant structures running through the carpal tunnel are the median nerve and the tendons of the flexors digitorum superficialis and profundus and the flexor pollicis longus (Figure 15–2). At the level of the carpal tunnel, the median nerve lies on top of the superficial flexor tendon of the index finger and underneath the palmaris longus tendon. The carpal tunnel is very compact; Takechi and Kono[1] measured an average area of 390 mm[2]. Changes within the tunnel can easily lead to increased pressure.[2] Carpal tunnel syndrome can be caused by a variety of disorders, which generally fall into two categories. Disorders such as thickening of ligaments and luxations of the carpal bones cause a decrease in the area of the tunnel. A disorder such as such as synovitis of the flexor tendon sheaths reduces space from within the tunnel because of an increase in the surface area of the contents.

Tendon and Tendon Sheaths at the Wrist

The tendon sheath around the tendons of the flexors digitorum profundus and superficialis is formed by a synovial membrane, which runs around the entire bundle of eight tendons. From the ulnar side, it "folds in" between the tendons of the superficial and deep flexors. This synovial membrane is connected palmarly with the flexor retinaculum and dorsally with the carpal bones. The tendon of the flexor pollicis longus has a separate tendon sheath.

Tendons of the wrist and finger extensors are found at the dorsal aspect of the wrist. These tendons lie underneath the extensor retinaculum, where "tunnels" for the various tendons are located (Figure 15–3).

BIOMECHANICS

An indication of the complexity of the motions in the carpus is the fact that even now there are no two identical descriptions of carpal movements. Various models have been suggested, only to be rejected eventually because of a variety of shortcomings.

Ranges of motions that occur in the wrist joint as a whole (radiocarpal, midcarpal, and carpometacarpal joints) can be determined from a number of different axes of reference. Various authors take the view that there is a difference in the motions of the proximal carpal row as a whole, compared with the distal row as a whole (the midcarpal joint[3]).[3–6]

For instance, Kapandji[3] states that the total flexion and extension in the wrist joint is approximately 85° in each direction. During flexion, 50° occurs in the radiocarpal joint and 35° is attributed to the midcarpal joint. In extension, the situation is exactly the opposite: 35° is attributed to the radiocarpal joint and 50° to the midcarpal joint. These midcarpal motions take place around an axis (the transverse), which runs between the lunate and capitate. The plane of reference is a plane in which the forearm, carpus, and metacarpus are in line with each other. Radial and ulnar deviation takes place around an axis that runs through the head of the capitate. The ranges of motion are 15° radial deviation and 45° ulnar deviation, measured from a line running through the radius and the middle of metacarpal III.[3]

An interesting study was performed by Berger et al.[7] with regard to the individual

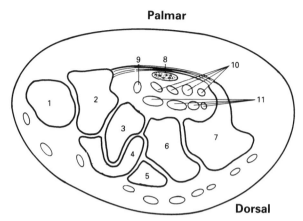

Figure 15–2 Cross-section of the left wrist at the level of the carpometacarpal joints. **1**, Metacarpal I; **2**, trapezium; **3**, trapezoid; **4**, base of metacarpal II; **5**, base of metacarpal III; **6**, capitate; **7**, hamate; **8**, median nerve; **9**, flexor carpi radialis tendon; **10**, flexor digitorum superficialis tendons; **11**, flexor digitorum profundus tendons.

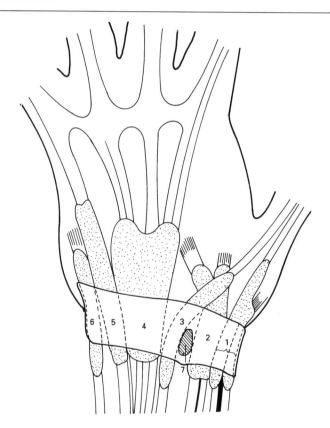

Figure 15–3 Tendon sheaths of the extensor tendons on the dorsal side of the right wrist. **1**, Abductor pollicis longus (radial) and extensor pollicis brevis; **2**, extensor carpi radialis longus (radial) and extensor carpi radialis brevis; **3**, extensor pollicis longus; **4**, extensor digitorum and extensor indicis; **5**, extensor digiti minimi; **6**, extensor carpi ulnaris; **7**, Lister's tubercle.

movements in the carpal bones. These researchers reconstructed three-dimensional relationships during movements of the carpus. With the help of a metal pin through metacarpal III in a fresh cadaver, motions were induced on the carpus (Table 15–1). It appeared that in some positions, there is unity of motion in the proximal carpal row in relation to the distal row; however, this does not hold true in every case.

Movement of the carpal bones is relatively individual. Of all of the carpal bones, the position of the lunate is the most difficult to predict.

The results of the analysis by De Lange et al.[4] were completely different from those of Berger et al.[7] The diagram of De Lange et al., represented in Table 15–2, appears to be the most applicable in the framework of our mobilization techniques. Note that Table 15–2 illustrates that the movement pattern of the proximal carpal bones in extension is very similar to that of ulnar deviation, except that in extension the accessory motions are very small, and in ulnar deviation the accessory motions are relatively large.

In extension, the movement pattern of the distal carpal bones is similar to that of radial deviation, with the exception that in radial deviation supination occurs. Furthermore, in extension, the extension motion is the largest component; in radial deviation, radial deviation is the largest component.

Extension with radial deviation occurs particularly in the midcarpal joint. Extension with ulnar deviation occurs particularly in the radiocarpal joint.

Legrand[8] postulated a model that was based on unified movement of the capitate and metacarpal III. This unit, which indeed has a strong mutual connection, moves as a whole in relation to the forearm.

Table 15–1 Results of the Research from Berger et al.[7] Regarding Movement of the Carpus

Carpal Bone	Radial Deviation to Neutral	Neutral to Ulnar Deviation	Flexion to Neutral	Neutral to Extension
Trapezium	Flexion Pronation	Flexion Supination	Supination	Supination
Trapezoid	Flexion Pronation	Flexion Supination	Pronation	
Capitate			Pronation	
Hamate		Extension Supination	Pronation	
Scaphoid	Extension Supination	Extension Supination	Counterclockwise	
Lunate		Extension Supination	Counterclockwise Pronation	Clockwise
Triquetrium		Extension Supination	Counterclockwise Pronation	

Table 15–2 Results of the Research by De Lange et al.[4] Regarding Movement of the Carpus

Wrist Motion from the Zero Position	Proximal Carpal Row	Distal Carpal Row
Flexion	Flexion Ulnar deviation Supination	Flexion Ulnar deviation
Extension	Extension Ulnar deviation Pronation	Extension Radial deviation
Radial deviation	Radial deviation Flexion Supination	Radial deviation Extension Supination
Ulnar deviation	Ulnar deviation Extension Pronation	Ulnar deviation Flexion Pronation

Source: Data from A. DeLange, J.M.G. Kauer, and R. Huiskes, Kinematic Behaviour of the Human Wrist Joint: A Rontgenstereophotogrammetric Analysis, *Journal of Orthopaedic Research*, Vol. 3, pp. 56–64, © 1985, Orthopaedic Research Society.

15.2   FUNCTIONAL ANATOMY OF THE HAND

The fingers, midhand, and connections of the carpus to the metacarpus all play a role in grasping motions.

JOINT MORPHOLOGY

Metacarpophalangeal Joints (Articulationes Metacarpophalangeae)

The metacarpophalangeal joints generally are described as being ellipsoid. Because movement is possible around three axes in this joint, the term *ellipsoid* is not completely correct.

The fibrocartilaginous palmar reinforcements of the joint capsules are very strong. These ligaments are connected to each other by means of a transverse collagenous structure. Terminal branches of the interdigital nerves run over these transverse ligaments.

Interphalangeal Joints (Articulationes Interphalangeae Manus)

The interphalangeal joints are considered to be "hinge" joints. The fibrous capsule of each joint is reinforced by collagenous ligaments.

MUSCULATURE

Flexion of the metacarpophalangeal joints is performed by the flexors digitorum superficialis and profundus, as well as the lumbrical and interosseous muscles. The flexor digitorum superficialis inserts on the middle phalanx of second through fifth fingers, while the profundus runs all the way to the end phalanx. The little finger also has a flexor digiti minimi. Flexion (or ulnar adduction) of the thumb is provided by the flexors pollicis longus and brevis, assisted by the first palmar interosseous muscle.

Extension of the second through fifth fingers is enabled by the extensor digitorum, whereby the index and little fingers also have their own extensor tendons—the extensor indicis proprius and extensor digiti minimi, respectively. Thumb extension (or radial abduction) is enabled by the extensor pollicis longus and brevis.

Adduction of the second through the fifth fingers in extension (in relation to a line through the long axis of the middle finger) is performed by the palmar interosseous muscles. In flexion, it is performed by the flexors digitorum superficialis and profundus. The thumb is adducted (dorsal adduction) by the adductor pollicis, first palmar interosseous, and opponens pollicis muscles.

Abduction is enabled by the dorsal interosseous muscles. In the little finger it is enabled by the abductor digiti minimi. Abduction (or palmar abduction) in the thumb is enabled by the abductor pollicis brevis.

The lumbrical muscles function to flex the carpometacarpal joints. Flexion in the interphalangeal joints is enabled by the flexors digitorum, extension by the extensor digitorum.

OTHER STRUCTURES

Palmar Aponeurosis

The palmar aponeurosis is a thick collagenous connective tissue plate, which is triangular in form. The tip of the triangle lies proximal to and is continuous with the flexor retinaculum and the palmaris longus tendon. The base is divided into four slips to the second through fifth fingers. Blood vessels and nerves travel to the finger regions between the four slips.

The aponeurosis is connected to the skin at its superficial aspect. The deep parts of the aponeurosis run parallel to the tendon sheaths of the flexors and to the deep transverse ligaments between the metacarpal heads.

The medial and lateral parts of the aponeurosis radiate to the fascia over the hypothenar and thenar regions, respectively.

BIOMECHANICS

From a biomechanical viewpoint, operation of the tendons and tendon sheaths of the hand is very interesting.[9] The tendons of both the flexors digitorum (profundus and superficialis) run in a fibrous tunnel at the level of the fingers, in which they are surrounded by a synovial membrane. The fibrous sheath is reinforced at different sites: at the metacarpophalangeal, proximal interphalangeal, and distal interphalangeal joints. Due to the form of the phalanx and metacarpal heads, a moment arm occurs in relation to the rotations of the corresponding joints.

Delattre et al.[9] postulated a twofold mechanism in full flexion of the fingers. The first mechanism is the working of the flexor digitorum superficialis on the middle pha-

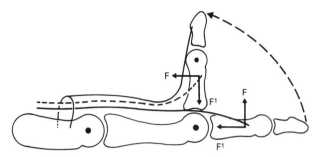

Figure 15–4 Effect of the leverage on the middle phalanx. Both components of the force (**F** and **F**¹) remain fairly constant during the flexion trajectory.

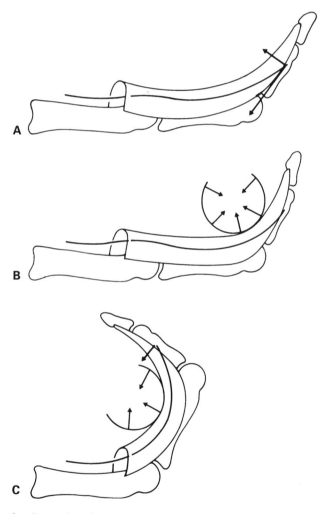

Figure 15–5 Effect of pulley action. **A**, In the first phase of the motion, there is only leverage; **B**, due to the curving of the tendon sheath, a pulley action occurs; **C**, the pulley shifts proximally, thereby having a greater effect on the distal phalanx.

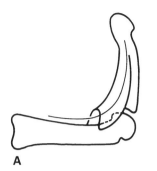 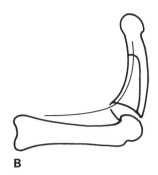

Figure 15–6 The shifting of the entrance of the tendon sheath (**A**) results in the tendon's entering the tendon sheath at a sharper angle (**B**).

lanx—leverage (Figure 15–4). Due to curving of the tendon sheath, a second effect occurs—pulley action (Figure 15–5). During increased flexion, the pulley shifts proximally, thereby having a greater effect on the distal phalanx.

Delattre et al.[9] also studied the course of the flexor tendons at the level of the meta-carpus. There the tendons enter the distal tunnels in such a way that the angle of entry into the sheath during flexion is fairly constant. If the entrance is shifted distally (as sometimes happens during surgery), the angle becomes sharper and increased flexion will occur in the metacarpophalangeal joint (Figure 15–6).

16

Surface Anatomy of the Wrist and Hand

PALPATION OF THE BONY STRUCTURES

In this description of the surface anatomy of the wrist, we discuss the area bordered proximally by the distal ends of the ulna and radius and distally by the distal end of the carpus. The borders of the area being examined should be marked in order to avoid mistakes in palpating the carpal bones. In so doing, the proximal and distal joint spaces are located.

Orientation of the carpal bones should be done by palpation from the dorsal aspect of the wrist. Palpation at the palmar aspect is made difficult by thick skin, strong palmar aponeurosis, and other soft tissue structures, such as the thenar and hypothenar eminences and the carpal tunnel.

Location of the Carpal Bones on the Dorsal Aspect of the Wrist

Ulnar Styloid Process

An important point of orientation at the dorsal aspect of the wrist is the head of the ulna at the distal end of the forearm. Just ulnar and distal to this structure, a pencil-shaped prominence—the ulnar styloid process—can be palpated (Figure 16–1). The ulnar styloid process is best located with the forearm in supination; in pronation the tendon of the extensor carpi ulnaris runs over the styloid process.

By beginning proximally at the olecranon process and following the posterior border of the ulna distally to its end, the styloid process

is also found. The location can be confirmed through active and passive wrist motions. During ulnar and radial deviation, the styloid process is stationary, unlike the distally located carpal bones.

Radial Styloid Process

The radial styloid process is larger and rounder than the ulnar styloid process (Figures 16–2, 16–7, and 16–10). It is best palpated at the most proximal point of the anatomical snuffbox, during radial abduction of the thumb. With simultaneous radial deviation of the wrist, this prominence becomes visible.

The anatomical snuffbox is bordered by the tendons of the abductor pollicis longus and extensor pollicis brevis on one side and the tendon of the extensor pollicis longus on the other side.

Lister's Tubercle

With the wrist in a neutral position, Lister's[*] tubercle can be located by sliding the palpating finger proximally from a point between the index and middle fingers to a small bony prominence on the distal end of the radius (Figures 16–3, 16–7, and 16–11). Just distal to Lister's tubercle is the joint line of the scaphoid and the radius.

The location can be confirmed by performing slight wrist flexion and extension. Unlike the distally located carpal bones, Lister's tu-

---

[*]Sir Joseph Lister, 1827–1912, English surgeon.

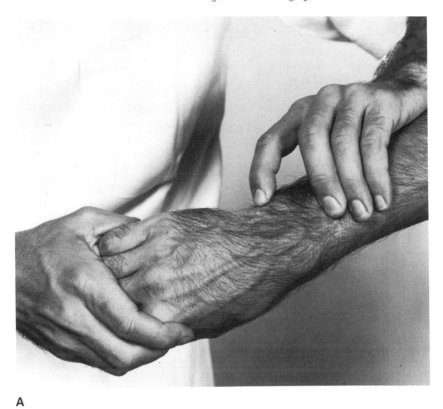

A

B

Figure 16–1 **A**, Right hand, palpation of the ulnar styloid process; **B**, sketched representation.

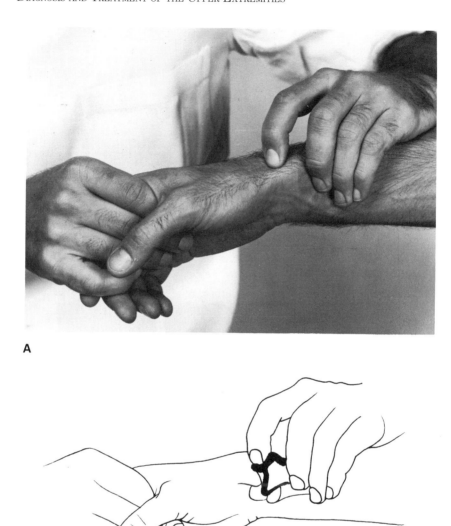

A

B

Figure 16–2 A, Right hand, palpation of the radial styloid process; **B**, sketched representation.

bercle is stationary during flexion and extension.

By connecting the ulnar styloid process, Lister's tubercle, and the radial styloid process, the proximal border of the carpus can be visualized.

Base of Metacarpal III

In wrist flexion, along an imaginary line connecting Lister's tubercle with the third ray, the prominent base of the third metacarpal can be palpated (Figure 16–4).

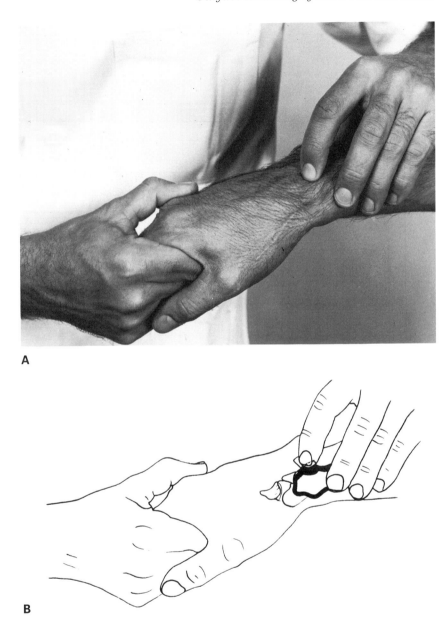

Figure 16–3 A, Right hand, palpation of Lister's tubercle; **B**, sketched representation.

In slight wrist extension, a small indentation can be palpated just proximal to the base. The capitate is located here (Figure 16–11).

Base of Metacarpal I

With the thumb in retroposition, the proximal end (or base) of the first metacarpal can

be palpated at the distal point of the anatomical snuff box (Figure 16–5).

Base of Metacarpal V

The base of the fifth metacarpal can be located by sliding the palpating finger proximally along the dorsoulnar aspect of the fifth

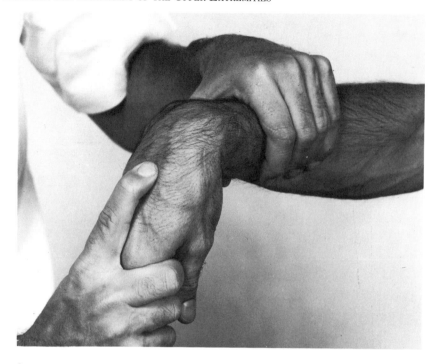

A

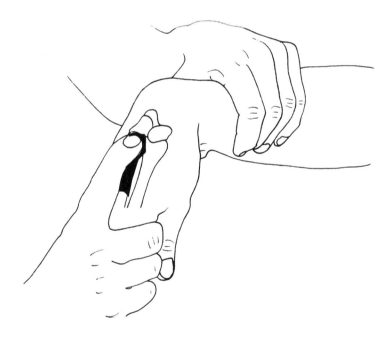

B

Figure 16–4 A, Right hand, palpation of the proximal end (base) of the third metacarpal; **B**, sketched representation.

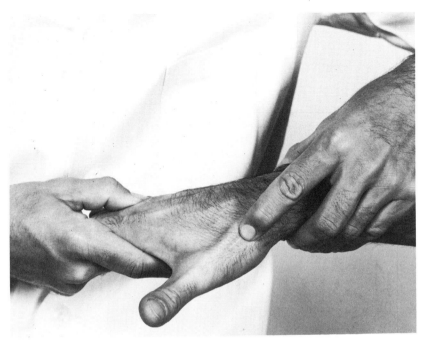

A

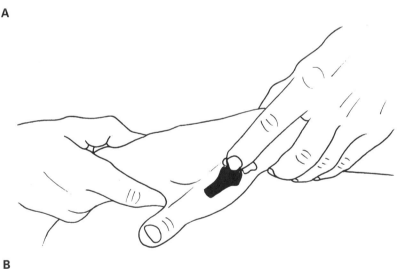

B

Figure 16–5 A, Right hand, palpation of the proximal end (base) of the first metacarpal; **B**, sketched representation.

metacarpal (Figure 16–6). In slight ulnar deviation, palpating the prominent base is made easier. Just proximal to this point is an indentation in which the hamate bone is found.

By connecting the bases of the first, third, and fifth metacarpals, the distal border of the carpus can be visualized. With both the proximal and distal borders of the carpus outlined,

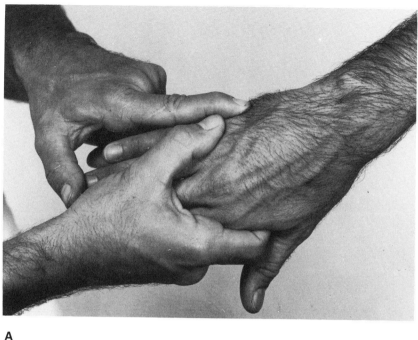

A

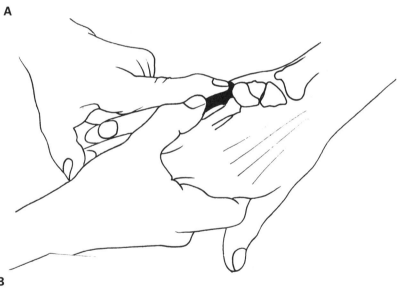

B

Figure 16–6 A, Right hand, palpation of the base of the fifth metacarpal; **B**, sketched representation.

systematic palpation of the individual carpal bones can begin (Figure 16–7).

Palpation in the Anatomical Snuffbox

The anatomical snuffbox is a triangular region observed during active radial abduc-tion of the thumb (Figures 16–8 and 16–9). One side (the base) is formed by the radial styloid process. The radial side of the tri-angle is formed by the abductor pollicis lon-gus and extensor pollicis brevis tendons, the ulnar side by the extensor pollicis longus tendon.

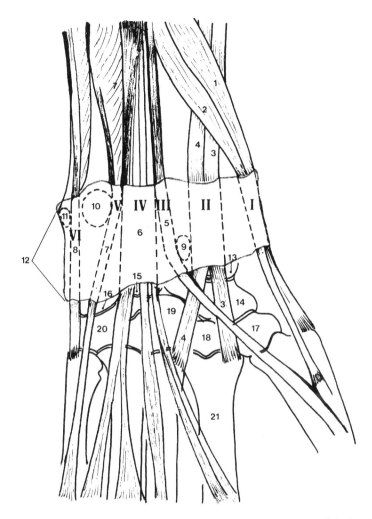

Figure 16–7 Right wrist, dorsal view. **1**, Abductor pollicis longus; **2**, extensor pollicis brevis; **3**, extensor carpi radialis brevis; **4**, extensor carpi radialis longus; **5**, extensor pollicis longus; **6**, extensor digitorum; **7**, extensor digiti minimi; **8**, extensor carpi ulnaris; **9**, Lister's tubercle; **10**, head of the ulna; **11**, ulnar styloid process; **12**, extensor retinaculum; **13**, radial styloid process; **14**, scaphoid; **15**, lunate; **16**, triquetrum; **17**, trapezium; **18**, trapezoid; **19**, capitate; **20**, hamate; **21**, metacarpal II.

Running along the floor of the anatomical snuffbox is the deep branch of the radial artery and the tendinous insertion of the extensor carpi radialis longus. Underneath these structures, the scaphoid and trapezium bones are found.

During alternating radial and ulnar deviation of the wrist, the radial styloid process can be palpated. Just distal to this prominence is the joint space between the scaphoid and ra-

dius. Here the clinically important, but nonpalpable, radial carpal collateral ligament is located.

With the wrist in radial deviation, the joint space between scaphoid and trapezium can be palpated approximately one fingerwidth distal to the radial styloid process.

The joint space between metacarpal I and the trapezium can be palpated by placing the palpating finger in the anatomical snuffbox,

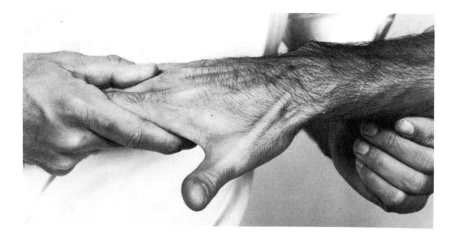

Figure 16–8 Right hand, the anatomical snuff box.

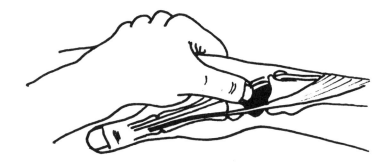

Figure 16–9 Right hand, palpation of the scaphoid bone in the anatomical snuffbox.

against the most proximal aspect of the base of the first metacarpal. Without moving the palpating finger, the thumb is brought into ulnar adduction. In so doing, the trapezium becomes palpable, and the palpating finger now rests in the joint space.

Scaphoid

At the midpoint of an imaginary line connecting the base of the third metacarpal with Lister's tubercle, an indentation is felt. In this "hole," the capitate is found. At its radial and proximal borders, the concave distal edge of the scaphoid can be felt (Figure 16–10). Because the extensor carpi radialis brevis tendon hinders palpation in this area, movement of the wrist should be done passively.

The scaphoid is also palpable in the anatomical snuffbox, just distal to the radial styloid process (Figure 16–9). During radial deviation of the wrist, the scaphoid pushes the palpating finger away.

Scaphoid fractures occur particularly during a fall from a great height or as the result of deflecting extreme mechanical forces with the hand. In such cases, the so-called nutcracker effect occurs whereby the scaphoid is cracked between the capitate and the radius.

Lunate

By now using an imaginary line between the base of the third metacarpal and the head of the ulna, the lunate can be located. At the distal half of this line, an indentation is felt. At

The border between the scaphoid and the lunate is located just distal to the midpoint of an imaginary line connecting Lister's tubercle and the distal radioulnar joint.

Like the scaphoid, the lunate tends to fracture when subjected to extreme mechanical forces. However, dislocations of this bone, which cause every movement of the wrist to be severely painful, are seen even more often. Once the diagnosis has been confirmed, the lunate is easily repositioned by means of wrist extension.

Triquetrum

Using the ulnar styloid process as an orientation point, the triquetrum can be palpated just distal to this prominence during ulnar deviation (Figure 16–7).

The palpation is made even easier by first locating the base of the fifth metacarpal and then sliding the palpating finger proximally. Just proximal to the base of the fifth metacarpal, the finger falls into a flat depression; the hamate is located further radial. Moving more proximal, the finger lands on the ulnarly prominent edge of the triquetrum. In so doing, the triquetrum cannot be mistaken for the more volar-lying pisiform.

Trapezium and Trapezoid

The border between the trapezium and trapezoid bones is found underneath the extensor pollicis longus tendon. The joint space can be palpated in the middle of the anatomical snuffbox at the radial side of the relaxed extensor pollicis longus tendon (Figures 16–7, 16–10, and 16–11).

Capitate

The borders of the largest carpal bone, the capitate, can be palpated in the already-mentioned indentation just proximal to the base of the third metacarpal (Figures 16–7 and 16–11). The joint space between the proximoradial side of the convex capitate and the concave part of the scaphoid is palpable to the experienced examiner during passive movements of the wrist.

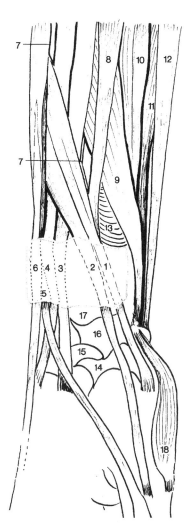

Figure 16–10 Right wrist, radial side. **1**, Abductor pollicis longus; **2**, extensor pollicis brevis; **3**, extensor carpi radialis longus; **4**, extensor carpi radialis brevis; **5**, extensor pollicis longus; **6**, extensor digitorum; **7**, part of the radius; **8**, brachioradialis; **9**, flexor pollicis longus; **10**, flexor digitorum profundus; **11**, flexor carpi ulnaris; **12**, flexor carpi radialis; **13**, pronator quadratus; **14**, trapezium; **15**, trapezoid; **16**, scaphoid; **17**, radial styloid process; **18**, abductor pollicis brevis.

the proximal and ulnar borders of this indentation (capitate), the lunate moves dorsally against the palpating finger during passive movement of the wrist (Figures 16–7 and 16–11).

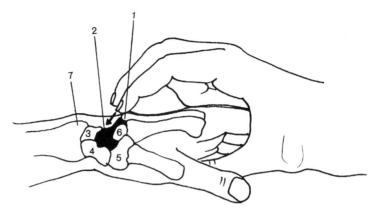

Figure 16–11 Left hand palpation of the capitate in the depression just proximal to the base of the third metacarpal. **1**, Tubercle of metacarpal III; **2**, capitate; **3**, lunate; **4**, scaphoid; **5**, trapezium; **6**, trapezoid; **7**, Lister's tubercle.

Like the lunate, the capitate can also luxate when subjected to extreme mechanical forces. The result is painful and limited wrist extension, which is quickly alleviated after repositioning the capitate. However, as a result of the dislocation, the ligaments between the capitate and the lunate are often sprained, causing residual pain. These structures respond very well to treatment of transverse friction. Although the ligaments, being part of the dorsal intercarpal ligaments, are not individually palpable, they are tender to palpation when injured. The capitate and the lunate are the reference points in localizing these ligaments.

Hamate

The hamate, which has a tip running to the lunate, is palpated between the triquetrum and tubercle of the fifth metacarpal (Figures 16–7 and 16–12).

Location of the Carpal Bones on the Volar Aspect of the Wrist

As already mentioned, inspection and palpation of the volar aspect of the wrist are difficult. However, there are four obvious bony prominences that can be used to determine the location of the flexor retinaculum (transverse carpal ligament), which, together with the deeper-lying skeletal structures, forms the carpal tunnel (Figure 16–12).

Even if the exact location of various structures in the carpal tunnel is difficult to determine, precise knowledge of their position is necessary. Lesions can be located by means of manual pressure, and the appropriate treatment can be administered precisely.

Tubercle of the Scaphoid

The prominent tubercle of the scaphoid is palpated by placing the palpating finger at the distal crease of the wrist on the tendon of the flexor carpi radialis (Figure 16–12). During ulnar deviation of the wrist, the tubercle is less prominent. During radial deviation the tubercle is more prominent.

Pisiform

The pisiform is found at the distal crease of the wrist on the volar-ulnar side of the proximal end of the hand (Figure 16–12). It is a round, sesamoid bone in the tendon of the flexor carpi ulnaris that is freely movable when the muscle is relaxed. Mobility of the bone can be assessed by holding the bone between thumb and index finger with the wrist in slight flexion.

Part of the flexor retinaculum is located between the pisiform and the scaphoid. Be-

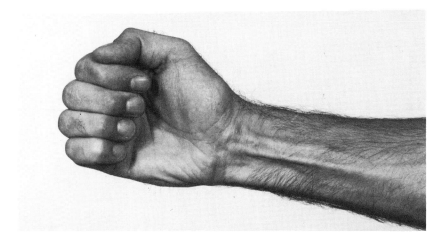

A

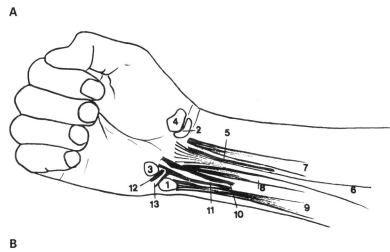

B

Figure 16–12 A, Right hand, volar aspect. **B**, Sketched representation; **1**, pisiform; **2**, tubercle of the scaphoid; **3**, hook of the hamate (between **1** and **3**, Guyon's tunnel); **4**, tubercle of the trapezium; **5**, median nerve; **6**, palmaris longus; **7**, flexor carpi radialis; **8**, flexor digitorum superficialis; **9**, flexor carpi ulnaris; **10**, ulnar artery; **11**, ulnar nerve; **12**, deep palmar ramus of the ulnar nerve; **13**, deep branch of the ulnar nerve.

cause of the insertion on the pisiform, tension in the proximal part of the flexor retinaculum is regulated by activity of the flexor carpi ulnaris. Distally, the flexor retinaculum runs between the hook of the hamate and the tubercle of the trapezium.

Two ligaments—actually the insertions of the flexor carpi ulnaris—run distally from the pisiform. With careful palpation, the pisometa-carpal and pisohamate ligaments can be felt.

Hook of the Hamate

The hook of the hamate can be palpated by placing the interphalangeal joint of the palpating thumb on the volar aspect of the pisiform. The end phalanx of the thumb is positioned along an imaginary line connecting the pisiform with the midpoint between thumb and index finger of the hand being palpated. On exerting pressure with the tip of the palpating thumb, a bony prominence is felt, the hook of the hamate. Palpation in this region is sometimes uncomfortable because a large branch of the ulnar nerve runs along the ulnar side of this bone (Figure 16–12).

Tubercle of the Trapezium

The tubercle of the trapezium is difficult to locate because it is partially covered by the muscles of the thenar eminence. The tubercle can be palpated 2 to 3 mm distal to the tubercle of the scaphoid, along an imaginary line connecting the scaphoid tubercle to the metacarpophalangeal I joint. During radial deviation of the wrist, the tubercle of the trapezium is less prominent. During ulnar deviation this tubercle is more prominent.

PALPATION OF MUSCLES AND OTHER SOFT TISSUE STRUCTURES ON THE VOLAR ASPECT OF THE WRIST

Carpal Tunnel

Tendons of the flexors digitorum profundus and superficialis, along with the flexor pollicis longus, run through the carpal tunnel (Figure 16–12). The only nerve running through the tunnel is the median nerve. In wrist fractures (eg, Colles* fracture), a volar dislocation of the lunate or tenovaginitis of the flexor digitorum profundus can compress the median nerve, leading to a carpal tunnel syndrome. Lesions of the flexor digitorum superficialis are rare.

The radial and ulnar arteries, as well as the radial and ulnar nerves, do not run through the carpal tunnel. The deep palmar ramus of the ulnar nerve is protected against mechanical forces as it runs between the pisiform and hook of the hamate (Guyon's† tunnel).

---

*Abraham Colles, 1773–1843, surgeon from Dublin.

†Jean Casimir Felix Guyon, 1831–1920, surgeon and urologist from Paris.

Palpation of the tendons on the volar aspect of the wrist is discussed in the section Palpation of the Flexors of the Forearm in Chapter 10, Surface Anatomy of the Arm, Elbow, and Forearm.

PALPATION OF MUSCLES AND OTHER SOFT TISSUE STRUCTURES ON THE DORSAL ASPECT OF THE WRIST

On the extensor side of the wrist, in contrast to the flexor side, a reinforced part of the forearm fascia (antebrachial fascia) serves as the extensor retinaculum for all of the hand and finger extensors together. It is 2.5 to 3.5 cm wide and is connected to the deep fascia in multiple areas as well as anchored to bones of the forearm and carpus. Thereby, six tunnels for an equal number of tendon sheaths are formed, through which one or more tendons run from the forearm to the hand (Figures 16–7, 16–10, and 16–13).

These tendons run parallel, except in one instance where two cross each other.

In this heavily trafficked area, in which not only tendons but also other structures can be found, exact location and precise identification of the various structures are possible only when based on a good knowledge of surface anatomy along with careful palpation techniques. Skilled palpation and a working knowledge of surface (as well as functional) anatomy are particularly necessary in order to recognize and differentiate among the numerous disorders and lesions in this region.

Extensor Tunnels

Tunnel I

Palpation of the extensor tunnels begins on the radial side of the wrist (Figures 16–7, 16–10, and 16–13). Running through the first tunnel are the fibrous tendon sheath and tendons of the abductor pollicis longus and ex-

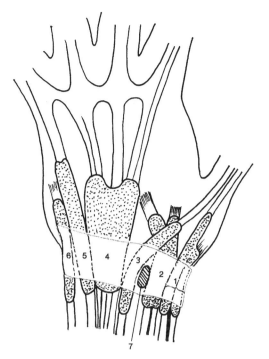

Figure 16–13 Left hand, extensor tunnels on the dorsum of the wrist. **Tunnel 1**, abductor pollicis longus and extensor pollicis brevis; **tunnel 2**, extensor carpi radialis longus and brevis; **tunnel 3**, extensor pollicis longus; **tunnel 4**, tendons of the extensor digitorum and the tendon of the extensor indicis proprius; **tunnel 5**, extensor digiti minimi; **tunnel 6**, extensor carpi ulnaris; **7**, Lister's tubercle.

tensor pollicis brevis; these go on to form the radial side of the anatomical snuffbox. These tendons are easy to palpate.

Look for tenderness and pain during resisted radial abduction and palmar abduction of the thumb. A tenosynovitis (inflammation of the tendon sheath) of these tendons is seen frequently. If the inflammation occurs at the level of the carpus, it is termed de Quervain* syndrome.

---

*Fritz de Quervain, 1868–1940, Swiss surgeon from Bern.

Tunnel II

The extensors carpi radialis longus and brevis run through the second extensor tunnel and can be palpated just radial to Lister's tubercle (Figures 16–7, 16–10, and 16–13).

The tendons can be followed further distally. With the wrist in slight extension and the hand making a fist, it is easy to see and palpate where the extensors carpi radialis longus and brevis separate, forming a V. Here the extensor carpi radialis brevis tendon is the easiest to follow. It runs to the bases of metacarpals II and III and inserts just beyond the clearly palpable carpometacarpal joint space. After locating the capitate bone proximal to the base of the third metacarpal, the extensor carpi radialis brevis is the first tendon found radial to this site.

The extensor carpi radialis longus tendon is best palpated with the thumb in maximal ulnar adduction, because otherwise the tendon from the third tunnel, the extensor pollicis longus, gets in the way. It inserts on the radial side of the base of the second metacarpal. Here, too, the insertion is palpated just beyond the trapezoid-metacarpal II joint space.

Tunnel III

The extensor pollicis longus is palpated at the ulnar side of Lister's tubercle. Its oblique course is particularly visible during active thumb retroposition and simplifies palpation considerably. After passing the tubercle, the tendon is easily recognizable as it runs to the end phalanx of the thumb (Figures 16–7, 16–10, and 16–13).

Sometimes after wrist fractures, Lister's tubercle is malpositioned and no longer functions as the turning point for the extensor pollicis longus tendon. This can eventually lead to mild pathology of the tendon sheath.

Tunnel IV

The tendons of the extensors digitorum and indicis proprius have a common sheath.

With the hand placed on a flat surface, the superficial tendons of the extensor digitorum can be palpated by individually extending the fingers from the index finger to the little finger, one after the other.

Tunnel V

The extensor digiti minimi is palpable just radial to the head of the ulna. Active extension of the little finger simplifies the palpation (Figures 16–7 and 16–13).

The distal radioulnar joint can also be found underneath the tendon of the extensor digiti minimi, just radial to the head of the ulna.

Tunnel VI

The extensor carpi ulnaris runs between the head and styloid process of the ulna, to the base of the fifth metacarpal. Active ulnar deviation with simultaneous slight wrist extension simplifies the palpation. The tendon is easiest to palpate just proximal or just distal to the head of the ulna (Figures 16–7 and 16–13).

Because of movement of the radius around the head of the ulna, the tendon is found at the ulnar aspect of the wrist in pronation and at the dorsal aspect of the wrist in supination.

PALPATION OF THE BONY AND LIGAMENTOUS STRUCTURES OF THE HAND

Even considering the frequency of hand lesions, palpation of the individual bony and ligamentous structures is rarely indicated. Many disorders, such as rheumatoid arthritis, affect the hand as a whole rather than its single parts. Thus, within the scope of the normal routine examination, detailed assessment generally is not performed. Palpation of the structures discussed below, however, may be necessary under certain circumstances, such as fractures, Dupuytren contracture, or dislocations.

Metacarpals

The metacarpals are easily palpable at the dorsal aspect of the hand, but they can be felt only indirectly at the palmar aspect (Figure 16–14). Their proximal ends consist of irregular cubistic bases. The base of metacarpal I forms a saddle joint with the trapezium, which is easily palpable distally, in the anatomical snuffbox. The tubercle of the first metacarpal, which is the proximal tip of the base, functions as an important orientation point in the wrist.

The base of metacarpal II articulates with the trapezoid and with a very small surface of the trapezium. In addition, like metacarpals III and IV, it has a connection with its neighboring metacarpals. Distal to the trapezoid, the immovable carpometacarpal II joint space can be palpated at the dorsal aspect of the hand.

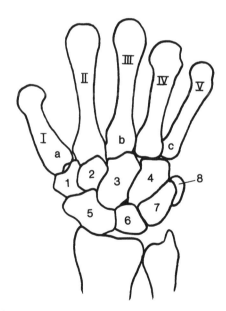

Figure 16–14 Right hand, dorsal aspect, metacarpals and carpus. **1**, Trapezium; **2**, trapezoid; **3**, capitate; **4**, hamate; **5**, scaphoid; **6**, lunate; **7**, triquetrum; **8**, pisiform. Orientation points: **a**, tubercle of metacarpal I; **b**, tubercle of metacarpal III; **c**, base of metacarpal V.

The base of metacarpal III is conspicuous because of the tubercle at its radial aspect. The bone has an immovable articulation with the capitate. At the dorsal aspect of the wrist, this joint is palpable just distal to the capitate.

The base of metacarpal IV has a joint surface in common with both the capitate and the hamate. This joint space can be palpated just distal to the capitate and hamate at the dorsum of the wrist. The small amount of motion in the joint is important for grasping functions.

The base of metacarpal V is used as an orientation point in the wrist. It articulates with the hamate, and the joint space can be palpated just distal to the hamate on the dorsal aspect of the wrist. In normal grasping motions, this joint has to be mobile. During grasping, the base of the fifth metacarpal simultaneously rotates and glides slightly in a palmar direction.

At the distal ends of the metacarpals are the metacarpal heads, which are palpable next to the long finger flexor tendons on the palmar aspect of the hand. The heads are round. Except for the first metacarpal, the metacarpal bones lie with bases and heads against each other, with open spaces between the shafts of the bones (metacarpal interosseous space). At the dorsal side of the hand, these spaces are largely taken up by the dorsal interosseous muscles.

If a fracture of one of the metacarpals is suspected, test to see whether axial pressure is painful. With the finger in flexion, pressure exerted in a proximal direction against the head of the metacarpal will provoke pain.

Palmar Aponeurosis

The triangular-shaped aponeurosis is found in the superficial region of the palm (Figure 16–15). It runs in line with the palmaris longus, or if the palmaris longus is absent, distal to the carpal tunnel (Figure 16–12). Its borders are difficult to delineate, due in part to the thick subcutaneous tissue of

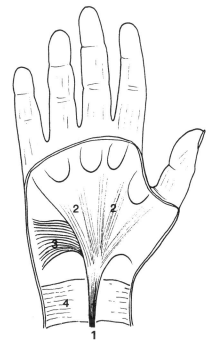

Figure 16–15 Right hand, palmar aponeurosis. **1**, Palmaris longus muscle; **2**, palmar aponeurosis; **3**, palmaris brevis; **4**, flexor retinaculum.

the palm. The edge of the palmar aponeurosis can be felt as a thickening, particularly on the radial side, when sliding the palpating finger ulnarly. On the ulnar side, the aponeurosis is interwoven with the palmaris brevis, a cutaneous muscle that cannot be palpated individually.

In elderly people, the aponeurosis can contract, leading to a flexion contracture of one or more fingers (Dupuytren's* contracture).

Metacarpophalangeal Joints

Palpation of the metacarpophalangeal joints is best performed during movement (Figures 16–16 and 16–17). With fingers and thumb flexed, the joint spaces are found *distal* to the knuckles. These sites can be con-

_____
*Guillaume Dupuytren, 1777–1835, surgeon from Paris.

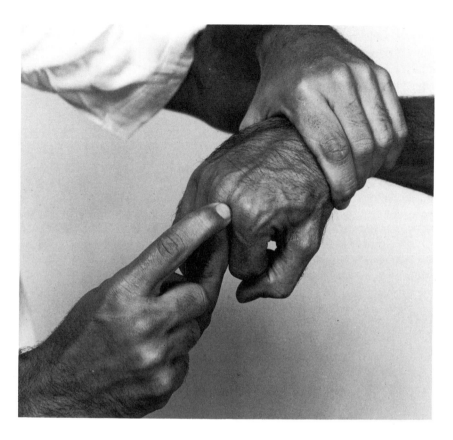

Figure 16–16 Palpation of the joint space between metacarpal III and the proximal phalanx of the middle finger.

firmed by performing a small amount of flexion and extension with the slightly bent thumb and fingers. Palpation of the joint spaces from the palmar aspect is much more difficult; it can be done, however, when performed during movement. In so doing, note that the joint spaces of metacarpals II through IV lie much more proximal than expected. Distal to the joint spaces, palmar skin folds are found between the phalanxes.

The metacarpophalangeal I joint is a saddle joint. The others are spheroid joints; however, because of the surrounding ligaments and the pull of neighboring muscles, the flexed fingers function as ellipsoid (hinge) joints. From a position of flexion, the fingers can straighten only actively. Extended fin-

gers also can actively abduct and adduct; passively, there is slight rotation in all of the joints. These motions are very important in the grasping function of the hand.

The superficial transverse metacarpal ligaments, which lie in the deep subcutaneous layer, are the only ligaments in this region that are palpable. They are felt as transversely running cords. Although dorsally metacarpals II through V are easily palpable, identification of ligaments in this region is not possible.

Phalangeal and Interphalangeal Joints

The interphalangeal joint of the thumb and both interphalangeal joints of the other fingers are well palpable from every side (Figure 16–17). They are ellipsoid (hinge) joints.

In examination of the fingers, attention is given to possible inflammatory processes (which should always be taken seriously) as well as to the condition of the nails. Irregularities observed in and around the nails can be due to certain systemic conditions, such as psoriasis or Reiter's disease.

PALPATION OF THE MUSCLES AND OTHER SOFT TISSUE STRUCTURES OF THE HAND

Flexor Digitorum Profundus and Superficialis Tendons

The tendons of the flexor digitorum superficialis can be palpated deeply in the palm by palpating transversely over the tendons (Figure 16–18). Alternating flexion and extension of the fingers with the wrist in slight extension will simplify the palpation.

Palpation of the little finger flexor tendon is performed just radial to the hypothenar eminence, which slightly interferes with the palpation.

In the hand, palpation of the flexor digitorum profundus tendons is impossible. The function of the muscle, however, can be

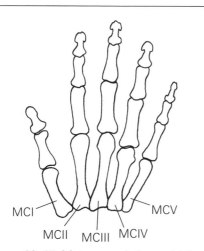

Figure 16–17 Metacarpophalangeal joints and interphalangeal joints.

assessed by flexing the end phalanx of each finger, one after the other.

On the palmar side of the thumb's proximal phalanx, the flexor pollicis longus is clearly palpable. Alternately bending and straightening the thumb will simplify the palpation.

Muscles of the Thenar Eminence

The muscle belly of the adductor pollicis is easily palpable with the thumb positioned in palmar abduction; the palpating finger is placed proximal to the metacarpophalangeal joint on the web space (between thumb and index finger), and the thumb is adducted (Figure 16–18).

Sometimes the opponens pollicis is visible directly palmar to metacarpal I. It is separated from the flexor pollicis brevis by a groove.

The junction between the flexor pollicis brevis and the abductor pollicis brevis is usually difficult to locate. The abductor pollicis brevis is most visible during active thumb abduction.

Fortunately, the ability to identify the individual muscles of the thenar eminence is of minimal practical significance.

Muscles of the Hypothenar Eminence

The muscles of the hypothenar eminence are easiest to palpate during grasping motions (Figure 16–18). Identifying the individual muscles (abductor digiti minimi, opponens digiti minimi, and flexor digiti minimi brevis) is nearly impossible and has almost no practical use.

Extensor Tendons

The tendons of the extensor digitorum, as well as the extensor digiti minimi tendon, are easy to see and palpate (transversely) on the dorsum of the hand.

Between the extensor tendons of the fourth and fifth rays, a strong intertendinous connection is almost always palpable proxi-

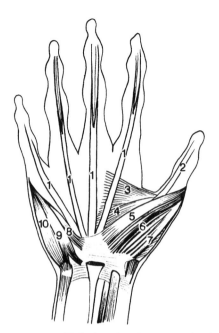

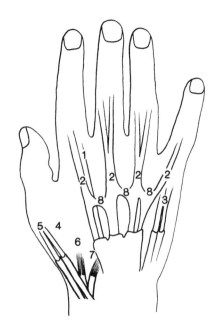

Figure 16–18 Right hand, palmar muscles (after removal of the interosseous and lumbrical muscles). **1**, Flexor digitorum superficialis tendons; **2**, flexor pollicis longus tendon; **3**, adductor pollicis, transverse head; **4**, adductor pollicis, oblique head; **5**, flexor pollicis brevis; **6**, abductor pollicis brevis; **7**, opponens pollicis; **8**, opponens digiti minimi; **9**, flexor digiti minimi brevis; **10**, abductor digiti minimi.

Figure 16–19 Right hand, finger extensor tendons. **1**, Extensor indicis proprius tendon; **2**, extensor digitorum tendons; **3**, extensor digiti minimi tendon; **4**, extensor pollicis longus tendon; **5**, extensor pollicis brevis tendon; **6**, extensor carpi radialis longus tendon insertion; **7**, extensor carpi radialis brevis tendon insertion; **8**, intertendinous connections (connexus intertendinei).

mal to the metacarpophalangeal joints (Figure 16–19). During alternating flexion and extension of the little finger, a connective tissue band springs back and forth underneath the palpating finger.

The tendons of the extensors pollicis longus and brevis are also easy to see and palpate. They border the anatomical snuffbox, which can be seen most clearly with the forearm pronated and the thumb actively held in retroposition.

Dorsal Interosseous Muscles

The muscle belly located on the dorsal aspect of the web space (between the first and second metacarpals) is the dorsal interosseous I muscle (Figure 16–20). By hold-

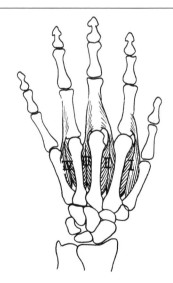

Figure 16–20 Left hand, dorsal interosseous muscles.

ing all of the fingers together, the muscle is pushed superficially and can be palpated easily.

The other dorsal interosseous muscles are difficult to palpate because of the finger extensor tendons and the intertendinous connections. They are found between the metacarpals and can best be reached on the dorsum of the hand while actively holding the fingers together.

If the muscles are atrophied (perhaps as the result of an ulnar nerve lesion) there are noticeable grooves between the metacarpals.

Radial Artery

Generally, the radial artery is palpated at the distal end of the forearm, between the flexor carpi radialis tendon and the radius or brachioradialis tendon (see Appendix A).

A deep branch of the radial artery can be palpated deep in the anatomical snuffbox. From there it runs further underneath the extensor pollicis longus tendon and penetrates the dorsal interosseus I muscle. Often, the branch can be palpated again further proximal to the dorsal interosseous I muscle, just next to the extensor pollicis longus tendon.

Ulnar Artery

The ulnar artery can be palpated at the distal forearm, just radial to the flexor carpi ulnaris tendon (see Appendix A). Its superficial branch can usually be palpated radial to the proximal part of the hypothenar eminence.

Radial Nerve

The superficial branch of the radial nerve can be felt on the dorsal aspect of the hand, directly proximal to the anatomical snuffbox (see Appendix A). Slightly further distally, the nerve crosses the extensor pollicis longus tendon at approximately the level of the carpometacarpal I joint. Through careful palpation, the nerve can be felt where it crosses the tendon.

Ulnar Nerve

In the hand region, branches of the ulnar nerve can usually be palpated in the palm, just radial to the hook of the hamate (see Appendix A).

Cutaneous Veins

Among individuals, the cutaneous veins vary greatly in their course. Their irregular patterns can be seen particularly on the dorsum of the hand. The veins on the radial side flow into the cephalic vein and, on the ulnar side, into the basilic vein.

17

Examination of the Wrist and Hand

FOREARM (ANTEBRACHIUM)

Zero Position

The arm is in the frontal plane; the elbow is in 90° flexion; the forearm is in the middle position between pronation and supination.

Maximal Loose-Packed Position

Proximal radioulnar joint: the elbow is in approximately 70° flexion; the forearm is in approximately 35° supination.

Distal radioulnar joint: the forearm is 10° supinated.

Maximal Close-Packed Position

The forearm is approximately 5° supinated.

Capsular Pattern

There is minimal to no limitation; pain is experienced at the end-range of pronation and supination.

WRIST

Zero Position

The longitudinal axis through the radius and the longitudinal axis through metacarpal III are in line with each other.

Maximal Loose-Packed Position

There is approximately 10° of wrist flexion and 10° of ulnar deviation.

Maximal Close-Packed Position

There is maximal wrist extension.

Capsular Pattern

Approximately equal limitations of motion are found in flexion and extension (Figure 17–1).

MIDHAND

Zero Position

The carpometacarpal I joint is in the middle position between maximal dorsal adduction (adduction) and palmar abduction (abduction).

The carpometacarpal II to V joints are in the same position as in the zero position of the wrist.

Maximal Loose-Packed Position

The carpometacarpal I joint is in the middle position between maximal dorsal adduction (adduction) and palmar abduction (abduction).

The carpometacarpal II to V joints are in the same position as in the zero position of the wrist.

Maximal Close-Packed Position

The carpometacarpal I joint is in maximal opposition.

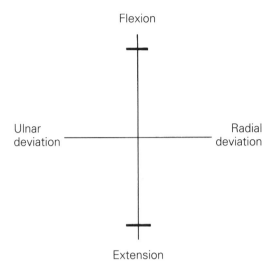

Figure 17–1 Capsular pattern of the wrist.

The carpometacarpal II to V joints are in the maximal close-packed position when the wrist is in maximal extension.

Capsular Pattern

In the carpometacarpal I joint, retroposition is limited (limitation of motion of radial abduction and dorsal adduction). In severe cases, opposition is sometimes also limited.

In the carpometacarpal II to V joints, extension and flexion are equally limited.

FINGERS

Zero Position

The longitudinal axes through the metacarpal and through the articulating proximal phalanx are in line with each other.

Maximal Loose-Packed Position

There is slight flexion in every joint. In the metacarpophalangeal joints II to V, there is slight ulnar deviation as well.

Maximal Close-Packed Position

All interphalangeal joints and the first metacarpophalangeal joint are in maximal extension; the metacarpophalangeal joints in II to V are in maximal flexion.

Capsular Pattern

Flexion is slightly more limited than extension (Figure 17–2).

OVERVIEW OF THE FUNCTIONAL EXAMINATION

Soft tissue lesions in the wrist-hand region generally cause very localized symptoms. The most well-known exceptions to this are the De Quervain and carpal tunnel syndromes.

When examining the wrist and hand, it should always be kept in mind that many neurological and other disorders can begin with symptoms in the hands, for example, paresthesia, muscle weakness, and edema.

General Inspection

The examining therapist can start to gather information as the patient enters the room. General posture, facial expression, and the use of assistive devices should be noted. At-

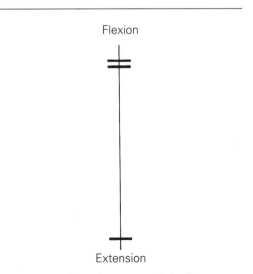

Figure 17–2 Capsular pattern of the fingers.

tention is paid to how the patient holds the affected arm and shakes hands. The use of a cast or a brace also should be noted.

History

Age, Occupation, Hobbies, Sports

Some disorders are age related. Lunate malacia, for example, is mostly seen in adolescents. Tendinitides and tenosynovitides are seen particularly in adults.

Other lesions are occupational or sports related. For instance, a ganglion of the wrist is seen mostly in persons such as masseurs and gymnasts who perform activities involving repeated loaded extension of the wrist. Many traumatic lesions of the hand, midhand, and fingers are specific to certain sports.

Chief Complaints

Depending on the type of pathology, complaints can consist of one or more of the following:

- pain during activities and/or at rest
- paresthesia
- loss of strength
- loss of sensation
- loss of range of motion
- locking of the wrist or fingers
- crepitation

The further distal a lesion is located in an extremity, the more the pain is localized. In other words, location of the pain and lesion at the same site occurs more often in the hand than is the case with lesions that are more proximal in the extremity.

If symptoms are also present at rest, the lesion is usually more severe than if the pain is experienced only during activities.

When paresthesia is diagnosed, differentiation should be made among pathologies of the cervical spine, thoracic outlet region, and peripheral nerve. The distribution of the pares-thesia is significant. Paresthesia due to compression of the median nerve in the carpal tunnel can be very misleading because it often radiates some distance proximally.

Locking of the wrist usually indicates carpal instability. Locking of the thumb or finger is usually an indication of a "trigger" thumb or finger (tendovaginitis stenosans).

In most cases, crepitation is an indication of a tenosynovitis. The crepitation is found at the same site as the lesion.

Onset

The following questions should be asked concerning the onset of symptoms:

- Were the symptoms insidious? Was the onset sudden or gradual?
- Was there a trauma? What was the nature of the injury?
- Has the extremity been overused? Were the symptoms immediate or experienced later?

Symptoms with an insidious nontraumatic onset can be due to arthritis, ganglion, or tendinitis. Particularly in the last two instances, microtrauma can play a causative role.

Many disorders in the wrist, midhand, and fingers have a traumatic onset. It is important to determine the type of trauma and compare the suspected diagnosis with the findings of the functional examination.

The prognosis is generally quite good when the symptoms arise immediately after activity. In these instances, if the lesion is treated in an appropriate and timely manner, the symptoms disappear quickly.

Duration

The duration of the symptoms also gives an indication of the prognosis. For instance, chronic instability is difficult to treat conservatively. Thus, the duration of the symptoms can be decisive in determining treatment and prognosis.

Other Complaints

Gaining information about other complaints is important, because the present symptoms can be based on an underlying systemic illness. Many systemic diseases start with an arthritis in the wrist or one of the small joints. This is characteristically true of rheumatoid arthritis and psoriasis.

Previous Incidents of the Symptoms

Information about the chronicity or recurrence of the problem should be obtained. For instance, a ganglion often has a history of disappearing spontaneously and then recurring.

Medication

If the patient is taking anticoagulants, caution should be exercised during injections, manipulations, and transverse friction. Many patients have been treated previously with nonsteroidal anti-inflammatory medication. In many instances, physical therapy results are poor because the patient has already received injections (unsuccessfully) of corticosteroids.

Previous Therapy and Results

Generally, it makes little sense to repeat a treatment that previously was unsuccessful, unless, of course, the previous treatment was incorrectly administered.

Specific Inspection

The examiner inspects the position of the wrist and the joints of the hand, looking for edema or local swelling and atrophy, particularly of the thenar and hypothenar muscles.

Changes in color can occur as the result of arterial or venous compression or pooling. Changes in the skin, such as shiny areas, pigmentation, peeling, and spots, should also be noted.

In addition, irregularities can be visible in and around the nails, such as in psoriasis and Reiter's disease.

Palpation

Before the functional examination, palpation for skin temperature and the nature of any visible swelling is performed.

Before the functional examination, the examiner determines whether the patient is experiencing symptoms *at that specific moment.* Per test, the examiner notes whether the symptoms change.

The affected side is always compared with the nonaffected side. The nonaffected side is always tested first to have an idea of what is "normal."

In the following description of the functional examination, the essential tests are indicated in ***boldface italic and underlined:*** these comprise the *basic functional examination.* The other tests are performed depending on the findings from the basic functional examination.

Functional Examination

DISTAL RADIOULNAR JOINT

Tests—Active Motions

17.1. Active forearm pronation
17.2. Active forearm supination

Tests—Passive Motions

17.3 Passive forearm pronation
17.4 Passive forearm supination

WRIST

Tests—Active Motions

17.5. Active supported wrist extension
17.6. Active supported wrist flexion
17.7. Active radial deviation
17.8. Active ulnar deviation

Tests—Passive Motions

17.9.   *Passive wrist extension*
17.10.   *Passive wrist flexion*
17.11.   *Passive wrist radial deviation*
17.12.   *Passive wrist ulnar deviation*

Tests—Resisted Motions

17.13.   *Resisted wrist extension with radial deviation*
17.14.   *Resisted wrist extension with ulnar deviation*
17.15.   *Resisted wrist flexion with radial deviation*
17.16.   *Resisted wrist flexion with ulnar deviation*

THUMB

Tests—Active and Passive Motions

17.17.   Active thumb retroposition
17.18.   *Passive thumb retroposition*

Tests—Resisted Motions

17.19.   *Resisted thumb radial abduction (extension)*
17.20.   *Resisted thumb palmar abduction (abduction)*
17.21.   *Resisted thumb dorsal adduction (adduction)*
17.22.   *Resisted thumb ulnar adduction (flexion)*

FINGERS

Tests—Passive Motions

17.23.   Passive metacarpophalangeal extension
17.24.   Passive metacarpophalangeal flexion
17.25.   Passive extension of the proximal interphalangeal joints
17.26.   Passive flexion of the proximal interphalangeal joints

17.27.   Passive extension of the distal interphalangeal joints
17.28.   Passive flexion of the distal interphalangeal joints

Tests—Resisted Motions

17.29.   Resisted abduction of the second and third fingers
17.30.   Resisted abduction of the third and fourth fingers
17.31.   Resisted abduction of the fifth finger
17.32.   Resisted adduction of the fifth finger
17.33.   Resisted adduction of the fourth finger
17.34.   Resisted adduction of the second finger

Palpation

After the functional examination, palpation is again performed for swelling and local skin temperature. In addition, the lesion that has been diagnosed by the functional examination is palpated to localize the injury accurately.

Additional Examination in Limitations of Motion

If a limitation of motion in a noncapsular pattern has been found, the appropriate joint-specific translatory tests should be performed to determine whether the limitation is indeed caused by the capsule.

Additional Examination for Hypermobility

If instability is suspected, apprehension tests, in addition to joint-specific translatory tests, are sometimes needed to confirm the diagnosis. Manipulatively, but with little force, the affected carpal bone is moved in the direction of the probable instability.

Other Examinations

If necessary, other examinations also can be performed to confirm a diagnosis or to gain further information when a diagnosis cannot be reached on the basis of the functional examination. These include the following:

- imaging techniques such as conventional radiographs, computed tomography (CT) scan, arthrography, arthro-CT, magnetic resonance imaging (MRI), and ultrasonography
- laboratory tests
- arthroscopy
- electromyography (EMG)

DESCRIPTION OF THE FUNCTIONAL EXAMINATION

The various joints in the wrist-hand region are examined by means of active and passive motions as well as isometrically resisted tests.

Active Motions

Active motions are assessed to determine the amount and trajectory of motion. The range of motion is compared with that in the passive motion. Pain provocation is also noted.

Passive Motions

As with the active motions, the amount of motion found during the passive evaluation is compared with that in the active motion.

In limitations of the passive motions, distinction is made between capsular and noncapsular patterns. Limitations of passive motion in a capsular pattern indicate arthritis or arthrosis (osteoarthrosis). Determining

pain provocation and interpreting the end-feel are also of great importance.

Resisted Motions

Contractile structures are tested for strength and pain provocation by performing isometrically resisted tests.

Surrounding the wrist are numerous tendons protected by tendon sheaths. The tendon sheath is a noncontractile structure, which means that it is not assessed during isometric resistance. In a pathology of the tendon sheath, passive motions are more significant; in a tenosynovitis, pain is provoked by means of stretch. Only in instances of severe tendon sheath inflammation, in which there are adhesions between the tendon sheath and the tendon, can isometrically resisted tests provoke pain.

DISTAL RADIOULNAR JOINT

Active Motions

17.1. Active Forearm Pronation

The patient rotates both forearms inward, in the horizontal plane, as far as possible without moving the upper arms. With this test, particularly, the mobility of the distal radioulnar joint is tested.

Pain in the wrist region usually indicates a lesion in the distal radioulnar joint, particularly if the supination is also painful. Motion in the distal radioulnar joint is seldom limited.

17.2. Active Forearm Supination

The patient rotates both forearms outward, in the horizontal plane, as far as possible without moving the upper arms. As in Test 17.1, mobility of the distal radioulnar joint is tested specifically.

Pain in the wrist region usually indicates a lesion in the distal radioulnar joint, particularly if the pronation is also painful. Motion in the distal radioulnar joint is seldom limited.

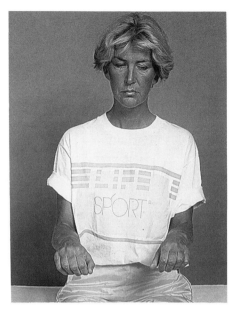

Test 17.1

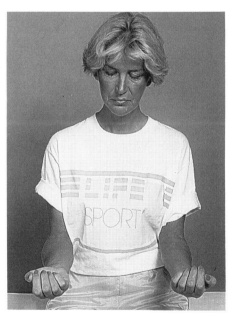

Test 17.2

A tenosynovitis of the extensor carpi ulnaris can cause pain during active and passive forearm supination.

Passive Motions

17.3. Passive Forearm Pronation

With the ipsilateral hand, the examiner grasps the radial side of the patient's forearm at the dorsal aspect, just proximal to the wrist. The other hand grasps the dorsal aspect of the patient's elbow.

The examiner moves the patient's forearm in pronation as far as possible. At the end of the motion, overpressure is exerted.

The range of motion is approximately 85°; the end-feel is rather firm.

Pain in the wrist region during passive pronation usually indicates a lesion in the distal radioulnar joint, particularly if the passive supination is also painful (capsular pattern). Motion in the distal radioulnar joint is seldom limited.

17.4. Passive Forearm Supination

With the ipsilateral hand, the examiner grasps the radial side of the patient's forearm at the volar aspect, just proximal to the wrist. The other hand grasps the dorsal aspect of the patient's elbow.

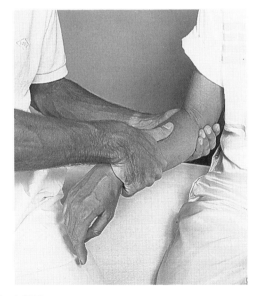

Test 17.3

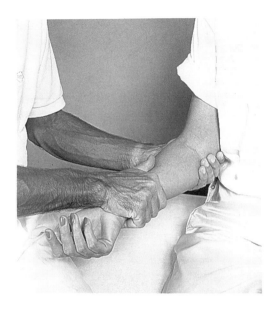

Test 17.4

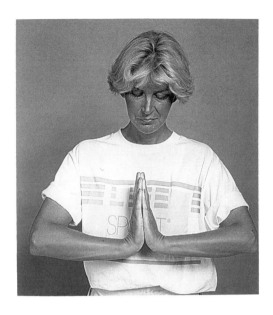

Test 17.5

The examiner moves the patient's forearm in supination as far as possible. At the end of the motion, overpressure is exerted.

Generally, the range of motion is approximately 90°; the end-feel is usually firmer than in passive pronation.

Pain in the wrist region during passive supination usually indicates a lesion in the distal radioulnar joint, particularly if the passive pronation is also painful (capsular pattern). Motion in the distal radioulnar joint is seldom limited.

A tenosynovitis of the extensor carpi ulnaris often causes pain during passive forearm supination, especially when the lesion is located at the level of the ulnar head.

WRIST

Active Motions

17.5. Active Supported Wrist Extension

The patient brings the volar side of both hands and fingers together and tries to bring both elbows as far as possible upward, without losing contact at the hands. In so doing, a general assessment is made about the wrist extension range of motion.

The range of motion is usually approximately 85° to 90°.

Pain or limitation of motion can have many causes, including the following:

- A ganglion at the level of the capitate usually causes painful and slightly limited extension.
- Instability of one of the carpal bones almost always causes pain in maximal flexion and/or extension.
- In limitations of motions in a capsular pattern, extension and flexion are equally limited and painful.

17.6. Active Supported Wrist Flexion

The patient places the dorsal sides of both hands and fingers against each other and attempts to bring the elbows as far as possible downward, without losing hand contact.

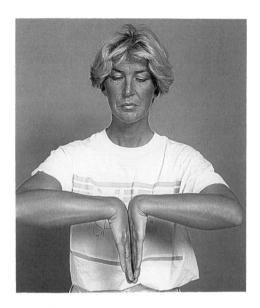

Test 17.6

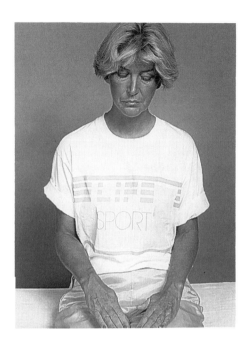

Test 17.7

Interpretation of pain or limitation of wrist flexion is, in many respects, the same as in Test 17.5. A ganglion can cause pain in flexion, but much less often causes a limitation of motion. If there is a lesion of the intercarpal ligaments (posttraumatic), passive wrist flexion is usually the most painful motion.

17.7. Active Radial Deviation

With the fingers together and the hands in line with the forearms, the patient attempts to move the fingers toward each other. In so doing, the mobility of the carpus is tested, and the ulnar carpal collateral ligament is stretched.

Limitation of motion and the presence of pain usually indicate a lesion of the carpus; pain without limitation of motion generally indicates a lesion of the ulnar collateral ligament.

17.8. Active Ulnar Deviation

With the fingers together and the hands in line with the forearms, the patient tries to move the fingers away from each other. Also here the mobility of the carpus is tested, but

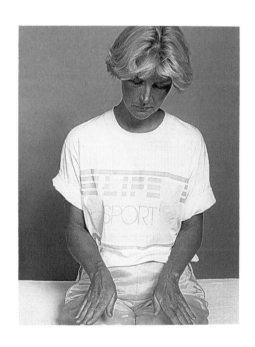

Test 17.8

in this instance, the radial carpal collateral ligament is stretched.

Limitation of motion and the presence of pain usually indicate a lesion of the carpus; pain without limitation of motion generally indicates a lesion of the radial collateral ligament.

Passive Motions

17.9. Passive Wrist Extension

With the ipsilateral hand, the examiner grasps the patient's hand, placing the fingers in the patient's palm. The patient's thumb rests between the examiner's thumb and index finger. With the other hand, the examiner grasps the patient's forearm just proximal to the wrist.

The examiner moves the patient's wrist as far in extension as possible. At the end of the motion, overpressure is exerted.

The end-feel is usually firm.

Interpretation of pain or limitation of motion is the same as described in Test 17.5.

17.10. Passive Wrist Flexion

Using the ipsilateral hand, the examiner grasps the patient's hand, with the fingers placed dorsally and the thumb placed volarly. With the other hand, the examiner grasps the patient's forearm just proximal to the wrist.

The examiner brings the patient's wrist as far as possible in flexion. At the end of the motion, overpressure is exerted.

The end-feel is usually firm.

Interpretation of pain or limitation of motion is the same as described in Test 17.6.

17.11. Passive Wrist Radial Deviation

With the ipsilateral hand, the thumb on the dorsum and the fingers on the volar aspect, the examiner grasps the patient's hand from the ulnar side. The examiner's index finger lies between the patient's index finger and thumb. With the other hand, the examiner grasps the patient's forearm at its dorsoradial aspect, just proximal to the wrist. The patient's wrist is in the neutral position.

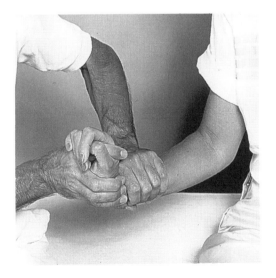

Test 17.9

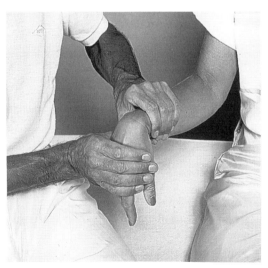

Test 17.10

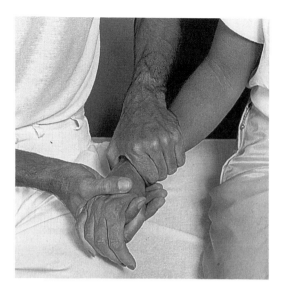

Test 17.11A

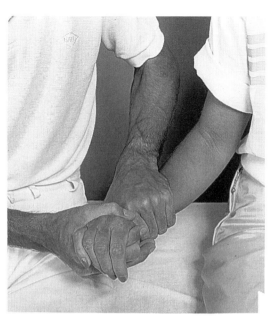

Test 17.11B Passive wrist radial deviation in slight extension.

The examiner moves the patient's hand in radial deviation as far as possible. At the end of the motion, overpressure is exerted.

The end-feel is usually firm. Interpretation of pain or limitation of motion is the same as described in Test 17.7.

In Test 17.11B, the examiner performs the same motion as described above, except that now the patient's wrist is first positioned in slight extension. At the end of the motion, overpressure is exerted. In so doing, specifically, the volar part of the ulnar carpal collateral ligament is tested. In addition, the tendon of the flexor carpi ulnaris is stretched.

In Test 17.11C, the examiner performs the same motion as described above, but now with the patient's wrist first positioned in slight flexion. In so doing, specifically, the dorsal part of the ulnar carpal collateral ligament is tested. In addition, the tendon sheath of the extensor carpi ulnaris is stretched.

17.12. Passive Wrist Ulnar Deviation

With the ipsilateral hand, the examiner grasps the patient's hand from the radial side of the second metacarpal; the thumb is placed

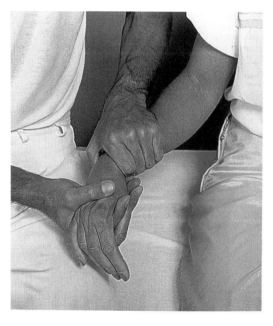

Test 17.11C Passive wrist radial deviation in slight flexion.

on the ulnar side of the patient's hand. The patient's wrist is in the neutral position. With the other hand, the examiner grasps the patient's forearm just proximal to the wrist.

The examiner moves the patient's hand in ulnar deviation as far as possible. At the end of the motion, the examiner exerts overpressure.

The end-feel is usually firm. The interpretation of pain or limitation of motion is the same as described in Test 17.8.

In Test 17.12B, the examiner performs the same motion as described above, but now the patient's wrist is first positioned in slight extension. In so doing, specifically, the volar part of the radial carpal collateral ligament is tested. In addition, the tendon sheath of the flexor carpi radialis is stretched.

In Test 17.12C, the examiner performs the same motion as described above, but now the patient's wrist is first positioned in slight flexion. In so doing, specifically, the dorsal part of the radial carpal collateral ligament is tested. In addition, the tendons and tendon sheaths of the extensors carpi radialis longus and brevis are stretched.

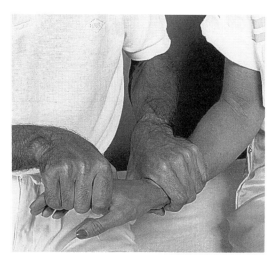

Test 17.12B Passive wrist ulnar deviation in slight extension.

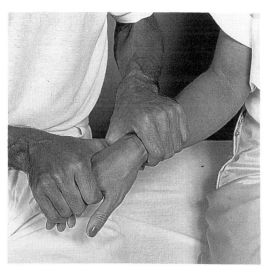

Test 17.12C Passive wrist ulnar deviation in slight flexion.

Resisted Motions

17.13. Resisted Wrist Extension with Radial Deviation

With the ipsilateral hand, the examiner grasps the patient's second metacarpal from

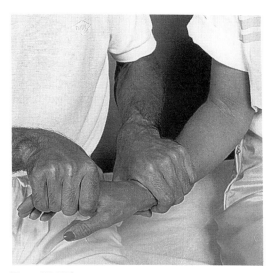

Test 17.12A

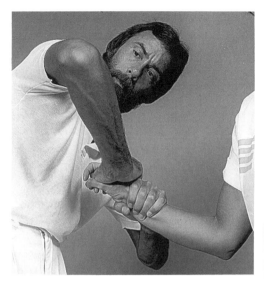

Test 17.13

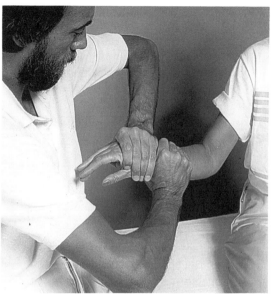

Test 17.14

the radial side. At the same time, the examiner's forearm is positioned in line with the direction of force. The examiner's elbow is higher than the hand.

With the other hand, just proximal to the wrist, the examiner fixes the patient's forearm; both of the examiner's forearms are in line with each other.

The patient's elbow is flexed 90°, and the dorsal aspect of the patient's forearm is in the horizontal plane.

The patient is asked to move the hand in the direction of the examiner's ipsilateral elbow. The examiner exerts isometric resistance.

In this test, the extensors carpi radialis longus and brevis are tested for strength and pain provocation.

17.14. Resisted Wrist Extension with Ulnar Deviation

With the contralateral hand, the examiner grasps the patient's hand (fifth metacarpal) from the ulnar side. At the same time, the examiner's forearm is positioned in line with

the direction of force. The examiner's elbow is higher than the hand. With the other hand, the examiner grasps the patient's forearm just proximal to the wrist. Both of the examiner's forearms are in line with each other.

The patient's elbow is flexed 90°, and the dorsal aspect of the forearm lies in the horizontal plane.

The patient is asked to move the hand in the direction of the examiner's contralateral elbow as the examiner exerts isometric resistance. In so doing, the extensor carpi ulnaris is tested for strength and pain provocation.

17.15. Resisted Wrist Flexion with Radial Deviation

With the ipsilateral hand, the examiner grasps the patient's second metacarpal from the radial side, whereby the examiner's forearm is positioned in line with the direction of force. The examiner's elbow is lower than the hand. With the other hand, the examiner fixes the patient's forearm, just proximal to the wrist; both of the examiner's forearms are in line with each other.

The patient's elbow is flexed 90°, and the dorsal aspect of the patient's forearm lies in the horizontal plane.

The patient is asked to move the hand in the direction of the examiner's ipsilateral elbow as the examiner exerts isometric resistance. The flexor carpi radialis is tested for strength and pain provocation.

17.16. Resisted Wrist Flexion with Ulnar Deviation

With the contralateral hand, the examiner grasps the patient's hand (fifth metacarpal) from the ulnar side, whereby the examiner's forearm is positioned in line with the direc-

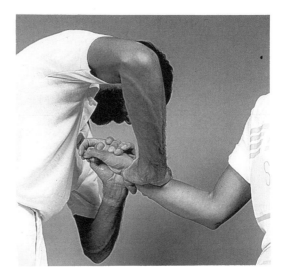

Test 17.16

tion of force. The examiner's elbow is lower than the hand. With the other hand, the examiner grasps the patient's forearm just proximal to the wrist. Both of the examiner's forearms are in line with each other.

The patient's elbow is flexed 90°, and the dorsal aspect of the forearm lies in the horizontal plane.

The patient is asked to move the hand in the direction of the examiner's contralateral elbow, while the examiner exerts isometric resistance. In so doing, the flexor carpi ulnaris is tested for strength and pain provocation.

THUMB

Active and Passive Motions

17.17. Active Thumb Retroposition

The patient places the volar aspects of both hands and fingers together, and brings the thumbs as far as possible in retroposition. In particular, the trapeziometacarpal I joint is tested.

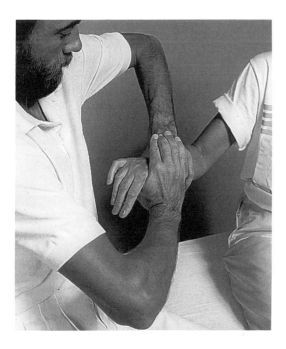

Test 17.15

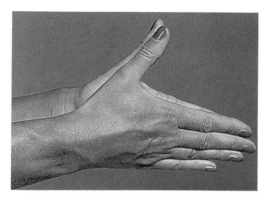

Test 17.17

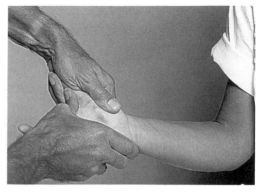

Test 17.18

A limitation of motion with pain is almost always due to an arthrosis or arthritis of the trapeziometacarpal I joint (capsular pattern).

17.18. Passive Thumb Retroposition

With the ipsilateral hand, the examiner grasps the patient's hand from the volar side; in essence, the examiner shakes the patient's hand. With the other hand, the examiner grasps metacarpal I between thumb (volar) and flexed index finger (dorsal), as close as possible to the carpometacarpal I joint.

The examiner then brings the thumb as far as possible into retroposition. At the end of the motion, overpressure is exerted.

A limitation of motion of the joint is almost always capsular, thus indicating arthritis or arthrosis. The normally firm end-feel is hardened.

The normal range of motion amounts to approximately 20° from the zero position.

Resisted Motions

17.19. Resisted Thumb Radial Abduction (Extension)

With the contralateral hand, the examiner grasps the patient's hand from the dorsal side in such a way that the distal phalanx of the examiner's thumb rests on the dorsal aspect

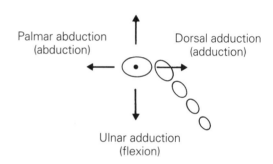

Diagram of Motions of the Thumb.

Radial abduction (extension)

Palmar abduction (abduction)

Dorsal adduction (adduction)

Ulnar adduction (flexion)

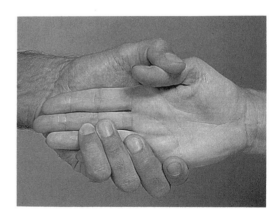

Test 17.19

of the interphalangeal joint of the patient's thumb. The patient's thumbnail should lie in the horizontal plane.

The patient tries to abduct (extend) the thumb radially while the examiner exerts isometric resistance. In so doing, the thumb extensors (extensors pollicis longus and brevis) are tested for strength and pain provocation.

Because resistance is exerted at the interphalangeal joint of the thumb, it is not possible to differentiate functionally between the two muscles.

17.20. Resisted Thumb Palmar Abduction (Abduction)

With the contralateral hand, the examiner grasps the patient's hand from the dorsal side in such a way that the distal phalanx of the examiner's thumb rests on the radial aspect of the interphalangeal joint of the patient's thumb. The patient's thumbnail should lie in the horizontal plane.

The patient tries to abduct the thumb palmarly while the examiner exerts isometric resistance. In so doing, the thumb abductors (pollicis longus and brevis) are tested for strength and pain provocation.

This test does not allow the examiner to differentiate between the abductor pollicis longus and the abductor pollicis brevis.

Note: The examiner can differentiate between these muscles by palpation. The insertion of the abductor pollicis longus is located just distal to the trapeziometacarpal I joint (brevis is rarely affected). Although the lesion may lie here, the functional examination is sometimes negative.

17.21. Resisted Thumb Dorsal Adduction (Adduction)

With the contralateral hand, the examiner grasps the patient's hand in such a way that the fingers are on the volar side and the thumb is on the dorsal side of the hand. The thumb of the other hand is placed between the patient's thumb and index finger.

The patient is asked to move the thumb toward the index finger while the examiner exerts isometric resistance. In so doing, the thumb adductors are tested for strength and pain provocation. The oblique head of the adductor pollicis is the most often affected, usually after an abduction trauma.

17.22. Resisted Thumb Ulnar Adduction (Flexion)

With the contralateral hand, the examiner grasps the patient's hand in such a way that the fingers are on the volar side and the thumb is on the dorsal side of the hand. The

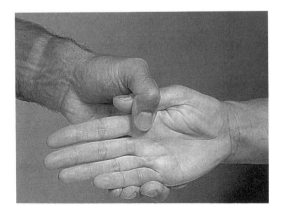

Test 17.20

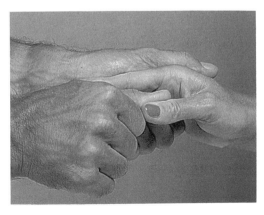

Test 17.21

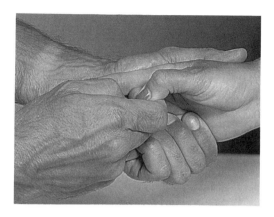

Test 17.22

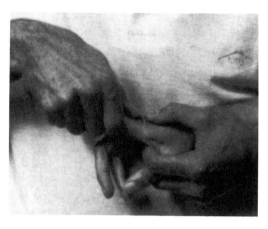

Test 17.23

examiner places the middle phalanx of the other hand's index finger against the volar aspect of the distal phalanx of the patient's thumb.

The patient is asked to flex the thumb while the examiner exerts isometric resistance. In so doing the thumb flexors are tested for strength and pain provocation. Of the flexors pollicis longus and brevis, sometimes only the longus is affected.

FINGERS

Passive Motions

17.23. Passive Metacarpophalangeal (MCP) Extension

With the ipsilateral hand, the examiner grasps the patient's proximal phalanx as close as possible to the MCP joint. The thumb is placed dorsally and the fingers are placed volarly on the phalanx. The examiner moves the MCP joint as far as possible into extension and exerts slight overpressure at the end of the motion.

The average range of motion in extension is between 30° and 45°. The end-feel is firm.

Lesions of these joints are usually caused by trauma or rheumatoid arthritis. In these

Range of motion: 30–45°
Firm end-feel

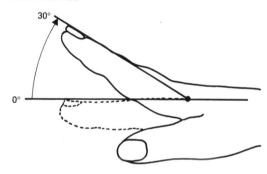

Diagram of movement in passive MCP extension.

instances, a capsular pattern of limitation is present; flexion is more limited than extension.

17.24. Passive Metacarpophalangeal Flexion

The examiner places the thumb of the ipsilateral hand on the dorsum of the patient's hand, just proximal to the MCP joint. The index finger, reinforced by the middle finger, is placed dorsally on the proximal phalanx, just distal to the MCP joint. The thumb (dorsal) and the fingers (volar) of the other hand fix the metacarpal bone. The examiner moves

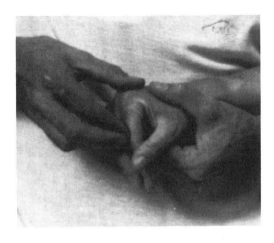

Test 17.24

Range of motion: 90°
Firm end-feel

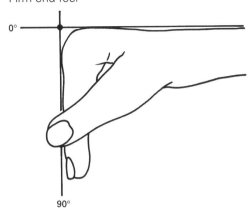

0°

90°

Diagram of movement in passive metacarpophalangeal flexion.

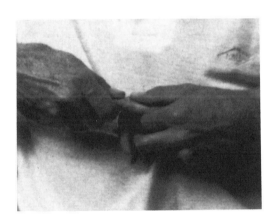

Test 17.25

Range of motion: 0–5°
Firm end-feel

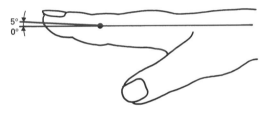

5°
0°

Diagram of movement in passive extension of
the PIP joints.

the MCP joint as far as possible into flexion,
and exerts slight overpressure at the end of
the motion.

The average range of motion in flexion is
approximately 90°. The end-feel is firm.

As mentioned in Test 17.23, lesions of
these joints are usually caused by trauma or
rheumatoid arthritis. In these instances, a
capsular pattern of limitation is present; flexion is more limited than extension.

17.25. Passive Extension of the Proximal Interphalangeal (PIP) Joints

With the ipsilateral hand, the examiner
grasps the patient's middle phalanx just distal
to the PIP joint; in so doing, the thumb is dorsal and the index finger is volar. The thumb
and index finger of the other hand fix the
proximal phalanx, just proximal to the PIP

joint. The examiner moves the PIP joint as far as possible into extension, and exerts slight overpressure at the end of the motion.

The average range of motion is 0° to 5°. The end-feel is very firm.

Lesions of these joints are usually caused by trauma or arthrosis, rheumatoid arthritis, or psoriatic arthritis. In these instances, there is a capsular pattern of limitation; flexion is more limited than extension.

17.26. Passive Flexion of the Proximal Interphalangeal (PIP) Joints

The thumb of the examiner's ipsilateral hand is placed just proximal to the PIP joint and the index finger, reinforced by the middle finger, just distal to the PIP joint. The thumb and the index finger of the other hand fix the proximal phalanx and metacarpal. The examiner moves the PIP joint as far as possible into flexion, exerting slight overpressure at the end of the motion.

The average range of motion is 100° to 120°. The end-feel is firm.

As mentioned in Test 17.25, lesions of these joints are usually caused by trauma or arthrosis, rheumatoid arthritis, or psoriatic arthritis. In these instances, there is a capsu-

lar pattern of limitation; flexion is more limited than extension.

17.27. Passive Extension of the Distal Interphalangeal (DIP) Joints

The thumb and index finger of the examiner's ipsilateral hand grasp the patient's distal phalanx just distal to the DIP joint. The thumb and index finger of the other hand fix the middle phalanx just proximal to the joint. The examiner moves the DIP joint as far as possible into extension, exerting slight overpressure at the end of the motion.

The average range of motion is 0° to 10°. The end-feel is very firm.

17.28. Passive Flexion of the Distal Interphalangeal (DIP) Joints

In order to test the passive flexion of the DIP joint, the PIP joint first must be flexed approximately 90°. The thumb and the index finger of the examiner's ipsilateral hand grasp proximal and distal to the DIP joint, respectively. The thumb and the index finger of the other hand fix the proximal phalanx and metacarpal. The examiner moves the DIP joint as far as possible into flexion, exerting slight overpressure at the end of the motion.

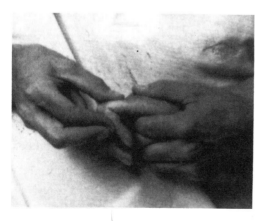

Test 17.26

Range of motion: 100–120°
Firm end-feel

0°

120°

Diagram of movement in passive flexion of the PIP joints.

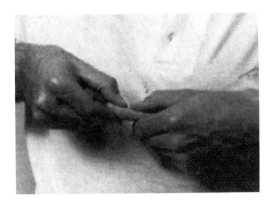

Test 17.27

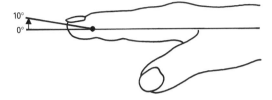

Range of motion: 0–10°
Hypertension
Firm end-feel

Test 17.27B Diagram of movement in passive extension of the DIP joints.

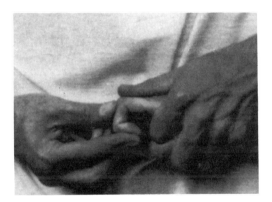

Test 17.28

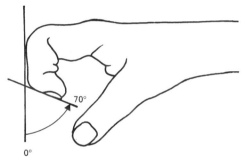

Range of motion: 70–90°
Firm end-feel

Diagram of movement in passive flexion of the DIP joints.

Resisted Motions

17.29. Resisted Abduction of the Second and Third Fingers

The patient holds the forearm pronated with the wrist in the neutral position. The fingers are extended and spread apart.

The examiner places the thumb and the index finger on the ulnar side of the third finger's DIP joint and on the radial side of the second finger's DIP joint, respectively. The patient is asked to move the index and middle fingers away from each other while the examiner exerts isometric resistance. In so doing, the dorsal interosseous muscles I and III are tested for strength and pain provocation.

Lesions of these muscles are rare.

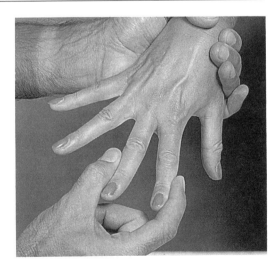

Test 17.29

Note: The placement of the fingers exerting isometric resistance is not actually anatomically correct for testing the interosseous muscles specifically. The "long lever" produced by this position, however, is the only way to test properly for pain provocation.

17.30. Resisted Abduction of the Third and Fourth Fingers

The positions of the patient and the examiner are essentially the same as those for Test 17.29, except that here resistance is given to the third and fourth fingers. In so doing, the dorsal interosseous II and IV muscles are tested for strength and pain provocation. See Test 17.29 for interpretation.

17.31. Resisted Abduction of the Fifth Finger

The position of the patient is the same as described in Test 17.29. The examiner exerts isometric resistance against the ulnar side of the little finger's DIP joint. In so doing, the abductor digiti minimi is tested for strength and pain provocation.

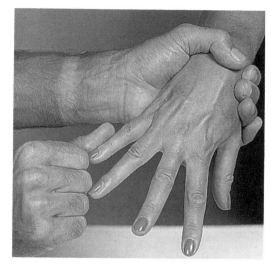

Test 17.31

17.32. Resisted Adduction of the Fifth Finger

The position of the patient is the same as described in Test 17.29. The examiner places the index finger against the radial side of the

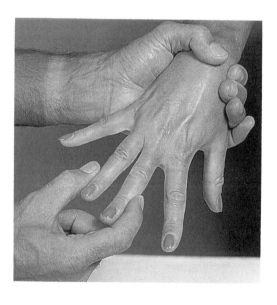

Test 17.30

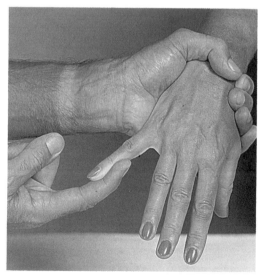

Test 17.32

little finger's DIP joint. The patient is asked to bring the little finger toward the middle finger while the examiner exerts isometric resistance. In so doing, the palmar interosseous III muscle is tested for strength and pain provocation.

Lesions of the palmar interossei are extremely rare.

17.33. Resisted Adduction of the Fourth Finger

The positions of the patient and the examiner are the same as in Test 17.32, but now isometric resistance is exerted against the ring finger. In so doing, the palmar interosseous II muscle is tested for strength

and pain provocation. See Test 17.32 for interpretation.

17.34. Resisted Adduction of the Second Finger

The position of the patient is the same as in Test 17.29.

The examiner places the tip of the index finger against the ulnar side of the patient's DIP joint. The patient is asked to move the index finger toward the middle finger while the examiner exerts isometric resistance. In so doing, the palmar interosseous I muscle is tested for strength and pain provocation. See Test 17.32 for interpretation.

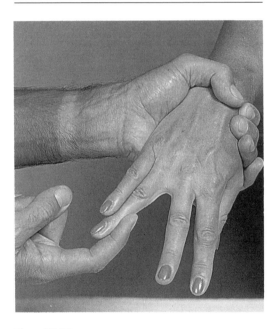

Test 17.33

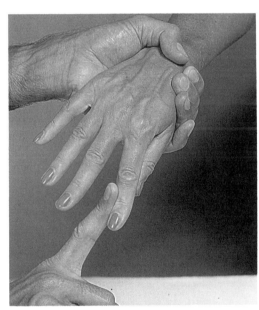

Test 17.34

18

Pathology of the Wrist

18.1 JOINT PATHOLOGY

PATHOLOGY WITH LIMITED MOTIONS IN A CAPSULAR PATTERN

Arthritis

Arthritis in General

In principle, every disease in which arthritides occur can cause an arthritis in the carpus; however, rheumatoid and traumatic arthritides are the most frequently seen.

Traumatic Arthritis

Local swelling occurs often, even after a mild trauma to the wrist. If the traumatic arthritis—pain, swelling, and limitation of motions—lasts longer than 1 week, one should expect a fracture of one of the carpal bones.

Clinical Findings. The patient complains of pain in the entire wrist region.

Functional Examination.

- Circular swelling is clearly visible.
- Active as well as passive flexion and extension of the wrist are painful and limited. Typically, the end-feel is caused by muscle spasm.

Treatment. Because it is almost impossible to rule out a carpal fracture in the first

several days after a trauma, the wrist should be immobilized, for the time being, in a sling. If the swelling and limitation of motion are still present after 1 week, the presence of a carpal fracture should be considered.

Nontraumatic Arthritis

Rheumatoid arthritis of the wrist is seen often. Many systemic diseases in which arthritides arise can also affect the wrist; however, this rarely happens.

In every limitation of motion that demonstrates a capsular pattern but does not have a traumatic or rheumatoid onset, laboratory testing should be performed.

Clinical Findings. There is gradual or sudden onset of a painful limitation of wrist motions in the capsular pattern.

Functional Examination.

- Both active and passive flexion and extension of the wrist are painful and limited (capsular pattern).
- In severe cases, various resisted tests are also painful when compression occurs in the joint.

Treatment. Treatment depends on the cause of the arthritis. In many cases, especially when oral medication does not provide adequate relief, an intra-articular injection is indicated.

Arthrosis (Osteoarthrosis)

Arthrosis of the wrist is usually the result of a previous severe trauma or chronic overuse, such as by persons whose work requires use of drills. Previous instances of infectious or rheumatoid disorders can also lead to arthrosis. In comparison with the incidence of arthrosis in the hip and knee joints, carpal arthrosis is much less common. Arthrotic changes are usually seen in the radial column, particularly between the radius and the scaphoid and between the trapezium and metacarpal I. The latter localization is discussed in Chapter 19, Pathology of the Midhand, Thumb, and Fingers.

Clinical Findings.
- In the early stages there is usually only a minimal limitation of motion. Often wrist movements are accompanied by crepitation.
- Pain arises in the later stages, when there are obvious limitations of motion in the capsular pattern with flexion and extension equally limited.
- Radiographs reveal the arthrotic changes, in which the often-seen cystic "bright spots" are particularly notable.

Treatment. Treatment is necessary when the patient complains of pain and, at the same time, synovial irritation of the joint is evident. Generally, the joint reacts very well to joint-specific mobilization. In addition, the most painful sites of the capsuloligamentous complex can be given injections of a corticosteroid in a dropwise fashion.

In some cases, for example, when there is extreme pain, a brace can be used to immobilize the wrist for several days or weeks.

Surgical arthrodesis is rarely indicated.

Fractures of the Carpal Bones

Although fractures are not discussed in this series of books, a short summary of the most frequently seen carpal fractures is discussed. A carpal fracture can be overlooked easily. In most cases, after what is apparently a minor trauma, a fracture is not visible on a radiograph. (Refer to Traumatic Arthritis.)

Fractures of the scaphoid are the most commonly seen carpal fractures; however, such diagnoses are missed frequently (Figure 18–1). Scaphoid fractures generally result from a fall on the extended wrist or, more rarely, from a fall on the hand with a flexed wrist. Direct force, such as a blow against the dorsum of the hand, can also cause a fracture. Fractures of the lunate, triquetrum, pisiform, capitate, and hamate are less common.

Clinical Findings

The patient often complains of a loss of strength in the hand.

Functional Examination

- The most classic finding of the scaphoid fracture is circumferential swelling around the wrist and tenderness to palpation in the anatomical snuffbox.
- The functional examination indicates a severe capsular pattern of limited motions and an extremely painful radial deviation. Axial compression through the thumb and index finger is painful.
- Directly after the trauma, the radiological examination is usually negative. Thus, radiographs should be repeated 8 to 10 days later.

Treatment

Treatment is generally conservative: immobilization in a cast for 10 to 16 weeks, depending on the location and type of fracture. Despite this, pseudoarthrosis develops in a number of cases (Figure 18–2).

PATHOLOGY WITH LIMITED MOTIONS IN A NONCAPSULAR PATTERN

Rupture of the Articular Carpal Disc

The articular disc is part of the triangular fibrocartilaginous (TFC) complex. Lesions of

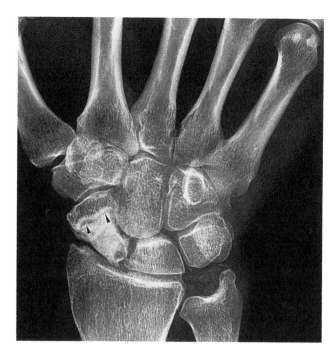

Figure 18–1 Conventional radiograph indicates the status after a scaphoid fracture. The fracture is still visible (***arrowheads***); there is necrosis of the proximal fragment. In addition, there is calcification of the soft tissue structures between the ulna and the triquetrum, as well as arthrosis of the radiocarpal joint.

the articular disc do not always involve a solitary structure. In such cases, each structure belonging to the TFC complex should be examined thoroughly.

Disc lesions can be the result of forceful repeated ulnar deviations that may occur in sports such as baseball and cricket.

The disc is even more vulnerable in the so-called positive ulna variant, a condition in which the ulna is relatively too long. This disorder is often accompanied by a rupture of the lunatotriquetral ligament.

Disc lesions can also be caused by the following:

- forced pronation and supination movements
- forced wrist extension combined with an axial working force
- forced wrist extension combined with forearm pronation

In certain sports, the motions listed above can lead to damage of the disc: basketball, volleyball, Olympic handball, water polo, tennis, gymnastics, boxing, and weight lifting.

Lesions of the disc are a well-known complication in most forearm fractures, and *always* occur in a dislocation of the distal radioulnar joint.

Clinical Findings

- Local swelling and pain are the most striking symptoms in fresh lesions.
- Making a fist is usually impossible because of pain. The patient has the feeling that the hand has lost strength.

Functional Examination

- Pronation and supination of the forearm, and particularly of the carpus, are pain-

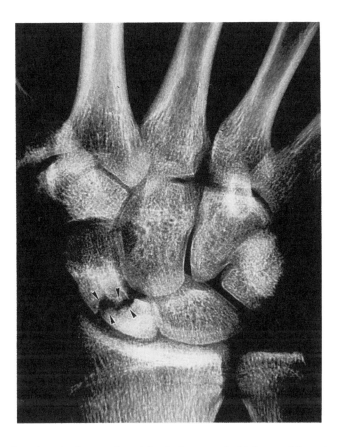

Figure 18–2 Pseudoarthrosis (**arrowheads**) of the scaphoid in an Olympic handball player. Conventional radiograph. This is the result of a fracture that went unrecognized.

ful and sometimes coupled with crepitation between the ulna and triquetral bone.

• Passive ulnar deviation and passive extension are sometimes painful; however, the combined motions of passive ulnar deviation, with either flexion or extension, are often the most painful tests.

• Arthrography and arthroscopy can help to confirm the diagnosis.

Treatment

The treatment of a symptomatic disc rupture generally is surgical. Currently the preferred method of treatment is arthroscopic disc resection.

In instances of a positive ulna variant, the ulna is shortened.

Lunatomalacia (Kienböck's Disease)

Lunatomalacia concerns an aseptic necrosis of the lunate based on a vascular disturbance of the bone. In this disorder, deformation of the lunate occurs easily, because bony tissue is replaced by fibrous tissue (Figure 18–3).

Kienböck's disease is seen particularly in adolescents, and more frequently in males.

Clinical Findings

The patient complains the most of pain at the dorsal aspect of the wrist, which can radiate proximally, sometimes to the elbow.

Functional Examination

Active and passive wrist extension is particularly limited and painful. The other wrist motions can also become limited after a while, or they may be only painful.

Treatment

Treatment consists of either immobilization (by means of a cast) or surgery.

LESIONS OF THE CAPSULOLIGAMENTOUS COMPLEX

Ligamentous Lesions without Instability

In this section, traumatic ligamentous sprains without subsequent clinical manifestations of instability are discussed. In principle, every carpal ligament can be sprained; however, lesions of the following five anatomical structures are seen most often:

1. dorsal intercarpal ligaments
2. radial carpal collateral ligament

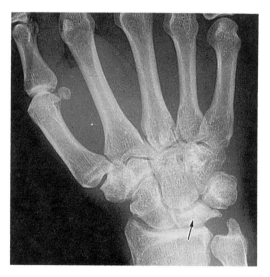

Figure 18–3 Conventional radiograph of lunatomalacia. The lunate is severely deformed (**arrow**).

3. ulnar carpal collateral ligament
4. lunatotriquetral ligament
5. pisiform-triquetral ligament

Dorsal Intercarpal Ligaments

A sprain of the dorsal intercarpal ligaments occurs especially as the result of a flexion trauma of the wrist. Usually, part of the ligamentous complex between the scaphoid and trapezium on one side and the triquetrum, lunate, and capitate on the other side are involved. The capitate-metacarpal III connections can also be sprained, often in combination with the just-mentioned lesions.

Chronic ligamentous stress can lead to a local synovitis. Because most of the dorsal ligaments are reinforcers of the joint capsule, traction osteophytes sometimes arise. This is particularly common with the scaphoid and lunate, which can compress against the radius during wrist extension. The result is an inflammatory reaction of the "pinched" soft tissue structures. (See also Carpal Boss [Carpe Bossu, Carpometacarpal Boss, Thrower's Wrist].)

Clinical Findings. The patient complains of local pain at the dorsal aspect of the wrist. Occasionally, in chronic cases, there is visible swelling due to the presence of osteophytes and the local soft tissue reaction.

Functional Examination. Passive wrist flexion is the most painful motion. If osteophytes are present, passive extension is also painful.

Treatment. Almost all uncomplicated sprains respond very well to local treatment of transverse friction. If there is a local synovitis, injection with a corticosteroid is indicated. Osteophytes may eventually have to be excised surgically.

Radial Carpal Collateral Ligament

Sprains of the radial carpal collateral ligament occur as the result of an ulnar deviation moment. Although a pure ulnar deviation trauma is rare, sprains generally occur during a combination trauma in which the wrist is in either flexion or extension with forced ulnar deviation. The result is a sprain of the dorsal or volar part of the ligament.

Clinical Findings. The patient complains of local pain at the radial aspect of the wrist.

Functional Examination.
- Depending on the trauma, passive ulnar deviation in slight wrist flexion or extension is the most painful motion.
- By palpation, the site of the lesion is located as precisely as possible. Predilection sites are the origin of the ligament on the radial styloid process and the insertion on the scaphoid.

Treatment. Transverse friction is usually very effective. The therapist should exercise caution regarding the cutaneous branches of the radial nerve and artery, which run through the anatomical snuffbox.

In those rare cases where therapy is not effective, a very small amount of corticosteroid can be injected, with utmost care taken to avoid the neurovascular structures.

Ulnar Carpal Collateral Ligament

Sprain of the ulnar carpal collateral ligament occurs as the result of a radial deviation trauma. This usually occurs in combination with flexion or extension of the wrist, during which the dorsal or volar parts of the ligament are injured. The lesion is frequently seen after a Colles fracture and after fractures of the ulnar styloid process.

During the functional examination, it should be kept in mind that this ligament is part of the TFC complex, and that lesions of other structures in the complex may also have occurred.

Clinical Findings. The patient complains of local pain at the ulnar aspect of the wrist.

Functional Examination.
- Passive radial deviation of the wrist is painful. By repeating the test in slight flexion and extension of the wrist, the dorsal and volar parts of the ligament can be differentiated.
- Using palpation, the therapist locates the site of the lesion as precisely as possible. Predilection sites are the origin of the ligament at the ulnar styloid process and the attachment at the triquetrum.

Treatment. Treatment of transverse friction is generally very effective, even in chronic cases. In those rare cases when therapy is not satisfactory, a small amount of corticosteroid can be injected.

Lunatotriquetral Ligament

Sprain of the lunatotriquetral ligament is almost always the result of a flexion trauma of the wrist with an accompanying radial deviation component. The lesion is seldom an isolated injury. Generally, the dorsal intercarpal ligaments are also affected, as well as the ulnar carpal collateral ligament, with or without a lesion of one of the other structures of the TFC complex.

Clinical Findings. The patient complains of local pain at the dorsoulnar aspect of the wrist. In instances of a complete tear, there is a subjective loss of strength and in many cases a click is experienced during some of the wrist movements.

Functional Examination.
- Passive wrist flexion, combined with radial deviation, is the most painful motion.
- Joint-specific translatory testing between the lunate and triquetrum is painful. In cases of a complete tear, a painful click can occur.

Treatment. In instances of an isolated sprain, transverse friction is very effective. If there is a complete tear, conservative treatment with a brace can be tried. In many cases, surgery is eventually required.

Pisiform-Triquetral Ligament

Sprains of the pisiform-triquetral ligament are usually the result of a direct trauma, such as a fall. Repeated trauma from sports or activities, such as karate, can also lead to problems with this ligament. Sometimes a tennis racket with a grip that is too thick is responsible for the lesion.

Sprains of the pisiform-triquetral ligament almost always cause a traumatic arthritis of the pisiformis joint, which is located between the pisiform and the triquetrum.

Differential Diagnosis.

- Insertion tendopathy of the flexor carpi ulnaris
- Lesion of one of the structures from the TFC complex

Clinical Findings. The patient complains of local pain at the volar aspect of the carpus at the level of the base of the hypothenar eminence. Pain is provoked during all motions in which the flexor carpi ulnaris is active.

Functional Examination. Passive wrist extension combined with radial deviation is painful. Resisted wrist flexion combined with ulnar deviation is painful. Pain and sometimes crepitation occur during passive translatory movement of the pisiform in relation to the triquetrum.

Treatment. The only effective treatment known is injection of a corticosteroid. If this therapy is not satisfactory, surgical removal of the pisiform, or fusion, is indicated.

Carpal Instability

The connection between the capitate and lunate is the weakest link in the wrist. Stability of the joint is provided by the following ligaments: (1) palmar ligaments between radius and capitate and (2) palmar ligament between capitate and triquetrum. The palmar radiocapitate ligament is the primary stabilizer of the distal carpal row in relation to the proximal carpal row. This ligament also connects the capitate and hamate. Every situation in which the tension in this ligament is decreased predisposes the capitate-lunate to a symptomatic instability.

The cause of an instability is often traumatic; one of these ligaments can be torn partially or completely, especially after a fracture of the distal radius or radial styloid process. As the result of a hyperextension trauma of the wrist, a sprain can also occur.

Poier's space (the triangle formed by the palmar ligaments between radius-capitate, radius-lunate-triquetrum, and capitate-triquetrum) is a weak point in the floor of the carpal tunnel.

Compared with the palmar ligaments, the dorsal radiocarpal ligaments are much thinner and weaker. They originate on the radius and insert on the lunate, triquetrum, and hamate; they are reinforced by the compartments of the finger extensor tendons.

Stability of the carpus is further enhanced by (1) the complex, multifaceted form of the articular surfaces of the carpal bones, (2) the capsuloligamentous complex, and (3) the wrist flexor and extensor tendons.

As mentioned, trauma is a common cause of carpal instability. Motor vehicle accidents and falls against the wrist are the most common traumas. All other causes are much less frequent. Of significance is the fall on the outstretched arm whereby the peak force acts on the thenar or hypothenar eminence. In this instance, a bony lesion (carpal fracture) often occurs as well.

Predisposing factors for wrist instability include the following:

- congenital general laxity
- neurological lesions in which there are deficits of the wrist flexors or extensors
- rheumatoid arthritis
- chronic microtraumata (prolonged stretch of the carpal

capsuloligamentous complex, seen in gymnasts, weight lifters, and boxers), leading to carpal instability.

Instability of the carpus is seen most often in the central column, less often in the radial column, and occasionally in the ulnar column. Injury to the ulnar column usually causes damage to the articular disc, and often to the distal radioulnar joint as well.

Because of the weak dorsal capsuloligamentous complex, dorsal instabilities are seen much more often than volar instabilities. If one or both of the carpal collateral ligaments rupture, lateral instability can also occur.

Taleisnik[10] makes a distinction between *static* and *dynamic* forms of carpal instability as the result of ligamentous laxity. The static form concerns permanent changes in the position of the carpal bones, which can be clearly diagnosed by radiographs. The dynamic form involves only abnormal intercarpal movements that occur during certain forced hand positions. This is difficult, if not impossible, to establish by radiography.

According to Dobyns et al.,[11] instability can be categorized into two main groups: *dissociative* (with widening between the concerned carpal bones) and *nondissociative*. Dissociative carpal instability is the result of ruptures of the intrinsic ligaments in the proximal row, particularly between the scaphoid and the lunate or between the lunate and the triquetrum. A scapholunate dissociation usually leads to a dorsal intercalated-segmental instability (DISI). Should a lunatotriquetrum dissociation occur, a volar intercalated-segmental instability (VISI) can result. In the nondissociative carpal instability, the intrinsic ligaments are intact.

Dynamic instability is frequently seen between the scaphoid and the lunate, less often between the lunate and the triquetrum, and least often between both carpal rows in the midcarpal joint.

Taleisnik[12] differentiates among instabilities according to their anatomical location:

- *lateral instability*, the most often seen, between the scaphoid and the lunate (Note that this lateral instability does not represent a lesion of the collateral ligament, which has little function in stabilization of the carpus.)
- *medial instability*, between the triquetrum and the hamate or the lunate (midcarpal instability)
- *proximal instability*, which is seen when an abnormal carpal alignment is a secondary result of a radius lesion or a massive radiocarpal rupture (ie, dorsal carpal subluxation, midcarpal instability as the result of poor healing of the distal part of the radius, or ulnar carpal shift).

Clinical Findings

- After a trauma, the patient complains of difficulties in the grasping function, for example, when lifting a heavy book or handling a tennis racket with one hand.
- Often there is chronic, vague pain in the wrist region of a more local character (radial or dorsal at the level of the distal radioulnar joint).
- During some motions, the patient experiences severe shooting pain in the wrist, sometimes coupled with "electric current" sensations and a paralyzed feeling: the "dead hand" syndrome.
- Sometimes a click is felt or heard during certain wrist motions.

Functional Examination

Findings in the functional examination depend on the severity of the instability and the clinical stage:

- Directly after a trauma, there is usually a significant capsular pattern of limited wrist motions (steps should be taken to rule out carpal fractures).

- In instances of chronic instability, the functional examination is often completely negative; only the apprehension test is positive.

Apprehension Test

The goal of the apprehension test is to force the carpal bones to move in the direction of the instability. Because the DISI is the most common form of instability, the test initially is directed toward causing a volar translation of the lunate, which occurs when the lunate moves in dorsal extension. In principle, this test can be performed for all of the carpal bones. In practice, however, the test is performed only with the lunate and the capitate, forcing them volarly.

Performance. With one hand, the examiner holds the patient's hand in the resting position (slight palmar flexion and ulnar deviation). The thumb of the other hand, reinforced by the other thumb, is placed against the dorsal aspect of the carpal bone being tested. Through a manipulative thrust, the carpal bone is moved volarly.

Assessment. The apprehension test is positive when the patient's "shooting" or "paralyzing" pain is provoked.

In addition to a positive apprehension test, and depending on the severity of the problem, the examiner can expect to see some or all of the following symptoms:

- A noncapsular pattern of limited motion(s) is present (usually the extension is limited with a pathological endfeel).
- A capsular pattern with pain is present as the result of a traumatic arthritis induced by poor control of carpal motions.
- A painful "click" occurs during one or more of the passive wrist motions. For instance, the passive radial deviation can produce a painful click at the ulnar side of the wrist, indicating an instability in the ulnar column (often between the tri-

quetrum and the hamate). A click produced at the ulnar side of the wrist during passive radiocarpal pronation usually indicates a lesion of the TFC complex.
- Shooting pain and the "dead hand" syndrome occur during the resisted wrist or thumb tests.

The joint-specific translatory tests generally demonstrate increased range of motion (particularly between scaphoid and lunate and lunate and triquetrum), during which a painful click of one of the carpal bones can also occur.

In some cases there are signs of irritation of the median nerve. Panting[13] saw median nerve lesions in 24 of 61 patients who had just suffered acute lunate dislocations. Occasionally, irritation of the radial nerve occurs.

Palpation for Tenderness. Sometimes there is tenderness at the joint space of the affected region (radiocarpal, midcarpal, or intercarpal).

Radiological Examination. In instances of a static instability, radiological examination is the most important diagnostic procedure. The current imaging techniques are as follows:
- anterior-posterior, lateral and oblique-lateral views
- functional views
  1. anteroposterior: in maximal radial deviation and maximal ulnar deviation
  2. lateral: in maximal extension and maximal flexion
- roentgen fluoroscopy, during which the above-described apprehension test is performed.

Treatment

If necessary—in limitations of motion due to a dislocation or subluxation—the appropriate repositioning manipulation can be performed. If the dislocation or subluxation immediately recurs during subsequent active motions, surgery is indicated.

Transverse friction can be applied to the affected ligaments to relieve pain.

Sometimes surgical treatment is unavoidable. In static instability, an intercarpal fusion is usually performed; in dynamic instability (often chronic), a ligamentous reconstruction is performed.[14]

A stabilizing brace is almost always indicated. First the brace is worn constantly, then tape is used, and later an elastic bandage can be applied. However, during vigorous activities (sports or activities requiring repeated firm grasping), the brace should be worn.

Dynamic stabilization exercises (initially performed with the brace on) can include the following:

- isometric
- isometric in the functional wrist patterns
- alternating concentric eccentric
- proprioceptive neuromuscular fascilitation patterns (particularly those in relation to grip function)

Strengthening and endurance exercises for the finger extensors and particularly the flexors should be performed. Instabilities in the central column are frequently found, because almost all of the compressive forces are guided through this column. Thus, initially, exercises should be performed in such a way that a pull is put on the carpus. An example would be for the patient to hang with the fingertips grasping a chin-up bar. In so doing, the compressive force of the exercise is neutralized by the pull of the body weight.

After both surgery and conservative treatment, therapy should be aimed at improving the "supportive" function of the wrist. Thus, stabilization exercises are performed during which the hand is engaged in slight supportive (weight-bearing) activities. These should first be done with the hand in the neutral position and later in various positions, gradually increasing to exercises in which the hand is maximally loaded.

Proprioceptive training for the supportive function of the wrist should also be part of the rehabilitation program. Such training can be done by using a handle that has been affixed to a balance board. The patient grasps the handle with the affected hand, holding the wrist in the neutral position, and exercises by trying to prevent the board from tipping. This exercise initially should be performed with the eyes open; later, with the eyes closed.

18.2 PATHOLOGY OF THE MUSCLE-TENDON UNIT

The disorders described in the following section are usually the result of relative overuse. In all of these disorders, the primary cause for the onset of the problem should be determined and, if possible, alleviated.

Many factors can lead to chronic overuse. For physicians and physical therapists, it is not always possible to trace the cause of the lesion, which is often biomechanical. Particularly in cases involving athletes, help should be obtained from experts, such as a trainer or a coach. For instance, an expert may be needed to assess a condition wherein string tension in a tennis racket is either too high or too low, leading to a tendopathy or tenosynovitis at the wrist. Advice may be needed to determine whether the grip of the racket handle is too thick or too thin, or whether improper technique is used when hitting the ball.

To prevent recurrent problems, causes must be identified and eliminated or, depending on the clinical stage, the activities provoking the wrist symptoms may have to be restricted.

TENDOPATHY OF THE EXTENSORS CARPI RADIALIS LONGUS AND BREVIS

The extensors carpi radialis longus and brevis are affected at the elbow much more frequently than at the wrist.

In racket sports the lesions at the wrist are almost always the result of poor technique, particularly when the player grasps the racket too forcefully during wrist extension. Lesions of these muscles are also seen in individuals who participate in fencing, canoeing, gymnastics, shot put, and weight lifting.

Sometimes problems are not caused by repeated contractions, but rather by chronic overstretching of the insertions.

Differential Diagnosis

- Carpal boss
- Ganglion
- Carpal instability

Clinical Findings

The patient complains of local pain at the dorsal aspect of the wrist.

Functional Examination

- In the functional examination, resisted wrist extension combined with radial deviation is the most painful test.
- Passive wrist flexion is often painful due to the subsequent stretch.

Treatment

Treatment is primarily causal. In addition, transverse friction and stretching exercises are usually very effective. Treatment should be given three to five times per week; generally 6 to 12 sessions are required to achieve full recovery.

In stubborn cases, the insertion(s) can be injected with a very small amount of corticosteroid. It is rarely necessary to administer more than two injections.

LESIONS OF THE EXTENSOR CARPI ULNARIS

The tendon of the extensor carpi ulnaris is loaded primarily in motions involving pronation with wrist extension and ulnar deviation. Such movements are made in tennis, for instance, when performing a topspin backhand.

Tendopathy

Tendopathies of the extensor carpi ulnaris usually occur at its insertion on the base of metacarpal V. Sometimes a tendinitis can occur just proximal to the insertion.

Differential Diagnosis

- Lesion of the TFC complex
- Sprain of the ulnar carpal collateral ligament
- Triquetrum-hamate compression syndrome

Clinical Findings

The patient complains of local pain at the ulnar side of the wrist.

Functional Examination

- Resisted wrist extension combined with ulnar deviation is painful. Passive flexion combined with radial deviation can be painful due to stretch.
- The exact site of the lesion is determined through palpation.

Treatment

Treatment is primarily causal, if possible. Transverse friction is usually very effective as local therapy.

In stubborn cases, the insertion can be injected with a very small amount of corticosteroid. Injection into the tendon itself is always contraindicated.

Tenosynovitis

An extensor carpi ulnaris tenosynovitis is usually located at one of two sites: (1) just distal to the ulnar head or (2) just proximal to the ulnar head.

Particularly in tennis players, and in females more often than in males, the lesion is located just proximal to the ulnar styloid process.

In rheumatoid arthritis, and in rare cases as the result of tuberculosis, a severe crepitating synovitis can occur.

Clinical Findings

The patient complains of pain at the ulnar or dorsoulnar aspect of the wrist.

Functional Examination

- If the lesion is localized just distal to the ulnar head, passive stretch (slight wrist flexion with maximal radial deviation) is the most painful test. If the lesion is just proximal to the ulnar head, passive forearm supination, in particular, is very painful.
- In severe cases, pain is also provoked during the resisted test (wrist extension with ulnar deviation), but generally only in the rheumatoid variant.

Treatment

Treatment is primarily causal. In tennis players, the pain-provoking stroke should be avoided. If necessary, the wrist can be taped appropriately to prevent maximal supination or pronation.

Transverse friction is usually effective, except in cases of crepitating rheumatoid or tuberculosis lesions.

In therapy-resistant cases, 0.5 mL of corticosteroid can be injected between the tendon and the tendon sheath. This injection, combined with a temporary reduction in activities, is usually very effective.

Dislocation

The tendon of the extensor carpi ulnaris can dislocate or subluxate from its fibroosseous tunnel as the result of strong forceful forearm supination with radial deviation of the wrist. This lesion is seen particularly in patients who play tennis, golf, baseball, or softball. Another possible cause for a dislocation or subluxation is the topspin backhand in tennis described earlier.

Clinical Findings

- There is a palpable and visible subluxation or dislocation of the tendon during active supination. During active pronation, the tendon generally clicks back into place again. This click is often audible. These active motions can be very painful.
- In passive pronation and supination, the symptoms are usually much less severe.

Treatment

After an acute dislocation, an immobilizing brace is usually worn for several weeks. The brace is usually applied with the forearm in pronation and the wrist in slight extension and ulnar deviation.

In a later phase, the use of a brace or taping is recommended during all sports activities requiring forearm rotation.

Surgery is indicated in cases of chronic dislocation and in recurring (symptomatic) dislocation when immobilization is not effective.

TENOSYNOVITIS OF THE EXTENSOR INDICIS

Extensor indicis tenosynovitis is an overuse lesion affecting the tendon at the dorsal aspect of the wrist where it runs together with the tendons of the extensor digitorum in the fourth extensor tunnel. The lesion is seen particularly in athletes who engage in crosscountry skiing, tennis, golf, or rowing.

A second location for this lesion is the tendon sheath at the level of the second metacarpophalangeal joint. Lesions at this site are seen almost exclusively in cross-country skiers whose sport is seasonally dependent. In cross-country skiing, the fingers are extended immediately after the push-off. In the normal diagonal stride, this occurs several hundred times per kilometer. If this movement is not performed throughout the entire year (such as in roller skiing), an overuse syndrome can occur easily.

Clinical Findings

- The patient is able to locate the pain precisely.
- In many instances, there is palpable crepitation during active movements.

Functional Examination

- Passive wrist flexion with simultaneous passive flexion of the index finger is the most painful test.
- In a tenosynovitis at the level of the metacarpophalangeal II joint, there can be adhesions from the tendon sheath to the surrounding subcutaneous tissue. This is always accompanied by obvious crepitation. In this instance, resisted extension of the index finger is also painful.

Treatment

Causal treatment of an extensor indicis tenosynovitis consists of better preparation before the onset of the seasonal sports activity. Thus, the patient should be given thorough information about the nature and cause of the lesion and instructed in preventive measures and exercises.

If the lesion is localized at the level of the wrist, daily transverse friction is very effective in most instances. Usually six to eight treatment sessions are required to achieve complete relief of pain.

In a tenosynovitis at the level of the MCP II joint, transverse friction is not very effective.

This lesion is best treated with an injection between the tendon and the tendon sheath, followed by 2 or 3 days of rest, during which the afflicted part is excluded from all activities.

TENOSYNOVITIS OF THE FLEXOR DIGITORUM PROFUNDUS

A tenosynovitis of the flexor digitorum profundus is seen most frequently in patients who do seasonal horticultural-type work and in cyclists who, during a vacation, ride in the mountains and thus make frequent use of the hand brakes. It is also a typical lesion in persons who participate in motocross events.

The typical site is just proximal to the volar wrist crease. The painful region usually extends to a length of approximately 4 cm.

As a complication, a carpal tunnel syndrome can arise.

As with the wrist extensor tendons, rheumatoid and tuberculotic tenosynovitides also can affect the flexor tendons.

Clinical Findings

The patient complains of pain at the volar aspect of the wrist, usually radiating proximally, rarely distally. If there is also a carpal tunnel syndrome, the patient will also complain of paresthesia in the hand.

Functional Examination

- Passive stretch is almost always more painful than contraction; passive wrist extension with simultaneous finger extension is usually the most painful test.
- Only in severe cases is resisted wrist flexion with simultaneous finger flexion painful.

Treatment

Along with causal treatment based on information regarding the source of the lesion, transverse friction should be tried. Because of the difficulty in reaching the tendons, however, this treatment is not always successful. In this instance, or in recurrent problems, an injection of 1 mL of corticosteroid between the tendon and the tendon sheath is the treatment of choice. Caution must be taken to avoid the median nerve.

Treatment can be enhanced by use of a brace, which limits extension and flexion motions in the wrist.

LESIONS OF THE FLEXOR CARPI RADIALIS

Lesions of the flexor carpi radialis are particularly common among tennis players, golfers, rowers, and canoeists. Motions leading to overuse include repeated palmar flexion of the wrist against resistance, as well as pronation and supination motions of the palmarly flexed wrist.

There are two predilection sites: (1) the teno-osseous insertion, at the level of the volar aspect of the base of metacarpal II (insertion tendopathy), and (2) the tendon sheath, at the volar aspect of the carpus (tenosynovitis).

Clinical Findings

The patient complains of local pain at the volar aspect of the wrist.

Functional Examination

- An insertion tendopathy is suspected more when pain is provoked during the resisted test (flexion with simultaneous radial deviation of the wrist) than during the stretch test (extension with simultaneously performed ulnar deviation of the wrist).
- In a tenosynovitis, distinctly the opposite is the case: the stretch test is more painful than the resisted test.

Treatment

Transverse friction is usually very effective. Occasionally it is necessary to inject the insertion with 0.5 mL of corticosteroid.

If it is necessary to inject a tenosynovitis, the corticosteroid is deposited between the tendon and the tendon sheath.

INSERTION TENDOPATHY OF THE FLEXOR CARPI ULNARIS

A flexor carpi ulnaris insertion tendopathy is almost always caused by repeated forceful ulnar deviation of the palmarly flexed wrist. Sometimes repeated forced stretch on the tendon leads to the disorder.

The lesion is usually sports related and is seen particularly in patients who engage in tennis, golf, rowing, or canoeing. High divers can also develop an insertion tendopathy if the water is contacted with the wrists in maximal extension.

There are three predilection sites: (1) proximal insertion on the pisiform, (2) distal insertion on the pisiform, and (3) insertion on the base of the fifth metacarpal.

Differential Diagnosis

- Distortion of the pisiform joint

Clinical Findings

The patient complains of pain on the volar-ulnar side of the wrist.

Functional Examination

The resisted test (resisted flexion with simultaneously performed ulnar deviation of the wrist) is more painful than the stretch test (passive wrist extension with simultaneously performed radial deviation).

Treatment

Our experiences with transverse friction and stretching exercises have been very good. Usually four to six daily treatment sessions are necessary to achieve complete recovery.

An injection of a corticosteroid is rarely indicated.

MYOTENOSYNOVITIS OF THE ABDUCTOR POLLICIS LONGUS, EXTENSOR POLLICIS BREVIS, AND EXTENSOR POLLICIS LONGUS

A myotenosynovitis (abductor pollicis longus bursitis, Wood's bursitis, intersection syndrome of the forearm) is a typical overuse lesion of the wrist extensors on the radial side. The tendons of the abductor pollicis longus and extensor pollicis brevis cross the tendons of the extensors carpi radialis longus and brevis just proximal to the extensor retinaculum. Sometimes, a small bursa (Wood's bursa) is found between these tendons.

It is not clear whether this lesion involves synovial irritation of the proximal continuation of the tendon sheaths or a true bursitis.

The lesion is seen particularly as the result of vigorous gardening.

In principle, the lesion is found in persons who get into and out of condition for certain kinds of sports or activities requiring repeated forceful wrist extension. Before 1975, the lesion was much more common because at that time tennis was still typically a summer sport. At the beginning of the tennis season, overuse occurred. Presently tennis is played the whole year through, and this lesion is seen much less frequently. Thus, if the person is not used to performing certain motions at a particular time, like the beginning of the season, he or she is at risk of doing damage. If the activity is done gradually, however, or for long periods of time, conditioning prevents harm.

Other sports in which this syndrome is seen include rowing, canoeing, and weight lifting.

Differential Diagnosis

- De Quervain syndrome

Clinical Findings

The patient complains of local pain and swelling approximately 4 cm proximal to Lister's tubercle.

Functional Examination

- Passive wrist flexion is painful because of stretch. The resisted tests generally are negative.
- Finkelstein's test will usually provoke pain, particularly when performed with the wrist in flexion.

Treatment

The patient should be given thorough information about what may be causing the lesion and how to prevent it from recurring.

Transverse friction is a very effective local treatment. During the first treatments there is often some increase in the symptoms. The patient should be warned about this. After three or four treatments, there is usually a significant reduction of pain. In the third week, the symptoms have usually completely disappeared.

Without treatment, the lesion will heal on its own in 6 to 8 weeks.

LESIONS OF THE ABDUCTOR POLLICIS LONGUS AND EXTENSOR POLLICIS BREVIS

The abductor pollicis longus and extensor pollicis brevis run together through the first extensor tunnel on the dorsal side of the wrist. Unfortunately, because of the location of this extensor tunnel, the tendons and the tendon sheath can be injured easily as a result of trauma. Another unfavorable factor is the rather sharp change in the angle of pull of the tendons—proximal to the radial styloid process, the tendons run in a proximoulnar direction.

It is interesting to note the variation in anatomy of the abductor pollicis longus tendon: In more than 50% of all individuals, there is an accessory tendon of the abductor pollicis longus. In approximately 20%, the tendons within the tendon sheath are separated by a fibrous wall, and in approximately 30%, each tendon has its own sheath.

Causes of pathology in this region are as follows:

- movements of the wrist (particularly extension or flexion combined with ulnar deviation) with the thumb fixed in a firm grip (for example, ringtoss, racket sports, and canoeing)
- repeated active muscle contractions
- acute and chronic punching trauma
- sometimes rheumatoid or tuberculotic disorders affecting these structures

There are three possible lesions:

1. tenosynovitis at the level of the carpus
2. tenovaginitis just proximal to the radial styloid process
3. insertion tendopathy of the abductor pollicis longus at the base of metacarpal I

Tenosynovitis at the Level of the Carpus

This lesion is also called de Quervain syndrome (de Quervain's disease) or, incorrectly, radial styloiditis.

Differential Diagnosis

- Radial styloid process syndrome
- Sprain of the radial carpal collateral ligament

Clinical Findings

A significant feature of this lesion is that the pain can radiate quite a distance—distally to the tip of thumb and proximally sometimes as far as the shoulder.

Functional Examination

- Finkelstein's test is the most painful test: A fist is made with the thumb in the palm, and the wrist is then brought into ulnar deviation from a position of slight wrist extension.

- Sometimes resisted radial abduction (extension) and palmar abduction (abduction) of the thumb are painful.
- During palpation, besides the tendon sheath at the level of the carpus, the radial styloid process is often very tender. The process itself is not affected, however, and under local anesthesia of the process' periosteum, the pain does not disappear. This is an example of the "misleading tenderness" phenomenon.

Treatment

It is very important that the patient be informed about possible causes and ways to prevent the disorder from recurring. Depending on the duration of symptoms, usually only one or two injections of (at the most) 1 mL of corticosteroid are necessary to relieve the symptoms completely within a few weeks (Figure 18–4).

Transverse friction can be tried, but numerous treatments are required before improvement is noticed. This treatment has to be applied during 15-minute sessions three times per week for at least 4 to 6 weeks.

Tenovaginitis Just Proximal to the Radial Styloid Process

This lesion is seen much less often than the de Quervain syndrome.

Clinical Findings

The patient complains only of local pain. The pain does not radiate as in the de Quervain syndrome.

Functional Examination

Finkelstein's test is the most positive test. Palmar and radial abduction of the thumb (abduction and extension, respectively) are sometimes painful against resistance.

Treatment

Refer to Tenosynovitis at the Level of the Carpus.

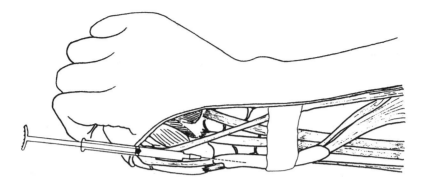

Figure 18–4 Injection between the tendon and the tendon sheath in a de Quervain syndrome.

Insertion Tendopathy of the Abductor Pollicis Longus at the Base of Metacarpal I

This lesion is rare.

Clinical Findings

The patient complains of pain at the radiovolar aspect of the wrist, at the level of the base of metacarpal I.

Functional Examination

In particular, resisted palmar abduction of the thumb is painful, as is, to a lesser degree, resisted radial abduction (extension).

Treatment

Only a few transverse friction treatments are needed to achieve complete relief of pain. In therapy-resistant cases, an injection of 0.5 mL of corticosteroid is indicated.

LESIONS OF THE FLEXOR POLLICIS LONGUS

The cause of this lesion is chronic overuse as the result of repeated forceful wrist flexion, whereby the thumb is also held in forceful flexion (such as in tennis serves and smashes, and Alpine and cross-country skiing). A tenosynovitis can also occur as the result of punching traumas.

There are three predilection sites:

1. tenosynovitis at the level of metacarpal I
2. tenosynovitis at the level of the carpus
3. tenovaginitis stenosans (trigger thumb) at the level of the head of metacarpal I

Tenosynovitis at the Level of Metacarpal I

Clinical Findings

The patient complains of pain at the volar aspect of the wrist or thenar eminence, which sometimes radiates slightly proximally.

Functional Examination

Passive retroposition of the thumb, with the wrist in extension, is the most painful test. In some cases, resisted thumb flexion is painful.

Treatment

The treatment of choice is transverse friction. The patient should be seen for 15-minute sessions, three times per week. Four to five weeks are usually required to achieve complete relief of pain.

Tenosynovitis at the Level of the Carpus

Clinical Findings

The patient complains of local pain, sometimes in combination with crepitation during thumb movements.

Functional Examination

As mentioned under Tenosynovitis at the Level of Metacarpal I, the passive stretch is more painful than contraction against isometric resistance.

Treatment

The treatment of choice is transverse friction. If minimal to no improvement is noted after six treatments, 0.5 mL of corticosteroid can be injected between the tendon and the tendon sheath. The needle is inserted between the tendons of the palmaris longus and flexor carpi radialis. If the palmaris longus is absent, the injection is administered just ulnar to the flexor carpi radialis tendon.

Tenovaginitis Stenosans (Trigger Thumb) at the Level of the Head of Metacarpal I

In this lesion, a traumatic etiology is suspected. There is a thickening of the tendon sheath, possibly due to scarring incurred after bleeding.

Clinical Findings

The patient complains of an inability to straighten the thumb from a bent position; it can be done passively, however, with help from the other hand. During passive extension from a bent position, a palpable click occurs and the motion is restored temporarily.

Functional Examination

Just proximal to the head of metatarsal I, a small, hard swelling is palpable on the volar side.

Treatment

A local injection of several drops of corticosteroid often is effective; however, the swelling does not disappear completely.

In repeated recurrence, surgery to split the tendon sheath is indicated.

18.3 OTHER PATHOLOGY

Please refer to Chapter 21, Peripheral Compression Neuropathies in the Wrist and Hand Region, for more information on neurological pathology.

SCAPHOID IMPACTION SYNDROME

The scaphoid impaction syndrome is caused by overuse of the wrist in extension. This is especially a problem for athletes such as weight lifters, shot putters, and gymnasts. A chondromalacia occurs at the dorsal aspect of the scaphoid, on the joint surface that articulates with the radius.

Differential Diagnosis

- Sprain of the dorsal ligaments
- Carpal instability
- Carpal boss
- Ganglion

Clinical Findings

- The patient complains of pain on the dorsal side of the wrist during loaded hyperextension. The patient often feels a loss of strength, which strongly resembles an instability.

- In the functional examination, passive wrist extension is the most painful motion. Sometimes passive radial deviation in slight wrist extension is also painful.
- Palpation of the scaphoid at the dorsal aspect of the wrist, with the wrist in slight flexion and ulnar deviation, is painful.
- Magnetic resonance imaging is diagnostic.

Treatment

Hyperextension is prevented by means of a brace. In more acute cases, a one-time injection of 0.5 mL of a corticosteroid may be indicated. Sometimes arthroscopic treatment is performed.

TRIQUETRUM-HAMATE COMPRESSION SYNDROME

Compression of what is presumed to be the capsuloligamentous complex, between the triquetrum and the hamate, can occur as the result of a one-time or chronic wrist extension with ulnar deviation.

Differential Diagnosis

- Lesion of the triangular fibrocartilaginous complex
- Tenosynovitis of the extensor carpi ulnaris
- Sprain of the ulnar carpal collateral ligament

Clinical Findings

- The patient complains of local pain and the feeling of a loss of strength in the wrist and hand, especially during firm grasping movements.
- In the functional examination, passive ulnar deviation in slight extension is the most painful test.
- Palpation produces local tenderness.

Treatment

Painful motions are prevented by means of a brace. A local injection of 0.5 mL of cortico-

steroid is often effective.

RADIAL STYLOID PROCESS SYNDROME

The radial styloid process syndrome consists of a very local periostitis in which the radial styloid process is compressed against the scaphoid as the result of a forced radial deviation of the wrist.

Differential Diagnosis

- De Quervain syndrome
- Sprain of the radial carpal collateral ligament

Clinical Findings

- The patient complains of local pain at the level of the radial styloid process.
- In the functional examination, passive radial deviation of the wrist is painful.
- Palpation of the most distal aspect of the radial styloid process is painful.

Treatment

If necessary, a brace can be used to prevent painful motions. A local injection of 0.5 mL of corticosteroid is often very effective.

CARPAL BOSS (CARPE BOSSU, CARPOMETACARPAL BOSS, THROWER'S WRIST)

Carpal boss consists of an irritation of the soft tissue between the base of metacarpal II or metacarpal III and the articulating carpal bones, the trapezoid and the capitate (Figure 18–5). The irritation occurs as the result of repeatedly performed forced extension of the wrist—overuse of the extensors carpi radialis longus and brevis, or it may be caused by a one-time traumatic extension of the wrist. Chronic microtraumas during forced extension can develop into an exostosis of the just-mentioned bony structures.

This thickening of the bone can be congenital, sometimes occurring in the form of an

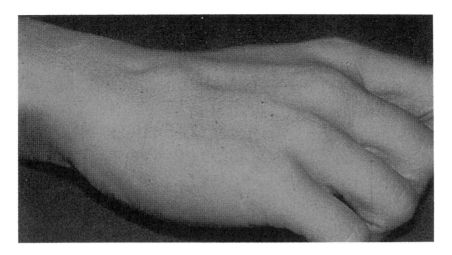

Figure 18–5 Clinical view of the carpal boss. There is visible swelling at the level of the bases of metacarpals II and III.

accessory bone. In these cases lesions of the local soft tissue structures are likely to occur earlier. A direct blow to the back of the hand or dorsal aspect of the wrist can lead to symptoms in an already existing carpal boss.

This lesion is seen particularly in athletes such as shot putters, gymnasts, tennis players, golfers, and those who engage in sports that feature throwing motions.

Differential Diagnosis

The therapist usually will need to differentiate between a ganglion and a carpal boss. In very rare instances, bony or soft tissue tumors or fractures can cause similar symptoms.

It is generally easy to differentiate a ganglion from a carpal boss. The capsule of a ganglion is often merged with the subcutaneous tissue. Thus, in movement of the wrist, a ganglion moves with it; in a carpal boss, the skin shifts over the exostosis.

Clinical Findings

- Initially there is only localized pain and tenderness at the dorsal side of the wrist. Depending on the etiology, local swelling may be present.

- In many cases, the patient complains of fatigue in the hand during activities.

- Sometimes a snapping can be felt during movement of the wrist extensor tendons over the carpal boss.

- The functional examination provokes painful and limited wrist extension. In some cases, flexion is also painful, likely due to stretch, but not limited.

- A radiograph of the wrist, from a lateral view with the wrist in maximal flexion, should reveal the exostosis. Sometimes an accessory bone can be seen.

Treatment

Treatment depends on the cause. Shot putters and weight lifters, who often force wrist extension, can be helped with a special brace to prevent maximal extension. If the cause is overuse of the extensors, effective treatments include stretching exercises, transverse friction, and limitation of pain-provoking movements.

The most difficult lesion to treat is the congenital variant. Sometimes injections of a local anesthetic are helpful, but occasionally improvement is achieved only through injections of a corticosteroid.

In persistent cases, surgical resection is indicated. If symptoms still remain, fusion of the carpometacarpal II and/or carpometacarpal III joint is indicated. This almost always provides excellent results.

GANGLION

A ganglion results from a mucoid degeneration of the capsule or tendon sheath with cyst formation. It is likely that these cysts produce ganglion symptoms even when they are still microscopically small and not yet visible or palpable.

A ganglion of the wrist is usually located on the dorsal side, especially between the radial finger extensors and the tendon of the extensor pollicis longus, or at the level of the capitate.

The lesion is seen particularly in persons who engage in professional or sports activities that load the wrist in extension. Masseurs are often afflicted with ganglions. The ganglion is seen most often in gymnasts, particularly young ones.

Differential Diagnosis

The therapist must gather enough information to differentiate between a ganglion and a carpal boss.

Clinical Findings

- Usually the patient is able to locate the pain precisely. If the ganglion is visible, it will be most easy to see when the wrist is in flexion (Figure 18–6).
- During the functional examination, the passive wrist extension in particular is markedly painful and often slightly limited. Passive flexion is usually mildly painful but not limited.
- In alternating wrist flexion and extension, the ganglion moves if connected to the subcutaneous tissue.
- It is not always easy to differentiate a ganglion coming from the joint capsule and one coming from the tendon sheath.

Sometimes the differentiation can be determined through palpation. In some cases, the ganglion from the tendon sheath is stretched painfully during resisted extension of the flexed fingers.

Treatment

Sometimes a ganglion is treated successfully by pressing it. This is best done through a manipulation; however, with this form of treatment the ganglion often recurs.

An attempt can be made to aspirate the ganglion and then inject 0.5 to 1 mL of corticosteroid; however, with this treatment also the ganglion often recurs.

Surgical treatment is the only method by which complete recovery, without recurrence, can be expected. It is very important, however, that the surgery be directed toward resecting the stem of the ganglion, where it is connected to the joint capsule.

PATHOLOGY OF THE DISTAL RADIOULNAR JOINT

Arthritis

In principle, the distal radioulnar joint can be affected as the result of every systemic disease by which arthritides can occur. The most frequent, however, is rheumatoid arthritis.

Usually the rheumatoid arthritis of the distal radioulnar joint does not respond well to medications. Because the other symptoms of the wrist and fingers are more prominent, the diagnosis of rheumatoid arthritis of the distal radioulnar joint is often missed.

Traumatic arthritis is by far the most frequent arthritis in the distal radioulnar joint. Often, trauma to the joint occurs as the result of forced pronation or supination. Traumatic arthritis is almost always seen in the distal radioulnar joint after forearm fractures.

Clinical Findings

- There is usually slight local swelling and local pain, which usually radiates slightly proximally.

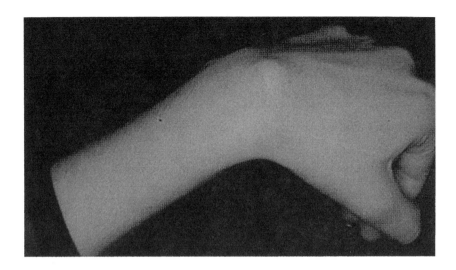

Figure 18–6 A ganglion on the dorsal side of the wrist is particularly visible in flexion.

- Active and (particularly) passive pronation and supination are painful at the end of the range of motion. The tests for the carpus do not produce symptoms. This applies to systemic types of arthritis, to which rheumatoid arthritis belongs, as well as to traumatic types of arthritis.

Treatment

An injection of corticosteroid is almost always effective. If a slight limitation of motion remains, joint-specific mobilization can be performed.

Subluxation or Dislocation

Dorsal dislocation of the distal radioulnar joint can be caused by forced hyperpronation or repeated forceful pronation movements. Typically it is a sports injury incurred by gymnasts and weight lifters, but it is also seen in tennis players, bowlers, and hockey players.

Distinction is made between dorsal and volar subluxation or dislocation. Volar subluxation or dislocation occurs as the result of forced supination movements and is rarely caused by sports activities.

Clinical Findings

- Symptoms include local pain and swelling. The patient complains of a feeling of a loss of strength in the wrist and hand, particularly during pronation movements.
- If there is volar subluxation, an indentation is visible at the level of the ulnar head.
- In a dislocation, both pronation and supination are impossible to perform. If the joint dislocates during movements, a painful click is often felt.
- The instability of the joint is palpable if the ulna is moved dorsally or volarly in relation to the radius.
- Palpation evokes local tenderness.
- The anteroposterior radiograph reveals a diastasis between the radius and ulna when compared with the other side. The examiner must look carefully to rule out the possibility of a fracture of the ulnar styloid process.

Damage to the articular disc always occurs when there is a dislocation of the distal radioulnar joint. In many cases there is also a lesion of the ulnar carpal collateral ligament.

Treatment

In an acute dorsal dislocation of the ulna, the joint can be repositioned by injecting local anesthesia and performing maximal forearm supination. After this procedure, an anti-rotation brace should be worn for at least 6 weeks. Later, the joint should be immobilized partially with tape during sports or other vigorous activities.

In a volar dislocation the ulna is manually repositioned from the volar aspect. After this procedure, an antirotation brace should be used for at least 4 weeks. A cast to stabilize the forearm in pronation is still often used for 4 weeks.

If repositioning procedures are unsuccessful, there is likely an impingement of the articular disc, requiring an open reposition. In this instance, the disc is resected and the capsuloligamentous complex is reattached both dorsally and volarly.

In chronic cases, both the dorsal and the volar instability can be immobilized partially by means of tape. (See also treatment under Rupture of the Articular Carpal Disc.)

Arthrosis

An arthrosis of the distal radioulnar joint is almost always the result of an earlier trauma, often a Colles fracture. An arthrosis can also be the result of a disease that causes an incongruence of the joint surfaces, occurring, for example, after an infection or a rheumatoid flare.

Clinical Findings

- The symptoms are similar to those in a traumatic arthritis of the distal radioulnar joint: painful passive pronation and supination.
- Sometimes there is also crepitation during pronation and supination.

Treatment

A firm bandage around the wrist usually decreases the severity of the symptoms. An injection of a corticosteroid sometimes provides good results. Joint-specific mobilization helps only in the early stages of the disorder.

19

Pathology of the Midhand, Thumb, and Fingers

PATHOLOGY OF THE TRAPEZIOMETACARPAL I JOINT

Pathology with Limited Motions in a Capsular Pattern

Traumatic Arthritis

A traumatic arthritis of the trapeziometacarpal joint is almost always the result of a hyperextension (radial abduction) or hyper-reposition trauma of the thumb. It involves an overstretch of the very strong volar capsuloligamentous complex.

In the differential diagnosis, joint dislocation and fracture of the first metacarpal have to be ruled out. Fractures are seen more often than dislocations.

Clinical Findings.

- Immediately after the trauma, severe pain is experienced at the volar side of the wrist, particularly at the proximal part of the thenar eminence.
- Generally there is an acute circumferential swelling at the level of the joint.
- A severe limitation in the capsular pattern is seen—retroposition of the thumb is painful and very limited, while the other thumb motions either are not limited or are minimally limited and painful.
- Sometimes various resisted tests also evoke symptoms due to compression in the joint or pull on the joint capsule.
- In cases of possible fracture or dislocation, radiographs should be made.

Treatment. Recovery from uncomplicated traumatic arthritis is very slow. Without treatment, symptoms can sometimes last for months. Very cautious joint-specific techniques, preceded by transverse friction of the volar capsuloligamentous complex, will accelerate the healing process significantly. Usually four to six treatments are necessary to achieve complete relief of pain.

In stubborn cases, an intra-articular injection of 1 mL of corticosteroid can be administered.

Nontraumatic Arthritis

In principle, the trapeziometacarpal joint can be the site of various arthritides; however, in practice, this is rarely the case. Rheumatoid arthritis and gout arthritis are some of the most frequent arthritides of this joint.

Clinical Findings.

- There is a painful limitation of thumb retroposition (capsular pattern) (Figure 19–1).
- In unknown etiology, blood and urine tests are indicated.

Treatment. Treatment depends on the severity of the disorder. Rheumatoid arthritis reacts very well to an intra-articular injection of 0.5 mL of corticosteroid.

Arthrosis

Arthrosis of the trapeziometacarpal I joint is seen particularly in women, often bilaterally. It usually concerns a form of primary ar-

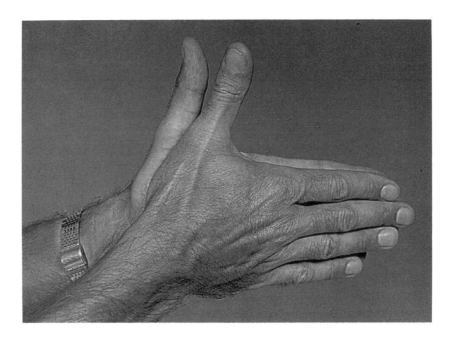

Figure 19–1 Clinical picture of a capsular pattern of limited motions of the trapeziometacarpal I joint in a patient with an idiopathic arthritis.

throsis, because there is no known history of an earlier pathology. The cause is unknown.

Sometimes this lesion is accompanied by arthrosis of the distal interphalangeal joints of the fingers.

Clinical Findings.

- The patient complains of pain and a limitation of motion. Specific activities of daily living, such as peeling potatoes, knitting, and crocheting, cause problems. The pain is localized to the region of the thenar eminence and sometimes radiates proximally.

- In the functional examination, retroposition of the thumb is limited (capsular pattern).

- A radiograph confirms the diagnosis (Figure 19–2).

Treatment. Transverse friction to the volar and radial aspects of the capsulo-

ligamentous complex, combined with joint-specific mobilization, often provides pain relief in the early stages of arthrosis. Through a home exercise program, it is very important that the patient maintain the range of motion gained by means of joint-specific mobilization in physical therapy.

An intra-articular injection of 0.5 to 1 mL of corticosteroid can provide pain-free periods ranging from months to years.

In severe cases that resist therapy, surgical treatment sometimes may be necessary.

Lesions of the Capsuloligamentous Complex

Dislocation of the Trapeziometacarpal Joint

Dislocation of the trapeziometacarpal joint is rare. When seen, it is primarily an affliction

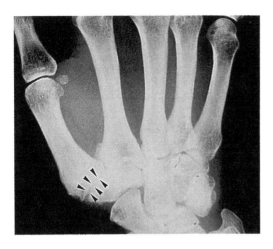

Figure 19–2 Conventional radiograph demonstrating arthrosis of the trapeziometacarpal I joint.

of skiers, boxers, Olympic handball players, and soccer goalies.

Fractures of the first metacarpal have to be considered in the differential diagnosis.

Clinical Findings.
- Dislocation of the first metacarpal usually occurs in a radiovolar direction. In an acute dislocation, the patient has severe pain at the level of the joint.
- Severity of pain makes functional examination impossible in cases of acute dislocations.

Treatment. Sometimes the patient repositions the dislocation by pulling on the thumb. Spontaneous repositions are also possible.

PATHOLOGY OF THE METACARPOPHALANGEAL I JOINT

Dislocation of the Metacarpophalangeal I Joint

In principle, a dislocation of the metacarpophalangeal (MCP) I joint can occur dorsally, volarly, or laterally. The dorsal dislocation is by far the most frequently seen. It is a typical sports injury of boxers and soccer goalies.

Clinical Findings
- The patient has severe pain and limitation of motion of the MCP I joint. The dislocation is usually visible.
- The functional examination cannot be made because of pain.
- Radiographs confirm the dislocation and provide details.

Treatment

The treatment for an acute dislocation is to reposition under radiographic control. Surgical treatment is indicated if the reposition cannot be performed—for instance, if interposition of soft tissue or of the sesamoid bones is found, or in cases of demonstrably severe instability.

Lesions of the Ulnar Collateral Ligament

This frequently seen sports injury occurs when the radially abducted thumb is forced further into a radial direction. This happens, for instance, during a fall in skiing when the ski pole forces the thumb into hyperradial abduction. If the pole is firmly held, however, the same lesion can occur because the pole itself then functions as a lever, forcing the ulnar collateral ligament to rupture. In both cases the injury is called a skier's thumb, which—after knee injuries—is the second most often seen ski injury.

Also, in water polo, Olympic handball, volleyball, and basketball, the retropositioned thumb can be forced into hyperradial abduction if the volar aspect of the thumb is forcefully struck by the ball. In addition, the injury is seen in contact sports or gymnastics, generally as the result of a fall on the outstretched thumb.

Clinical Findings

- There is pain and swelling of the MCP I joint. Often there is discoloration as the result of a hematoma.
- Both active and passive flexion and extension are limited and painful (capsular pattern) due to the traumatic arthritis. Passive radial abduction is very painful in a partial tear, whereas in a complete tear there is often no pain at all during this test.
- In a complete tear, the instability is obvious.
- An avulsion fracture can be ruled out by a radiograph. Stress views show the instability when compared with views of the other side. Arthrography is an alternative radiological diagnostic.

Treatment

Conservative treatment usually is appropriate only for sprains and partial tears. Surgical treatment is indicated in complete tears of the ulnar collateral ligament.

Lesions of the Radial Collateral Ligament

Lesions of the radial collateral ligament are rare; they occur when the dorsally adducted thumb is forced in an ulnar direction.

Clinical Findings

For the most part, the symptoms are similar to those of lesions of the ulnar collateral ligament. It must be understood, however, that in this instance the pain (sprain) and the instability occur when the MCP I joint of the thumb is put in ulnar adduction.

Treatment

Refer to treatment for lesions of the ulnar collateral ligament.

PATHOLOGY OF THE METACARPOPHALANGEAL AND INTERPHALANGEAL JOINTS OF THE FINGERS—LIMITED MOTIONS IN A CAPSULAR PATTERN

Traumatic Arthritis

Traumatic arthritis in the MCP II to V joints and in the interphalangeal (IP) finger joints is commonly seen. It is often incurred from participation in sports such as skiing, ballplaying, and those that feature body contact. Phalangeal fractures have to be considered in the differential diagnosis.

Clinical Findings

- Circumferential swelling is seen around the joint shortly after the trauma.
- The functional examination discloses a painful limitation of motion, with flexion usually slightly more limited than extension (capsular pattern).

Treatment

Without treatment, symptoms can last for a long time (sometimes up to a year). An intra-articular injection of 0.5 mL of corticosteroid is usually very effective. Immobilization is strongly discouraged because it usually leads to the permanent formation of contractures.

Nontraumatic Arthritis

The most frequent type of nontraumatic arthritis of the finger joints is rheumatoid arthritis. Although the other metacarpophalangeal joints can be affected, it usually starts in the MCP II joint. In some cases, only the IP joints are affected.

Psoriatic arthritis often begins in the distal interphalangeal joints. The differential diagnosis should consider arthrosis.

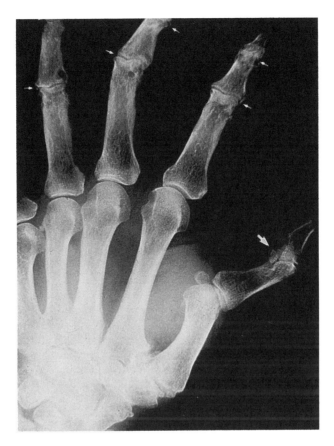

Figure 19–3 Conventional X-ray showing rheumatoid arthritis of the interphalangeal joints and a deformation of the metacarpophalangeal I joint.

Clinical Findings

- The patient has pain and circumferential swelling around the affected joints.
- In cases of rheumatoid arthritis, deformation of the hand ultimately occurs, whereby the fingers are positioned in ulnar deviation in the metacarpophalangeal joints (Figure 19–3).
- The functional examination demonstrates a larger limitation of flexion than of extension (capsular pattern).

Treatment

Treatment depends on the cause of the arthritis. In rheumatoid arthritis, the initial treatment is medication. Depending on the stage of the disorder, medication can be enhanced by physical therapy.

Sometimes one or more joints remain very painful despite medication. In such cases, an intra-articular injection of 0.5 to 1 mL of corticosteroid provides good results.

Surgical treatment is indicated in therapy-resistant cases.

Arthrosis

Arthrosis of the finger joint is seen particularly in middle-aged women. A typical extra-articular fibrous thickening usually is seen, mainly located at the level of the distal interphalangeal joints (the so-called Heberden's nodules). When these nodules are located at the level of the proximal interphalangeal joints, they are called Bouchard's nodules.

During the differential diagnosis, it is important to consider psoriatic arthritis, a disorder that often begins in the distal interphalangeal joints. Also, rheumatoid arthritis occasionally appears first in the interphalangeal joints.

Clinical Findings

- Patients generally experience the most pain in the periods when the nodules develop. Sometimes, one or more nodules develop overnight.
- The functional examination demonstrates the typical capsular pattern of limited motions, with flexion slightly more limited than extension.

Treatment

In most instances, the symptoms are not severe enough to warrant treatment. Medication is usually more effective than physical therapy.

During the painful periods, the patient is encouraged to perform all normal hand activities with as much respect as possible for the pain. Usually the process stabilizes after a few years. The patient should be counseled thoroughly and reassured that continued normal use over time is the best treatment.

LESIONS OF THE CAPSULOLIGAMENTOUS COMPLEX

Subluxation or Dislocation of the Metacarpophalangeal Joints II to V

Subluxations or dislocations of the MCP II to V joints usually occur as the result of a fall on the extended hand. They can occur either dorsally or palmarly. The latter is the most commonly seen.

Clinical Findings

- The acute subluxation or dislocation is characterized by severe local pain, to an extent that the functional examination cannot be performed.
- Radiological examination confirms and provides detail on the dislocation.

Treatment

Interposition of the palmar fibrocartilaginous plate may make it impossible to reposition the joint. In these cases, open reposition with restabilization of the joint is the only therapeutic possibility.

Rupture of the Collateral Ligaments of the Metacarpophalangeal Joints

Rupture of the collateral ligaments of the metacarpophalangeal joints usually involves the index and little fingers. The ulnar collateral ligament of the index finger is particularly affected as the result of a radial abduction trauma. The radial collateral ligament of the little finger is particularly affected as the result of an ulnar abduction trauma.

These are often sports-related injuries.

Clinical Findings

- There is pain and swelling at the level of the affected joint.
- The stability examination is best performed with the joint in 90° flexion; in this position, the collateral ligaments are the most taut.
- Radiographs are necessary to rule out an avulsion fracture.

Treatment

If the radiograph does not show an avulsion fracture, the best treatment is conservative—immobilization in a brace for 3 to 4 weeks in 70° flexion. In instances of an avulsion fracture, surgery is indicated.

Dislocations of the Interphalangeal Joints

Dislocations of the proximal interphalangeal joints are seen more often than dislocations of the very stable distal interphalangeal joints. Dislocations of the proximal interphalangeal joints can occur in a dorsal, palmar, or sideways direction. Dislocations of the distal interphalangeal joints almost always occur dorsally.

Dorsal dislocations are not always paired with a rupture of one or both collateral ligaments. In sideways dislocations, the collateral bands almost always rupture. Ulnar dislocations, with a rupture of the radial collateral ligament, are seen much more often than radial dislocations, with rupture of the ulnar collateral ligament. Palmar dislocations are the least often seen.

A radiograph should be obtained to rule out avulsion fractures.

Clinical Findings

- Severe local pain, limitation of motion, and visible deformity as a result of the dislocation are characteristics of this lesion.
- The functional examination *should not be performed* without the benefit of a radiograph.

Treatment

If there is not a fracture, the dislocated phalanx is repositioned under traction and immobilized in a brace for 2 to 3 weeks in 20° to 30° of flexion. Afterward, the finger should be immobilized partially by means of tape until the function has returned completely and there is no longer any pain.

In an avulsion fracture, stability is tested carefully after reposition. If there is an instability, surgery is indicated. Once stability is restored, the finger is conservatively treated.

In rare instances of a palmar dislocation, the lesion is treated surgically.

PATHOLOGY OF THE MUSCULOTENDINOUS COMPLEX

Dislocation of the Tendon of the Extensor Digitorum Communis at the Level of the Metacarpophalangeal Joint

Dislocation of the tendon of the extensor digitorum communis at the level of the metacarpophalangeal joint is seen most frequently in patients with rheumatoid arthritis of the hands. Spontaneous dislocation in the absence of rheumatoid arthritis is rare. In most instances, a trauma is concerned, and in some cases it is congenitally or idiopathically acquired.

In traumatic etiology, a sports injury is usually involved.

Clinical Findings

- An acute dislocation is usually accompanied by severe local pain.
- The tendon of the middle finger is affected much more often than the tendons of the other fingers.
- Usually, the dislocation occurs in an ulnar direction.
- The visible dislocation occurs at the metacarpophalangeal joint during flexion of the finger.

Treatment

Treatment can be either conservative or surgical. Conservative treatment consists of 3 weeks of immobilization of the finger in extension by use of a brace.

Boutonniere (Buttonhole) Deformity

A rupture of the middle part of the tendon of the extensor digitorum communis, which inserts at the base of the middle phalanx, can occur as a result of forced flexion of the proximal interphalangeal (PIP) joint. This may result, for example, from a fall on the hand with flexed fingers or while playing sports wherein the fingers of the hand may be struck by the ball.

The index finger is the one most frequently traumatized.

Clinical Findings

- Initially, the patient has little pain and minimal loss of function. There is local swelling and tenderness at the dorsal side of the base of the middle phalanx.
- The finger's PIP joint is held in flexion. Extension in the joint is no longer possible.
- Because the ulnar and radial expansions of the extensor tendon usually also rupture, the tendon shifts palmarly and works then as a palmar flexor. The head of the proximal phalanx pokes dorsally between the lateral parts of the extensor tendon as through a buttonhole (Figure 19–4).
- The distal interphalangeal (DIP) joint is hyperextended, and a slight hyperextension of the MCP joint occurs as well. This is caused by the direction of pull of the lateral expansions of the extensor digitorum communis in conjunction with the direction of pull of the interossei.
- A radiograph should be obtained to rule out avulsion fractures.

Treatment

In acute cases, surgery is preferred over conservative treatment.

Conservative treatment consists of immobilization by means of a finger brace, whereby the PIP joint is maximally extended, while the DIP and MCP joints remain mobile. Immobilization should last at least 5 weeks.

Swan Neck Hyperextension Deformity

This deformity results from a traumatic hyperextension of the PIP joint or as the result of a dorsal dislocation, whereby the palmar fibrocartilaginous plate of the joint ruptures (Figure 19–5). This allows for hyperextension of the joint through the pull of the extensor digitorum communis.

The lesion is seen particularly in volleyball and Olympic handball players.

Clinical Findings

- In the acute stage, it is sometimes difficult to make an exact diagnosis. The patient has swelling and pain localized at the level of the PIP joint.
- During the functional examination, flexion of the PIP joint is very painful and limited.
- Radiographs should be used to rule out an avulsion fracture.

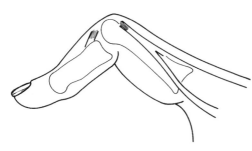

Figure 19–4 Illustration of the so-called buttonhole deformity showing dorsal dislocation of the head of the proximal phalanx. Flexion in the interphalangeal joint and hyperextension in the DIP joint are present.

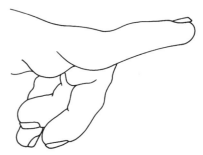

Figure 19–5 Illustration of the so-called swan neck deformity showing traumatic hyperextension of the PIP joint as a result of a rupture of the palmar fibrocartilaginous plate.

Treatment

Immobilization of the finger usually achieves full recovery. Immobilization by means of a brace should last at least 2 weeks, and is done with the MCP joint in 90° flexion and the PIP and DIP joints in 10° flexion.

Surgery is necessary to treat avulsion fractures.

Lesion of the Tendon of the Extensor Digitorum Communis at the Level of the Distal Interphalangeal Joint (Hammer Finger, Mallet Finger)

A traumatic hyperflexion or hyperextension of the DIP joint is regularly seen in volleyball players. The result is a partial or complete tear of the extensor aponeurosis and sometimes an avulsion fracture or total fracture of the distal phalanx. The latter lesion occurs as the result of hyperextension.

Clinical Findings

- There is local pain and severe tenderness between the nail and the DIP joint.
- The patient is unable to extend the DIP joint actively.

Treatment

If an uncomplicated rupture of the extensor aponeurosis has occurred, conservative or surgical treatment is appropriate. Conservative treatment consists of immobilization of the DIP joint in hyperextension and the PIP joint in 90° flexion. Operative reconstruction is more effective than immobilization.

Rupture of the Tendinous Insertion of the Flexor Digitorum Profundus

A rupture of the tendinous insertion of the flexor digitorum profundus is a typical sports injury seen particularly in rugby, football, hockey, and contact sports wherein it is the result of a traumatic overstretch of the DIP joint.

This type of rupture can be combined with an avulsion of part of the base of the distal phalanx. In some cases, the tendon can retract as far as the palm of the hand.

Clinical Findings

- Pain and swelling of the entire finger are experienced.
- Active flexion of the DIP joint is impossible. Usually the patient can no longer extend the PIP joint maximally.
- In many cases, the lateral view on radiographs discloses an avulsion fracture.

Treatment

Treatment is surgical, consisting of re-fixation of the tendon on the base of the distal phalanx. With severe swelling, surgery is not indicated but may be performed when the swelling has disappeared. The hand is placed in a sling during the presurgery period.

Tenovaginitis Stenosans of the Flexors Digitorum Profundus and Superficialis (Trigger Finger)

Tenovaginitis stenosans of the flexors digitorum profundus and superficialis concerns a very local thickening of the flexor tendons of the fingers, just proximal to the MCP joint.

The cause of these lesions is unknown. It is possible that multiple microtraumas play a role in this disorder.

Clinical Findings

- The patient generally complains of the inability to flex or extend maximally the finger actively.
- Just proximal to the MCP joint, a hard bump can be felt in the tendon. Palpation of this bump is usually painful.
- If the lesion has been present for a long time, the patient often can bend or straighten the finger but only with the help of the other hand.

Treatment

Sometimes a local injection of 0.5 mL of corticosteroid is effective. Usually this treatment provides only temporary relief, if any. Surgical splitting of the tendon sheath is then indicated.

Sprain of the Origin of the Adductor Pollicis, Oblique Head

A sprain of the origin of the oblique head of the adductor pollicis is considered a traumatic lesion. It is rarely a solitary lesion and is almost always seen in conjunction with a lesion of the trapeziometacarpal joint or metacarpophalangeal I joint.

Clinical Findings

- There is local pain at the volar aspect of the capitate at the base of the thenar eminence. This painful site is found proximally, in line with the third metacarpal.
- Resisted thumb adduction is the most painful test. Passive thumb retroposition can be painful because of stretching.

Treatment

Transverse friction is usually very effective. Four to six treatments generally are necessary to achieve complete relief of pain.

Lesions of the Interosseous Muscles

Lesions of the interosseous muscles of the hand are rare. When a lesion is seen, it is usually in a person who performs a significant amount of fine work with the fingers, such as a typist or a musician playing a string or key instrument.

The dorsal interosseous muscles are much more often affected than the palmar interosseous muscles.

The lesion can be localized in the muscle belly, tendon, or teno-osseous insertion.

Clinical Findings

- If the lesion concerns a dorsal interosseous muscle, as is usually the case, the pain is felt particularly on the dorsal aspect of the midhand region. Sometimes the pain radiates proximally.
- In the functional examination, abduction of the fingers against resistance is painful:
  1. radial abduction of the index finger = dorsal interosseus I
  2. radial abduction of the middle finger = dorsal interosseus II
  3. ulnar abduction of the middle finger = dorsal interosseus III
  4. ulnar abduction of the ring finger = dorsal interosseus IV
- The exact site of the lesion can be localized by palpation.
- In lesions of the palmar interosseous muscles, closing the fingers against resistance is painful:
  1. ulnar abduction of the index finger = palmar interosseous I
  2. radial abduction of the ring finger = palmar interosseous II
  3. radial abduction of the little finger = palmar interosseous III

Treatment

Irrespective of the site of the lesion, transverse friction is very effective in almost every case. If the muscle belly is affected, usually only two or three treatments are necessary for complete recovery. If the lesion lies in the tendon or at the insertion, four to six treatments generally are required to achieve complete relief of pain.

Dupuytren's Contracture

Dupuytren's contracture concerns a fibrous hypertrophy with contracture of the palmar aponeurosis. Initially there are fibrous bumps that, in later stages, spread out into cords. The result is a flexion contracture of one or more fingers, which is usually localized at the level of the fourth and fifth rays of the hand.

The disorder is seen particularly in men over age 40.

The cause is unknown. It is possible that chronic microtraumas play a role. For instance, in horse and carriage days this disorder was a rather common problem for coachmen—the so-called coachman's hand.

Hereditary factors also seem to play a significant role. In addition, some antiepileptic medications can contribute to the disorder, and it is seen in epileptics comparatively often.

Clinical Findings

- The patient does not have pain, but has an early inability actively, and later passively, to straighten the fourth and fifth fingers.
- The fibrous cords of the palmar aponeurosis are palpable.

Treatment

This disorder is extremely difficult to treat. Physical therapy treatments are rarely effective. If there is improvement with physical therapy, the effect is generally only temporary.

Unfortunately, surgical treatments are not always satisfactory either.

OTHER DISORDERS

Aseptic Necrosis

Kienböck's disease, aseptic necrosis of the lunate, is discussed in Chapter 18. This disorder is based on a vascular disturbance in the bone. Deformation of the affected bone can occur easily because, in this disease, the bone tissue is replaced by fibrous tissue.

This disorder is seen particularly in children and adolescents, and in males more frequently than females. Juvenile aseptic necrosis of bone—or osteochondrosis—in the hand is occasionally also seen in one of the metacarpal heads (Burns' disease) or in the proximal interphalangeal joints of the fingers (Thiemann's disease).

Ganglia

A ganglion can occur at several places in the hand. A common site is between the heads of the second and third metacarpals. It is important to differentiate a ganglion in this area from a beginning rheumatoid arthritis of the MCP II and III joints.

Clinical Findings

- There is a fluctuating swelling palpable between the heads of the metacarpals II and III. The joint itself does not appear to be swollen.
- The functional examination usually produces no symptoms.

Treatment

Aspiration and injection of a ganglion in this region is usually effective. In contrast to a ganglion at the level of the carpus, a ganglion in the metacarpus rarely recurs.

Please see Chapter 21, Peripheral Compression Neuropathies in the Wrist and Hand Region, for a discussion of neurological disorders.

*   *   *

For an overview of the common pathologies of the wrist and hand, refer to Appendix B, Algorithms for the Diagnosis and Treatment of the Upper Extremities.

20

Treatment Techniques in Lesions of the Wrist and Hand

DISTAL RADIOULNAR JOINT ARTHRITIS

Functional Examination

- Passive pronation and supination are painful and sometimes slightly limited at end-range.

Intra-articular Injection

Traumatic arthritis, rheumatoid arthritis, and other arthritides that are rheumatoid in nature are the most significant indications for an intra-articular injection (Figure 20–1).

Position of the Patient

The patient sits at the short end of the treatment table with the pronated forearm resting on the table.

Position of the Physician

The physician sits diagonally across from the patient, next to the long side of the treatment table.

The physician palpates the tendon of the extensor digiti minimi, which lies directly radial to the ulnar head (the patient extends the little finger). This tendon runs directly over the distal radioulnar joint (Figure 20–2).

Performance

A syringe is filled with 0.5 to 1.0 mL of triamcinolone acetonide, 10 mg/mL. A 2-cm long needle is inserted vertically (the tendon

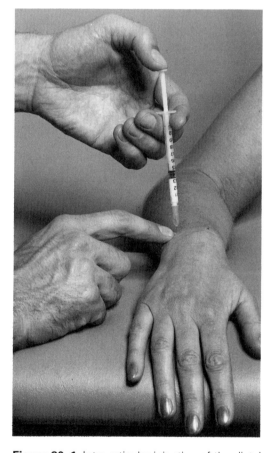

Figure 20–1 Intra-articular injection of the distal radioulnar joint.

does not hinder the injection). After approximately 1.5 cm, if the needle comes into contact with bone, the direction of the needle can be altered slightly so that it can go deeper

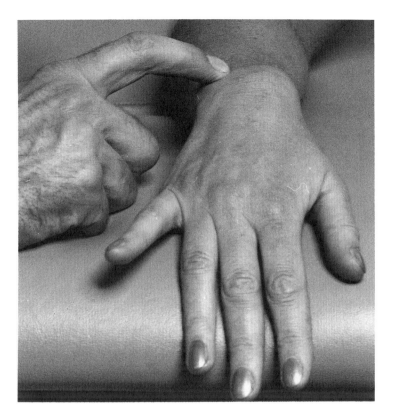

Figure 20–2 Localization of the distal radioulnar joint by palpating the tendon of the extensor digiti minimi.

without any resistance. Because the needle is only 2 cm long, there is no danger of going through the joint to the other side.

Follow-Up

Activities should be limited for 1 week. The patient should be reassessed in 2 weeks. Usually, one or two injections are sufficient to achieve complete relief of pain.

SPRAIN OF THE TRIQUETRO-PISIFORM JOINT

Functional Examination

- Resisted palmar flexion and ulnar deviation of the wrist are usually painful.

- Passive extension and radial deviation of the wrist can be painful.
- Pain and crepitation can be elicited by passive movement of the pisiform against the triquetrum.

Injection

Differentiation between a sprain of the triquetro-pisiform joint and an insertion tendopathy of the flexor carpi ulnaris is not always easy. Injection of a local anesthetic can help to confirm the diagnosis.

Position of the Patient

The patient sits next to the short end of the treatment table. The forearm rests in maximal supination on the table.

Position of the Physician

The physician sits diagonally facing the patient, next to the long side of the treatment table.

If the right side is being treated, the physician grasps the patient's hand from the radial aspect with the left hand. The patient's hand is held in slight palmar flexion and ulnar deviation, with the forearm positioned in supination. Using the middle finger, the physician shifts the pisiform ulnarly.

Performance

A syringe is filled with 0.5 to 1.0 mL of triamcinolone acetonide, 10 mg/mL. Directly dorsal to the pisiform, a 2- to 3-cm long needle is inserted horizontally between the triquetrum and pisiform (Figure 20–3).

With the pisiform shifted in an ulnar direction, the joint surface of the bone is partially palpable.

Note: The pisiform bone is often larger than expected.

GANGLION AT THE DORSAL ASPECT OF THE WRIST

Functional Examination

- Passive extension of the wrist is painful and sometimes limited.
- Passive palmar flexion of the wrist is usually painful.

Aspiration/Injection

A ganglion on the dorsal aspect of the wrist is not always visible or palpable. Differentiation between a ganglion and a subluxation of a carpal bone or a ligamentous lesion is necessary, but not always easy.

In making a prognosis, it is significant to note whether the ganglion comes from the joint capsule or from a tendon sheath. Ganglions coming from the joint have a stronger tendency to recur.

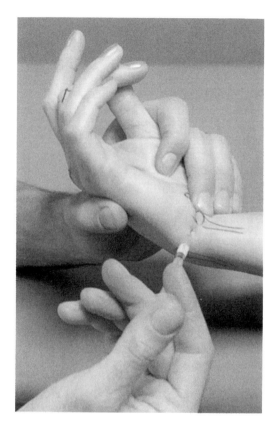

Figure 20–3 Injection of the joint between the pisiform and the triquetrum.

If the patient has significant complaints, aspiration and subsequent injection are indicated.

Position of the Patient

The patient sits next to the short end of the treatment table with the forearm supported on the table in a pronated position. The hand hangs over the edge of the table with the wrist in palmar flexion.

Position of the Physician

The physician sits diagonally facing the patient next to the long side of the treatment table. With one hand the physician grasps the patient's hand, holding it in slight palmar flexion.

Performance

A large syringe (to provide better suction) with a thick injection or aspiration needle is used. After inserting the needle horizontally, the ganglion is aspirated (Figure 20–4).

Triamcinolone acetonide (0.5 to 1.0 mL of 10 mg/mL) is injected after the aspiration, using either the same needle or another, thinner, needle (Figure 20–5). This injection after aspiration is necessary even if there is no aspirated fluid. When there is only a very small ganglion, the area where the patient locates the pain should be injected.

Sometimes a ganglion can be treated successfully by using manipulative pressure. However, in most of these cases, the problem recurs.

If the ganglion recurs after aspiration and injection of a corticosteroid, the procedure can be repeated, but with a stronger concentration of corticosteroid. In these instances, the results are usually permanent. What probably happens here is an irreversible drying out of the ganglion.

Follow-Up

Activities that may have an impact on the affected area are reduced for 1 week. The patient's condition is reassessed after 2 weeks.

Surgery may be indicated if more than three injections are needed or if the condition recurs too frequently.

SPRAIN OF THE RADIAL COLLATERAL LIGAMENT

Functional Examination

- Passive ulnar deviation of the wrist is painful.
- If the volar part of the radial collateral ligament is affected, passive ulnar deviation in slight extension will be the most painful motion. If the dorsal part is affected, passive ulnar deviation in slight flexion will be the most painful motion.

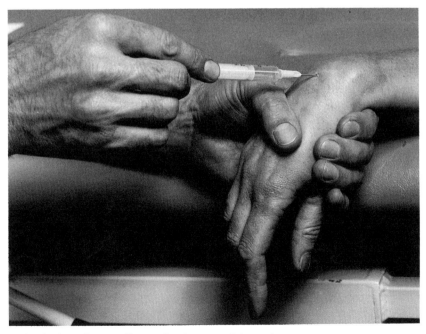

Figure 20–4 Aspiration of a ganglion at the dorsum of the wrist.

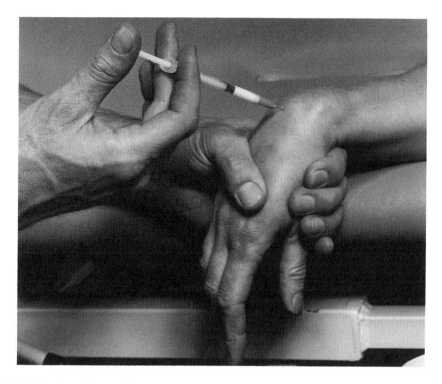

Figure 20–5 Injection of a ganglion.

Both radial and ulnar collateral ligaments of the wrist have a specific volar and dorsal part; each collateral ligament has a V shape.

Transverse Friction for the Volar Part of the Radial Collateral Ligament

Position of the Patient

The patient sits next to the short end of the treatment table with the forearm resting in slight pronation on the table. The hand hangs over the edge of the table.

Position of the Therapist

The therapist sits next to the treatment table, diagonally in front of the patient. If the right hand is being treated, the therapist uses the right hand to hold the patient's hand in slight ulnar deviation and extension (Figure 20–6).

The most tender site is localized by palpation. There are three possible sites for the lesion:

1. the insertion on the styloid process of the radius
2. the ligament itself (which is rare)
3. the insertion on the volar aspect of the scaphoid

The therapist places the left index finger, reinforced by the middle finger, on the most painful site; the thumb is placed on the ulnar side of the wrist.

Site 1. If the origin on the radius is affected, the patient's hand is placed in a more neutral position in order to relax the ligament slightly. The therapist's thumb is placed more proximal in relation to the index finger. For the transverse friction, pressure is exerted medially and proximally against the styloid

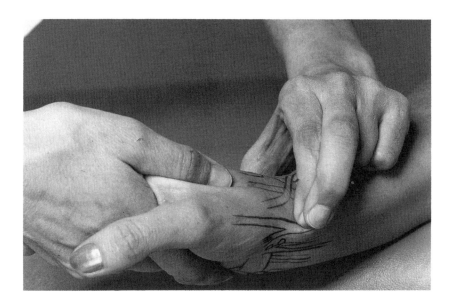

Figure 20–6 Transverse friction of the volar part of the radial collateral ligament.

process, and the index finger moves volar to dorsal, transverse to the fibers of the ligament.

Site 2. If the ligament itself is affected, the hand is placed in slight ulnar deviation and extension in order to put a slight stretch on the ligament. The therapist's thumb is placed directly opposite to the index finger. Pressure is exerted medially, and the index finger is moved volar to dorsal, transverse to the fibers of the ligament.

Site 3. If the insertion at the scaphoid is affected, the hand is placed in slight ulnar deviation and extension in order to put a slight stretch on the ligament. The therapist's thumb is placed more distal in relation to the index finger. Pressure is exerted medially and slightly distally against the scaphoid, and the index finger is moved volar to dorsal, transverse to the fibers of the ligament.

Performance

The active phase of the transverse friction occurs through an extension of the therapist's wrist in conjunction with a slight abduction of the arm.

Duration of Treatment

Treatment should be administered three to five times per week, with the transverse friction lasting approximately 15 minutes per session. In almost all cases, the problem is resolved within 3 to 4 weeks of treatment.

If there is little or no improvement, however, an injection of a corticosteroid may be indicated.

Transverse Friction for the Dorsal Part of the Radial Collateral Ligament

Position of the Patient

This technique is the same as that described for the volar part of the ligament, except that the wrist is placed in ulnar deviation and *slight flexion* in order to put the ligament in a stretched condition (Figure 20–7).

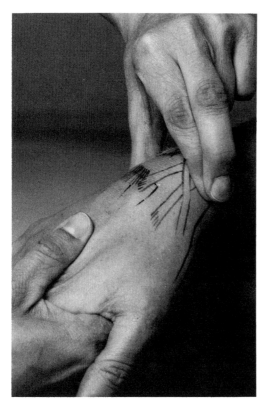

Figure 20–7 Transverse friction of the dorsal part of the radial collateral ligament.

Performance

Refer to the procedure for the volar part of the ligament.

Duration of Treatment

Transverse friction should be performed for approximately 15 minutes, and the patient should be seen three to five times weekly. Two to four weeks are generally required for good results. If the treatments bring little or no relief, an injection of corticosteroid, 10 mg/mL, may be indicated.

Injection

An injection of the radial collateral ligament is indicated only when transverse fric-

tion is not effective or it is impossible for the patient to receive physical therapy.

Position of the Patient

The patient sits next to the short end of the treatment table. The forearm rests on the table in a neutral position (between pronation and supination) with the wrist in ulnar deviation and the hand hanging over the edge of the table.

Position of the Physician

The physician sits next to the long side of the table, diagonally facing the patient. By means of palpation, the affected site of the ligament is carefully located.

First the palmar aspect of the ligament is palpated with the patient's hand positioned in slight extension and ulnar deviation. The hand is then positioned in slight palmar flexion and ulnar deviation in order to palpate the dorsal aspect of the ligament. In each position, three possible sites for the lesion exist:

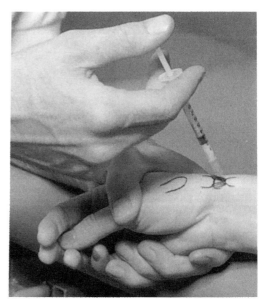

Figure 20–8A Injection of the radial collateral ligament at its insertion on the styloid process of the radius.

(1) the origin at the radial styloid process (Figure 20–8A), (2) the ligament itself (which is rare), and (3) the insertion at the scaphoid (Figure 20–8B).

Performance

A syringe containing 0.5 to 1.0 mL of triamcinolone acetonide, 10 mg/mL, and a 2-cm long needle are used to inject the lesion in a dropwise fashion, guided by where the patient indicates there is pain.

Follow-Up

The arm should be placed in a sling for 3 days, and the patient should limit activities that may have an impact on the affected area for the following 3 to 4 days. The patient's condition is reassessed after 2 weeks.

A second injection is rarely necessary to achieve complete relief of pain.

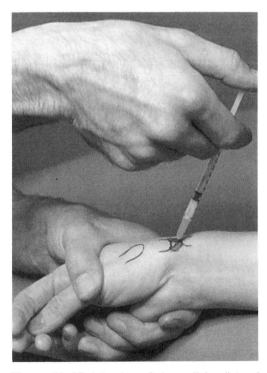

Figure 20–8B Injection of the radial collateral ligament at its insertion on the volar aspect of the scaphoid.

SPRAIN OF THE ULNAR COLLATERAL LIGAMENT

Functional Examination

- Passive radial deviation of the wrist is painful.
- If the volar part of the ligament is affected, radial deviation in slight extension will be the most painful passive motion. If the dorsal part of the ligament is affected, radial deviation in slight flexion will be the most painful motion.

Transverse Friction

A sprain of the ulnar collateral ligament is usually the result of a Colles' fracture. Transverse friction generally is very effective, requiring only three or four treatments, as is the case with lesions of the radial collateral ligament.

When performing the transverse friction, the patient's forearm is first placed in supination to move the extensor carpi ulnaris tendon away from the ulnar collateral ligament. Positioning the patient's hand and the administration of the friction massage is the same as described for the radial collateral ligament, but takes the ulnar structures into consideration.

Injection

In rare cases, however, when no improvement is seen after six treatments of transverse friction, an injection is indicated.

Position of the Patient

The patient sits next to the short end of the treatment table with the pronated forearm, supported by a small towel or a pillow, resting on the table.

Position of the Physician

The physician sits next to the long side of the treatment table, diagonally facing the patient.

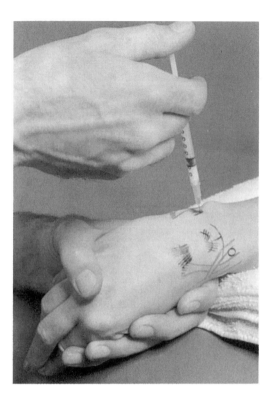

Figure 20–9 Injection of the ulnar collateral ligament at its insertion on the styloid process of the ulna.

The physician grasps the patient's hand and positions it in radial deviation and—depending on which part of the ligament is affected—either slight extension or slight flexion.

Performance

The most tender site is located by palpation. Three possible sites for the lesion exist: (1) the origin at the ulnar styloid process (Figure 20–9), (2) the ligament itself (which is rare), and (3) the insertion at either the dorsal or volar aspect of the triquetrum.

A syringe containing 0.5 to 1.0 mL of triamcinolone acetonide, 10 mg/mL, and a 2-cm long needle are used to inject the lesion in a dropwise fashion, guided by where the patient indicates there is pain.

Follow-Up

The arm should be placed in a sling for 3 days, and the patient should limit activities that may have an impact on the affected area for the following 3 to 4 days. The patient's condition is reassessed after 2 weeks.

In most cases, only one injection is needed to achieve the desired results.

SPRAIN OF THE DORSAL INTERCARPAL LIGAMENTS

Functional Examination

- Passive wrist flexion is painful due to stretch.
- Passive wrist extension can be painful due to compression.

Transverse Friction

A lesion of the intercarpal ligaments must be differentiated from a ganglion and a thrower's wrist.

Position of the Patient

The patient sits at the short end of the treatment table with the pronated forearm resting on the table. The hand hangs in slight wrist flexion over the edge of the table.

Position of the Therapist

The therapist sits next to the long side of the treatment table, diagonally facing the patient. If the right wrist is being treated, the therapist grasps the patient's hand from the volar aspect with the left hand.

After careful palpation for the most tender site of the various ligaments on the dorsal aspect of the wrist, the therapist places the tip of the right thumb or the tip of the right index finger on the site of the lesion.

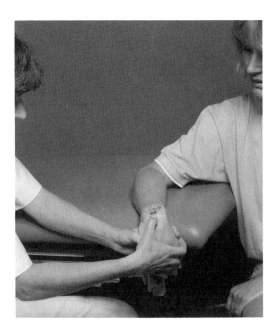

Figure 20–10 Transverse friction of the ligament between the capitate and the third metacarpal.

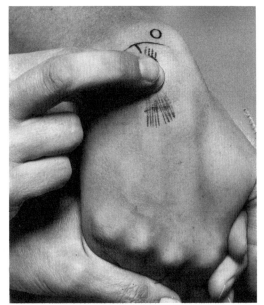

Figure 20–11 Transverse friction of the insertion of the ligaments that run from the lunate and scaphoid to the capitate.

Performance

With the Thumb. The active phase of the transverse friction technique is performed through a slight adduction of the thumb with simultaneous extension of the wrist (Figure 20–10). At the same time, the upper arm is slightly adducted.

During the treatment, the therapist ensures that the patient's extensor tendons remain on either side of the thumb.

With the Index Finger. The tip of the index finger, reinforced by the middle finger, can also be used to perform this technique. Placement of the index finger depends on which ligament and which part of the ligament is affected.

Example 1. The lesion is located at the level of the distal insertion of the ligament between the capitate and the third metacarpal. The fingernail of the thumb is almost horizontal as the tip of the thumb is positioned against the base of the third metacarpal; pressure is exerted distally (Figure 20–10).

Example 2. The lesion is located on the capitate, at the insertion of the ligaments that run from the lunate and the scaphoid to the capitate (Figure 20–11). The transverse friction is performed from radial to ulnar by means of a slight extension of the wrist and simultaneous slight adduction of the upper arm. Here the fingernail is almost vertical.

Duration of Treatment

The patient should be seen three to five times per week, and the transverse friction be performed for approximately 15 minutes. Generally, the results of the treatment are very good, and within 6 to10 treatments the patient has complete relief of pain.

INSERTION TENDOPATHY OF THE EXTENSOR CARPI RADIALIS BREVIS

Functional Examination

- Passive wrist flexion can be painful due to stretch.
- Resisted wrist extension with radial deviation is painful at the wrist.

Transverse Friction

Although an extensor carpi radialis brevis tenosynovitis does exist, insertion tendopathies are far more common. Thus, treatment for an insertion tendopathy of the extensor carpi radialis brevis is discussed here.

Position of the Patient

The patient sits next to the short end of the treatment table with the forearm supported in pronation on the table. The wrist is positioned in flexion and ulnar deviation with the hand hanging over the edge of the table.

Position of the Therapist

The therapist sits next to the long side of the treatment table, diagonally facing the patient.

If the patient's right hand is being treated, the therapist grasps the patient's hand from the volar aspect with the left hand. With either the tip of the thumb or the tip of the index finger, the therapist carefully locates the site of the lesion, at the bases of the second and third metacarpals.

Performance

With the Thumb. The active phase of the transverse friction technique is performed by means of a slight thumb adduction, slight wrist extension, and simultaneous arm adduction (Figure 20–12).

With the Index Finger. With the index finger reinforced by the middle finger, pressure is exerted against the base of the metacarpal. By means of slight wrist extension and slight arm adduction, the index finger is moved in a radial to ulnar direction, transverse to the fibers of the insertion (Figure 20–13).

Duration of Treatment

The patient should be seen for treatment three to five times per week. Transverse friction should be performed for approximately 15 minutes.

If little or no improvement is noted after six sessions of transverse friction, an injection of corticosteroid, 10 mg/mL, is indicated.

Injection

An injection of the insertion of the extensor carpi radialis brevis is indicated only if transverse friction treatments are unsuccessful.

Position of the Patient

The patient sits next to the short end of the treatment table. The forearm rests on the table in a pronated position with the hand hanging over the edge of the table and the wrist in flexion.

Position of the Physician

The physician sits next to the long side of the treatment table, diagonally facing the patient.

If the right side is being treated, the physician grasps the patient's hand from the volar aspect with the left hand. By means of careful palpation, the site of the lesion is located at the ulnar aspect of the base of metacarpal II or the radial aspect of the base of metacarpal III. If preferred, the physician can mark the affected site.

Performance

With a syringe containing 0.5 mL of triamcinolone acetonide, 10 mg/mL, and a 2-cm

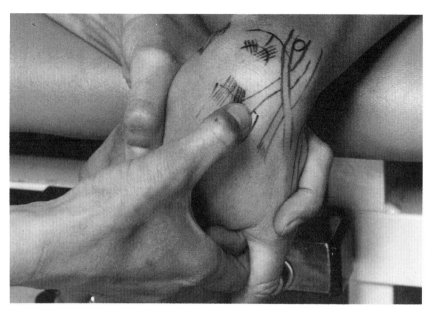

Figure 20–12 Transverse friction of the insertion of the extensor carpi radialis brevis.

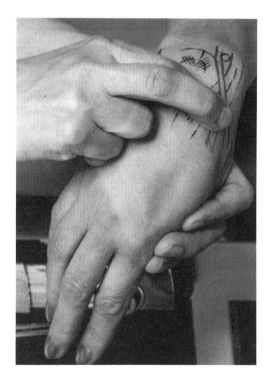

Figure 20–13 Transverse friction of the extensor carpi radialis brevis with the index finger.

long needle, the lesion is injected in a dropwise fashion guided by the patient's indications of pain (Figure 20–14).

Follow-Up

The patient should wear a sling for 3 days and should limit activities that may have an impact on the affected area for the following 3 to 4 days. After 2 weeks the patient's condition is reassessed.

Occasionally a second injection is necessary to achieve complete relief of pain. In rare instances a third injection is required.

INSERTION TENDOPATHY OF THE EXTENSOR CARPI RADIALIS LONGUS

Functional Examination

- See Insertion Tendopathy of the Extensor Carpi Radialis Brevis.

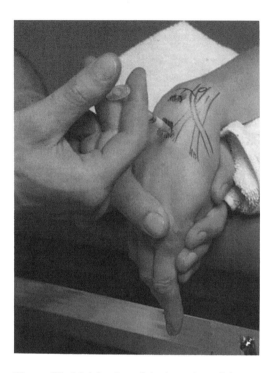

Figure 20–14 Injection of the insertion of the extensor carpi radialis brevis.

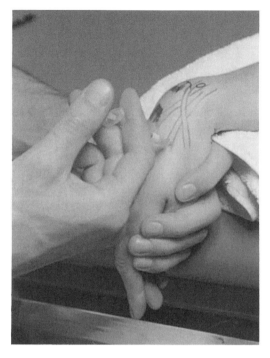

Figure 20–15 Injection of the insertion of the extensor carpi radialis longus.

Transverse Friction

The application of this technique is identical to that described under Insertion Tendopathy of the Extensor Carpi Radialis Brevis except that here the location of the lesion is at the radial aspect of the base of the second metacarpal.

Injection

The injection is administered in the same way as that described under Insertion Tendopathy of the Extensor Carpi Radialis Brevis except that here the location of the lesion is at the radial aspect of the base of the second metacarpal (Figure 20–15).

INSERTION TENDOPATHY OF THE EXTENSOR CARPI ULNARIS

Functional Examination
- Resisted wrist extension with ulnar deviation is painful.
- Passive wrist palmar flexion, usually combined with radial deviation, can be painful due to stretch.

Transverse Friction

Position of the Patient
The patient sits next to the end of the long side of the treatment table. The forearm rests on the table in pronation with the wrist positioned at the edge of the table.

Position of the Therapist

The therapist sits next to the short end of the treatment table.

If the patient's right hand is being treated, the therapist uses the right hand to grasp the patient's hand from underneath, coming from the radial aspect. The patient's hand is held in slight extension and ulnar deviation in order to relax the extensor carpi ulnaris tendon.

The tip of the index finger of the other hand is placed against the base of the patient's fifth metacarpal, and the thumb is placed as distally as possible on the radial side of the second metacarpal.

Performance

With the index finger, reinforced by the middle finger, pressure is exerted in a radiodistal direction against the base of the fifth metacarpal. The therapist performs the transverse friction in a palmar to dorsal direction by means of wrist extension and simultaneous arm adduction (Figure 20–16).

Duration of Treatment

The patient should be seen three to five times per week, and the transverse friction should last approximately 15 to 20 minutes. Usually 6 to 10 treatments are required in order to achieve complete relief of pain. If there is little or no improvement after six treatments, an injection of a corticosteroid is indicated.

Injection

If results are unsatisfactory after six treatments of transverse friction, an injection of a corticosteroid is indicated.

Position of the Patient

The patient sits next to the short end of the treatment table. The forearm rests in maxi-

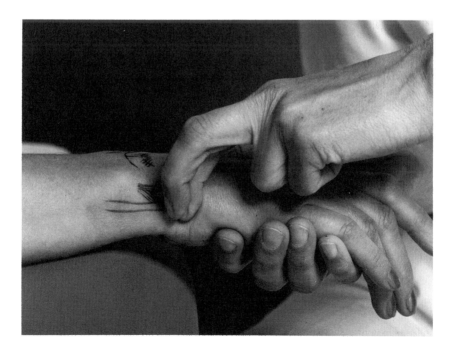

Figure 20–16 Transverse friction of the insertion of the extensor carpi ulnaris.

mal pronation on the table, and the hand and wrist hang over the edge of the table.

Position of the Physician

The physician sits next to the long side of the treatment table, diagonally facing the patient. One hand fixes the patient's hand in slight palmar flexion and ulnar deviation.

Performance

After first carefully palpating to locate the exact site of the lesion, a 2-cm long needle is used to inject the insertion of the extensor carpi ulnaris at the base of the fifth metacarpal. Guided by the patient's pain, 0.5 to 1.0 mL of triamcinolone acetonide, 10 mg/mL, is injected in a dropwise fashion. With the patient positioned as shown in Figure 20–17, the needle is inserted almost vertically.

Follow-Up

The arm should be partially immobilized in a sling for 3 days. After that, activities that may have an impact on the affected area are limited for the next 3 to 4 days. The patient's condition is reassessed after 2 weeks.

A second injection is rarely necessary to achieve complete relief of pain.

TENOSYNOVITIS OF THE EXTENSOR CARPI ULNARIS

Functional Examination

- Passive palmar flexion, particularly when combined with radial deviation, can be painful due to stretch.
- In severe cases, resisted wrist extension with ulnar deviation can be painful.

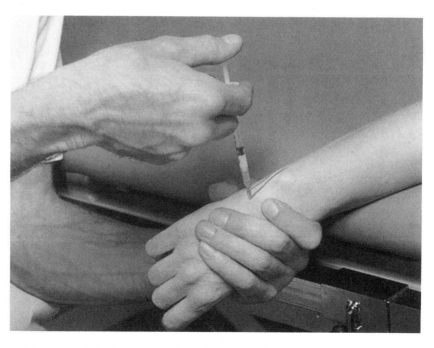

Figure 20–17 Injection of the insertion of the extensor carpi ulnaris.

- If the lesion is localized at the level of the ulnar head, passive supination will also be painful (sometimes this is the only pain-provoking test).

Transverse Friction

In a tenosynovitis of the extensor carpi ulnaris, the lesion can be located at the level of the carpus, directly proximal to the styloid process of the ulna, or proximal to the head of the ulna.

Position of the Patient

The patient sits next to the treatment table with the forearm resting in maximal supination on the table.

Position of the Therapist

The therapist sits diagonally facing the patient.

If the right side is being treated, the therapist uses the right hand to grasp the patient's hand from the ulnar aspect. The tendon sheath is now stretched by placing the forearm in supination and the wrist in radial deviation.

The tip of the index finger of the other hand locates the most painful site of the lesion. Approaching the lesion from the volar aspect, the tip of the index finger is now placed on the dorsoradial side of the lesion.

Note: With the forearm in pronation, the extensor carpi ulnaris tendon lies at the ulnar aspect of the ulna. With the forearm in supination, the tendon lies at the dorsal aspect of the ulna.

Performance

The therapist's index finger is reinforced by the middle finger. The thumb exerts counterpressure at the radial side of the wrist (Figure 20–18). The active phase of the trans-

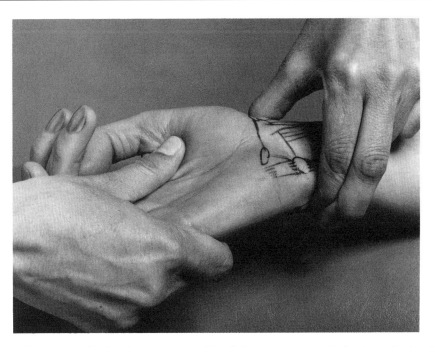

Figure 20–18 Transverse friction in a tenosynovitis of the extensor carpi ulnaris at the level of the most distal part of the ulna.

verse friction is performed by means of wrist extension and slight arm adduction.

If positioning the forearm in supination and wrist in radial deviation is too painful, the forearm can be positioned in pronation and the wrist in slight flexion and radial deviation for the transverse friction (Figure 20–19). In this instance, the active phase of the transverse friction also consists of wrist extension and slight arm adduction.

Duration of Treatment

The patient should be seen three times per week for treatment, and the transverse friction should be performed for approximately 15 minutes. Generally, 6 to 12 treatments are required for relief of symptoms.

If the patient is a tennis player or an athlete participating in other racket sports, the treatment can be supplemented by taping.

If improvement is unsatisfactory after six treatments, an injection of corticosteroid, 10 mg/mL, between the tendon and the tendon sheath should be considered.

Taping

In addition to the transverse friction in treatment of the extensor carpi ulnaris tenosynovitis, taping the wrist can be very beneficial, especially for athletes participating in racket sports. The application described below restricts the painful supination of the forearm.

Position of the Patient

The patient sits next to the treatment table and rests the arm on the table. The elbow is positioned in 90° flexion with the forearm in pronation and the wrist in the resting position (maximal loose-packed position).

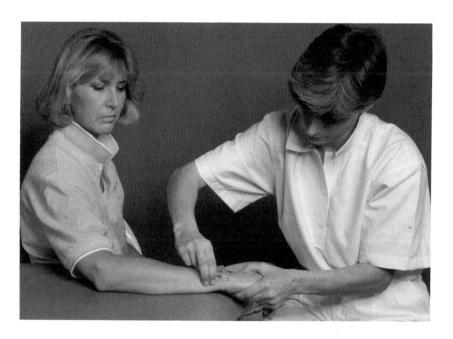

Figure 20–19 Transverse friction of the extensor carpi ulnaris with the forearm in pronation.

Position of the Therapist

The therapist stands opposite to the patient's arm that is to be taped.

Performance

With a 7-cm wide elastic wrap, the taping is begun at the level of the dorsal side of the third metacarpal. The tape is slit for the thumb, and is then wrapped in a circular manner in the direction of pronation via the volar aspect of the wrist. The wrap ends at the ulnar side of the wrist or the forearm, after going once around the entire wrist or forearm (Figure 20–20A).

The initial wrap is reinforced with 2- to 2.5-cm wide nonelastic tape. The tape is placed starting at the dorsal side of the third metacarpal and runs between the index finger and the thumb, via the palm of the hand, to the dorsal side of the distal forearm (Figure 20–20B).

A second strip of tape is placed, beginning at the dorsal side of the third metacarpal, running over the trapeziometacarpal joint, and then to the distal-dorsal aspect of the forearm, ending on the first strip of tape (Figures 20–21A and 20–21B).

This simple tape application can be used as a preventive measure during training and competition, even when the athlete does not have any symptoms.

Injection

The lesion can be located either at the level of the carpus or directly proximal to the styloid process of the ulna.

When transverse friction does not bring the desired results after six treatments, an injection of a low concentration of corticosteroid

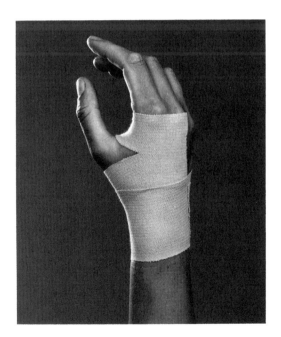

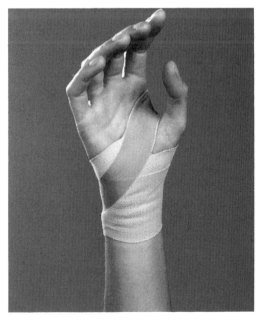

Figure 20–20A Taping for a tenosynovitis of the extensor carpi ulnaris.

Figure 20–20B Reinforcement of the initial wrap.

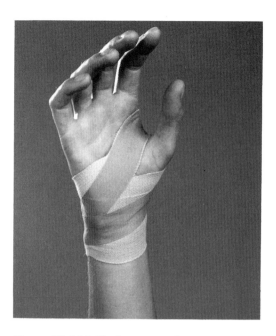

Figure 20–21A Final wrap, palmar view.

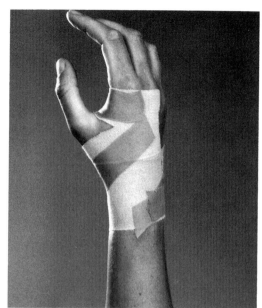

Figure 20–21B Final wrap, dorsal view.

between the tendon and the tendon sheath is indicated.

Position of the Patient

The patient sits next to the short end of the treatment table with the arm in approximately 90° abduction. The forearm is in maximal pronation and rests on the table. The wrist and hand hang over the edge of the table.

Position of the Physician

The physician sits next to the short end of the table, diagonally facing the patient. With one hand, the physician grasps the patient's hand and positions the wrist in maximal radial deviation.

Performance

A syringe is filled with 0.5 mL of triamcinolone acetonide, 10 mg/mL. If the lesion is located at the level of the carpus, a 3-cm long needle is inserted almost horizontally at the level of the base of the fifth metacarpal (Figure 20–22). In instances when the lesion is located in the region of the ulnar groove, the needle is inserted at the level of the distal edge of the ulnar head.

The needle is pushed in until it contacts the tendon (greater resistance); it is then pulled back slightly and redirected parallel to the tendon. At first only part of the solution is injected. If there is a longitudinal swelling without fluid dispersion (indicating that the solution is indeed between the tendon and the tendon sheath), the remainder of the solution is injected.

Follow-Up

The wrist should be immobilized partially in a sling for 3 days, and activities that might have an impact on the affected area are limited for the following 3 or 4 days. The patient's condition should be reassessed after 2 weeks.

A second injection is usually necessary for complete recovery.

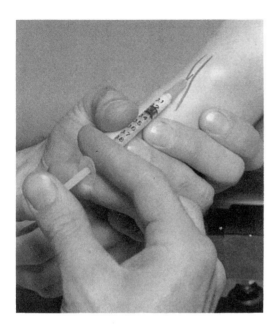

Figure 20–22 Injection between the tendon and the tendon sheath of the extensor carpi ulnaris.

TENOSYNOVITIS OF THE EXTENSOR INDICIS

Functional Examination

- Often, active extension of the index finger elicits crepitation.
- Passive flexion of the index finger is painful due to stretch.
- Resisted extension of the index finger can be painful.

Injection

This lesion is most frequently seen in cross-country skiers. It usually occurs at the level of the metacarpophalangeal II joint. Occasionally it is observed at the level of the carpus. The patient is usually unable to tolerate transverse friction, even with prior administration of cryotherapy or other pain-relieving measures.

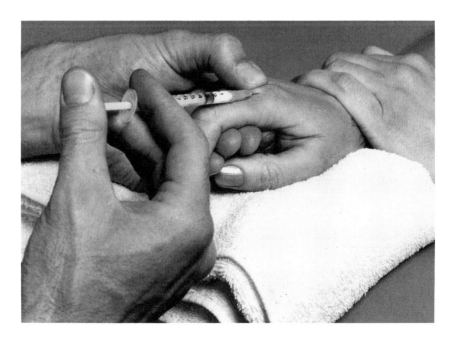

Figure 20–23 Injection between the tendon and the tendon sheath of the extensor indicis at the level of the metacarpophalangeal II joint.

Position of the Patient

The patient sits next to the short end of the treatment table with the forearm resting in pronation on the table.

Position of the Physician

The physician sits next to the long side of the treatment table, diagonally facing the patient.

With one hand, the physician holds the patient's metacarpophalangeal II joint in slight flexion and locates the site of the lesion with the thumb.

Performance

With a 2-cm long needle, 0.5 mL of triamcinolone acetonide, 10 mg/mL, is injected between the tendon and the tendon sheath. The needle is inserted horizontally directly distal to the site of the lesion (Figure 20–23).

Once the needle is correctly positioned, the solution is injected slowly. There should be a longitudinal swelling along the length of the tendon.

Follow-Up

Activities that could have an impact on the affected area should be limited for 1 or 2 days. Afterward the patient can resume full activities.

TENOSYNOVITIS OF THE FLEXOR DIGITORUM PROFUNDUS

Functional Examination

- Passive wrist extension with finger extension is painful due to stretch.
- Resisted wrist flexion with resisted finger flexion can be painful.

Transverse Friction

Transverse friction is the treatment of choice for a deep finger flexor tenosynovitis. An injection is administered only if the problem is so severe that a carpal tunnel syndrome develops. Strangely enough, the superficial finger flexors are seldom affected.

Position of the Patient

The patient sits at the short end of the treatment table with the forearm resting in slight supination on the table.

Position of the Therapist

The therapist sits next to the long side of the treatment table, diagonally facing the patient.

If the right hand is to be treated, the therapist grasps the patient's hand with the right hand. The patient's hand is positioned in slight flexion. With the wrist in extension, the tendons become taut, making it difficult or impossible to reach the tendon sheaths of the deeper-lying tendons.

The therapist places the index and middle fingertips of the other hand just ulnar to the midline of the wrist; the medial tendons are most often affected.

Performance

By means of wrist extension and slight arm adduction, the therapist moves the index and middle fingers in an ulnar to radial direction, transversely over the tendons (Figure 20–24).

Duration of Treatment

The patient should be seen three to five times per week for treatment. The transverse friction should be performed for approximately 15 minutes per treatment. Usually, about 10 treatment sessions are necessary to achieve complete relief of pain.

INSERTION TENDOPATHY OF THE FLEXOR CARPI RADIALIS

Functional Examination

- Resisted wrist flexion combined with radial deviation is painful.

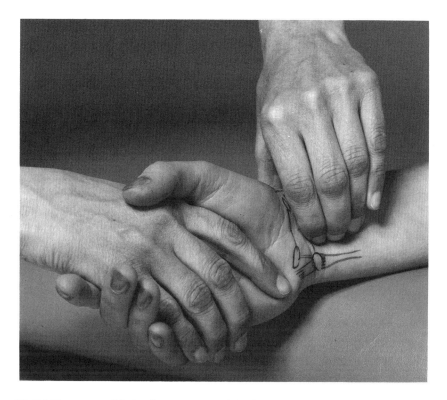

Figure 20–24 Transverse friction in a tenosynovitis of the flexor digitorum profundus.

- Passive wrist extension together with ulnar deviation can be painful due to stretch.

Transverse Friction

An insertion tendopathy of the flexor carpi radialis is an injury typically resulting from throwing and racket sports. It is rarely seen in nonathletes.

Position of the Patient

The patient sits next to the short end of the treatment table with the maximally supinated forearm resting on the table and the hand hanging over the edge.

Position of the Therapist

The therapist sits next to the long side of the table, diagonally facing the patient.

With either the right or left hand, and considering the patient's pain, the therapist grasps the patient's hand, positioning it in extension and ulnar deviation. The tip of the index finger of the other hand locates the most painful site of the insertion at the base of the metacarpal II.

Performance

By means of wrist extension, the index finger, reinforced by the middle finger, performs the active phase of the transverse friction in an ulnar to radial direction (Figure 20–25).

Duration of Treatment

Daily 15-minute sessions of transverse friction usually lead to full recovery after three to six treatments. During the treatment period, the patient should continue to stay active but

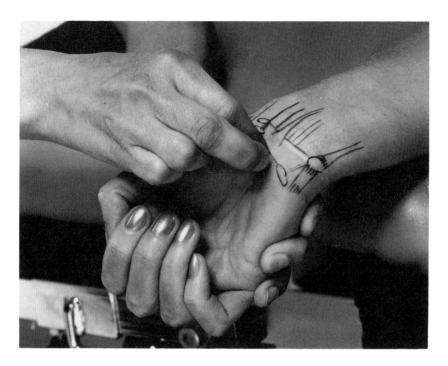

Figure 20–25 Transverse friction of the insertion of the flexor carpi radialis.

should avoid pain-provoking activities found particularly in throwing and racket sports.

Injection

Transverse friction is preferred over injection as treatment for an insertion tendopathy of the flexor carpi radialis. Occasionally, however, an injection is necessary.

Position of the Patient

The patient sits next to the short end of the treatment table with the maximally supinated forearm resting on the table.

Position of the Physician

The physician sits next to the long side of the table, diagonally facing the patient.

With one hand, the physician grasps the patient's hand, holding the wrist in slight extension. During transverse friction, the wrist is positioned in *maximal* extension. For the

injection, however, maximal extension puts too much tension on the fibers to be infiltrated, making the injection more difficult.

With the index finger or thumb of the other hand, the physician locates the site of the lesion.

Performance

A syringe is filled with 0.5 mL of triamcinolone acetonide, 10 mg/mL (local anesthetic is ineffective in this lesion).

At the site of the lesion, a 2-cm long needle is inserted vertically (Figure 20–26). The solution is injected in a dropwise fashion, taking into consideration the patient's pain.

Follow-Up

The hand and wrist should be immobilized partially in a sling for 3 or 4 days. During the next 4 days, the patient should perform as few problem-provoking activities as possible. Af-

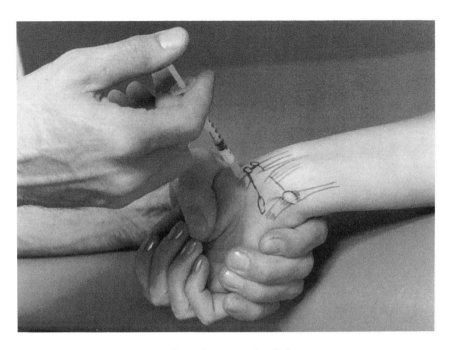

Figure 20–26 Injection of the insertion of the flexor carpi radialis.

ter 1 week activities can be increased slowly. The patient's condition should be reassessed after 2 weeks.

More than one injection is rarely necessary to achieve full recovery.

TENOSYNOVITIS OF THE FLEXOR CARPI RADIALIS

Functional Examination

- Passive wrist extension with simultaneous ulnar deviation is painful due to stretching of the tendon sheath.
- In severe cases, resisted wrist flexion combined with radial deviation is painful.

Transverse Friction

When the tendon sheath of the flexor carpi radialis is affected, it is usually at the level of the carpus.

Position of the Patient

The patient sits next to the short end of the treatment table with the forearm resting in maximal supination on the table and the hand hanging over the edge.

Position of the Therapist

The therapist sits next to the long side of the treatment table, diagonally facing the patient.

If the right side is to be treated, the therapist grasps the patient's hand with the right hand, holding it in submaximal extension and ulnar deviation. Using the tip of the index finger of the other hand, the therapist locates the most painful site of the lesion.

Performance

Because the tenosynovitis generally occurs over a distance of 1.5 to 2.0 cm, the index and middle fingers, placed next to each other, are used to perform the transverse friction (Figure 20–27). During the active phase of the technique, the wrist extends in order to move

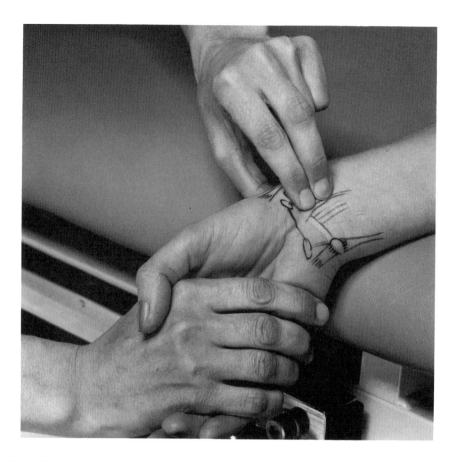

Figure 20–27 Transverse friction of a flexor carpi radialis tenosynovitis.

the fingers in an ulnar to radial direction over the tendon sheath.

Duration of Treatment

Although more treatments generally are needed than are needed for an insertion tendopathy, this lesion reacts very well to transverse friction. The patient should be seen daily, or at least three times per week, for 15 minutes of transverse friction each session.

Between 5 and 10 treatments usually are required to reach full recovery. If there is no obvious improvement after six treatments, an injection is indicated.

Injection

As with the flexor carpi radialis insertion tendopathy, transverse friction in the flexor carpi radialis tenosynovitis generally provides excellent results. In the rare case when six treatments do not provide satisfactory results, an injection between the tendon and the tendon sheath is indicated.

Position of the Patient

The patient sits next to the short end of the treatment table with the forearm resting in maximal supination on the table.

Position of the Physician

The physician sits next to the long side of the treatment table, diagonally facing the patient.

With one hand the physician grasps the patient's hand and holds it in slight wrist extension. With the other hand, the physician palpates the tuberosity of the scaphoid and then, just ulnar to it, the tendon of the flexor carpi radialis.

Performance

A 2-cm long needle is used to inject 0.5 mL of triamcinolone acetonide, 10 mg/mL, between the tendon and the tendon sheath. The needle is inserted almost horizontally, just medial to the tuberosity of the scaphoid, and pushed in until a firm resistance is felt; the tendon has been reached (Figure 20–28). At this point, the needle is withdrawn slightly and repositioned even more horizontally before being pushed in further. If minimal resistance is encountered, a small amount of solution is injected. Longitudinal swelling should be visible, indicating that the needle is positioned properly between the tendon and the tendon sheath. The remainder of the solution is then injected.

Follow-Up

The hand and wrist should be immobilized partially in a sling for 3 or 4 days. During the next 4 days, the patient should perform as little activity involving the affected areas as possible. After 1 week activities can be increased slowly. The patient's condition should be reassessed after 2 weeks.

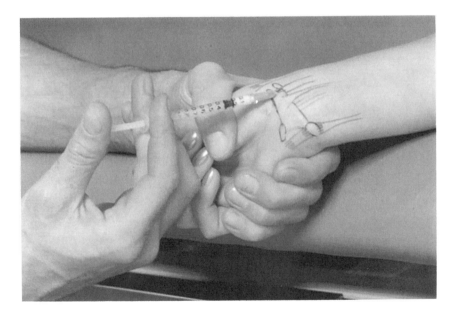

Figure 20–28 Injection between the tendon and the tendon sheath of the flexor carpi radialis at the level of the carpus.

More than two injections are rarely necessary to reach full recovery.

INSERTION TENDOPATHY OF THE FLEXOR CARPI ULNARIS

Functional Examination

- Resisted wrist flexion combined with ulnar deviation is painful.
- Passive extension of the wrist combined with radial deviation is painful because of stretching.

Transverse Friction

Differentiation between an insertion tendopathy of the flexor carpi ulnaris and a sprain of the triquetrum-pisiform joint is not always easy if the lesion lies at the level of the pisiform. Sometimes an injection of local anesthetic can aid in confirming the diagnosis. If pain still can be provoked after an injection of the triquetrum-pisiform joint, the lesion most likely lies at the insertion of the flexor carpi ulnaris.

Position of the Patient

The patient sits next to the short end of the treatment table. The maximally supinated forearm rests on the table; the hand hangs over the edge of the table with the wrist in extension.

Position of the Therapist

The therapist sits next to the long side of the treatment table, diagonally facing the patient. If the right side is being treated, the therapist grasps the patient's hand with the right hand, holding it in extension and radial deviation.

With the thumb of the other hand, the therapist palpates the area to locate the site of the lesion. Likely sites include (1) the proximal insertion on the sesamoid pisiform, (2) the distal insertion on the pisiform, and/or (3) the insertion at the base of metacarpal V.

Performance

The therapist places the tip of the thumb just ulnar to the lesion. By means of radial deviation of the wrist, the thumb is moved in an ulnar to radial direction over the affected structure (Figure 20–29).

Duration of Treatment

The patient should be seen daily, or at least three times per week, and the transverse friction is performed for 15 to 20 minutes each session. As soon as it can be tolerated, the pressure exerted during the transverse friction is increased. Without a relatively large amount of pressure, the treatment usually is not successful.

Usually six to eight treatments are necessary to achieve complete relief of pain. An injection of triamcinolone acetonide, 10 mg/mL, is indicated when transverse friction treatments prove ineffective.

Injection

See comments under transverse friction.

Position of the Patient

The patient sits next to the short end of the treatment table. The maximally supinated forearm rests on the table. The hand hangs over the edge of the table with the wrist in extension.

Position of the Physician

The physician sits next to the treatment table, diagonally facing the patient.

With one hand, the physician grasps the patient's hand and holds it in extension. With the other hand, the physician locates the site of the lesion.

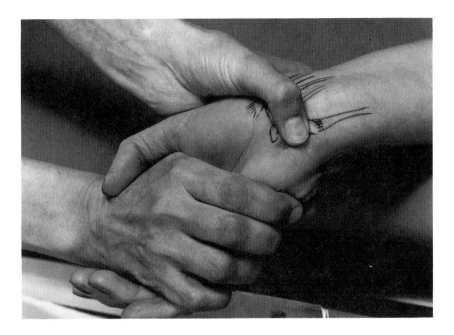

Figure 20–29 Transverse friction of the flexor carpi ulnaris at the distal insertion on the pisiform.

Performance

A syringe filled with 0.5 mL of triamcinolone acetonide, 10 mg/mL, and a 2-cm long needle are used for the injection.

If the lesion is located at the proximal or distal aspect of the pisiform, the needle is inserted at an angle of approximately 45° to the pisiform (Figure 20–30). If the insertion at the base of the fifth metacarpal is affected, the needle is inserted vertically with relation to the skin.

Corresponding to when the patient feels pain, the superficial and deep fibers are injected in a dropwise fashion.

Follow-Up

The hand and wrist should be immobilized partially in a sling for 3 or 4 days. During the next 4 days, the patient should perform as little activity involving the affected area as possible. After 1 week activities can be increased slowly. The patient's condition should be reassessed after 2 weeks.

In most cases, only one injection is needed to achieve full recovery.

TENOMYOSYNOVITIS OF THE ABDUCTOR POLLICIS LONGUS AND EXTENSORS POLLICIS LONGUS AND BREVIS

Functional Examination

- Passive wrist flexion is painful, especially when combined with flexion of all of the thumb joints.
- Resisted radial abduction and palmar abduction of the thumb are painful.
- Usually there is severe pain as well as crepitation.

Transverse Friction

This lesion is located at the musculotendinous junction of the thumb extensors and long abductor of the thumb, approximately 3

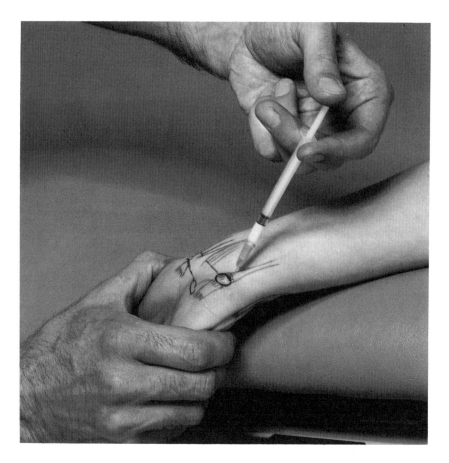

Figure 20–30 Injection of the proximal insertion of the flexor carpi ulnaris on the pisiform.

to 4 cm proximal to Lister's tubercle. There is a synovial sheath at this site, which is also affected.

Position of the Patient

The patient sits next to the short end of the treatment table with the forearm supported in pronation on the table. The hand hangs over the edge of the table.

Position of the Therapist

The therapist sits next to the long side of the treatment table, diagonally facing the patient. Two different techniques can be used for this transverse friction.

Technique 1: *Treatment Using the Thumb.* If the patient's right hand is to be treated, the therapist grasps that hand with the left hand, positioning the hand in flexion. The thumb of the other hand is placed directly ulnar from the site of the lesion. The thumb points in a proximal direction.

Technique 2: *Treatment Using the Fingers.* With this method, the patient's hand is grasped with the therapist's right hand. The tips of the index, middle, and ring fingers of the other hand are placed directly radial to the site of the lesion (fingertips point in a radial direction).

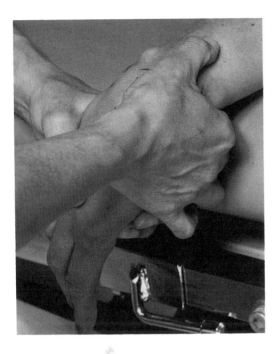

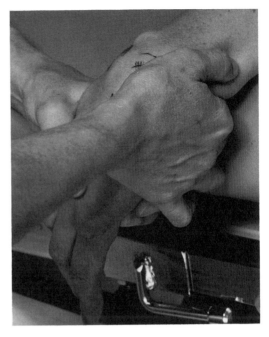

Figure 20–31A Initial position in transverse friction of the musculotendinous junction of the abductor pollicis longus and extensor pollicis longus and brevis.

Figure 20–31B End position in the transverse friction technique that uses the thumb.

Performance

Technique 1. The active phase of the transverse friction is performed by means of thumb adduction with simultaneous slight wrist extension. In so doing, the thumb moves in an ulnar to a radial direction over the lesion (Figures 20–31A and 20–31B).

Technique 2. The transverse friction is performed by means of wrist extension with simultaneous slight shoulder adduction. In this way, the fingers are moved in a radial to an ulnar direction over the affected fibers (Figures 20–32A and 20–32B).

Duration of Treatment

Patients generally respond very well to the transverse friction, and in three to four treatments significant improvement is noted. The transverse friction should be performed for approximately 15 minutes, and the patient should be seen three times per week for treatment.

In some cases, the patient enjoys pain relief within the first minutes of transverse friction, only to have the pain increase to an even greater level after the treatment. This phenomenon can be observed with the first two to four sessions of transverse friction. Although the therapist may be inclined to discontinue this form of treatment, continuation of the treatments beyond this stage almost always results in a very sudden drastic improvement. In our experience, patients have reacted very well to transverse friction of this lesion, and the treatment should not be abandoned because of a temporary setback. Occasionally, it takes 2 to 3 weeks to achieve complete relief of pain.

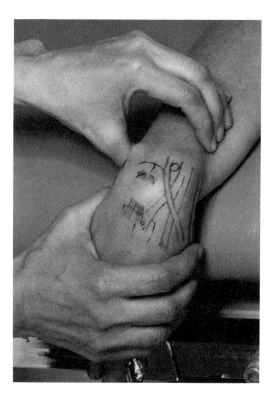

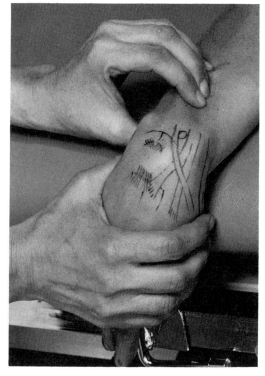

Figure 20–32A Initial position in transverse friction technique that uses the fingers.

Figure 20–32B End position of the technique using the fingers.

TENOSYNOVITIS OF THE ABDUCTOR POLLICIS LONGUS AND EXTENSOR POLLICIS BREVIS (DE QUERVAIN SYNDROME)

Functional Examination

- The Finkelstein test, during which the patient makes a fist and the therapist brings the wrist into slight extension and ulnar deviation, is very painful.
- Only in severe cases are resisted palmar abduction and resisted radial abduction (extension) of the thumb painful.

Transverse Friction

Generally the treatment of choice in a de Quervain syndrome is a single injection of a corticosteroid, 10 mg/mL. Transverse friction can be used when injection is not possible. Although treatment with transverse friction ultimately leads to good results, many sessions are needed. Compared with the use of transverse friction in the treatment of other lesions, a very long time is needed before the pain is reduced enough to allow for any amount of pressure to be exerted during the friction.

The lesion is located at the level of the carpus, just distal to the styloid process of the radius.

Position of the Patient

The patient sits next to the short end of the treatment table with the forearm supported on the table. The forearm is supinated ap-

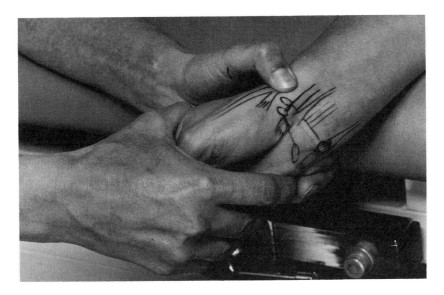

Figure 20–33 Transverse friction in the de Quervain syndrome.

proximately 10°, bringing the affected area into a horizontal position.

Position of the Therapist

The therapist sits next to the long side of the treatment table, diagonally facing the patient.

If the patient's right hand is being treated, the therapist grasps the patient's hand from the radial aspect with the right hand. The patient's thumb is positioned in ulnar adduction and the wrist in slight extension with ulnar deviation, taking care to avoid pain or muscle splinting.

The therapist places the thumb of the other hand just volar to the lesion.

Performance

The active phase of the transverse friction is performed in a volar to dorsal direction by means of wrist extension and slight arm adduction (Figure 20–33).

Duration of Treatment

The transverse friction should be performed for approximately 15 to 20 minutes per treatment. The patient should be seen three times per week for 4 to 7 weeks.

During the treatment period, if possible, activities that provoke the symptoms should be avoided.

Injection

Injection of triamcinolone acetonide between the tendons and the tendon sheath is the treatment of choice in a de Quervain syndrome.

Position of the Patient

The patient sits next to the treatment table with the forearm resting in slight supination on the table. The wrist is positioned in slight extension and ulnar deviation, and the fingers grasp the thumb.

Position of the Physician

The physician sits diagonally facing the patient. One hand supports the patient's hand and wrist (with the thumb positioned in ulnar adduction and the wrist in slight extension with ulnar deviation). The other hand locates the site of the lesion and the joint space of the trapeziometacarpal joint.

Performance

A syringe is filled with 1 mL of triamcinolone acetonide, 10 mg/mL. At an angle of approximately 30° to the horizontal, a 2-cm long needle is inserted at the level of the trapeziometacarpal joint, pointing in the direction of the styloid process of the radius (Figure 20–34).

As soon as the needle contacts firm resistance (the tendon), it is withdrawn slightly, repositioned almost horizontally, and pushed in further. At this point, part of the solution is injected. If the needle is correctly positioned, a longitudinal swelling arises along the tendon, indicating that the solution lies between the tendons and the tendon sheath. The remaining 0.5 to 1 mL of solution is now injected.

Follow-Up

The hand and wrist are immobilized partially in a sling for 3 days, and activities involving the affected extremity should be reduced

significantly for the next 3 or 4 days. After approximately 1 week, activities can be increased gradually. The patient's condition should be reassessed in 2 weeks.

In most cases, one or two injections are needed to achieve full recovery.

TENOVAGINITIS OF THE ABDUCTOR POLLICIS LONGUS AND EXTENSOR POLLICIS BREVIS

Functional Examination

- The Finkelstein test provokes pain, but not as much as in the de Quervain syndrome.
- In severe cases, resisted radial abduction and resisted palmar abduction of the thumb are painful.

Transverse Friction

This lesion is located just proximal to the radial styloid and responds very well to transverse friction.

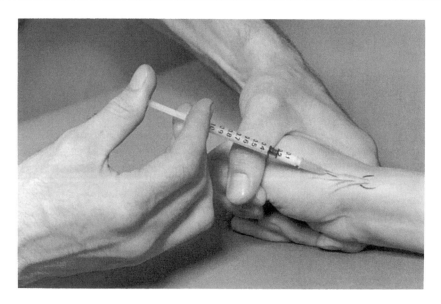

Figure 20–34 Injection between the tendons and the tendon sheath in the de Quervain syndrome.

Position of the Patient

The patient sits next to the short end of the treatment table. The forearm rests on the table and is positioned in very slight pronation in order to bring the affected area into a horizontal position. The wrist and hand hang over the edge of the table.

Position of the Therapist

The therapist sits next to the long side of the treatment table, diagonally facing the patient.

If the right side is affected, the therapist uses the right hand to grasp the patient's hand, positioning the patient's thumb in ulnar adduction and the wrist in extension and ulnar deviation. The tip of the thumb of the therapist's other hand is placed just volar to the site of the lesion.

Performance

As in treatment of the de Quervain syndrome, transverse friction is performed in a volar to dorsal direction during the active phase by means of radial deviation of the wrist and slight adduction of the arm (Figure 20–35).

Duration of Treatment

In contrast to the de Quervain syndrome, this lesion reacts very well to transverse friction. The patient should be seen three to five times per week for 2 to 4 weeks. Transverse friction should be performed for 15 minutes per session.

Injection

An injection of triamcinolone acetonide, 10 mg/mL, is also very effective in the treatment of a tenovaginitis of the abductor pollicis longus and extensor pollicis brevis.

The technique is performed in a manner similar to that described for the de Quervain syndrome, except that the forearm is positioned in very slight pronation instead of supi-

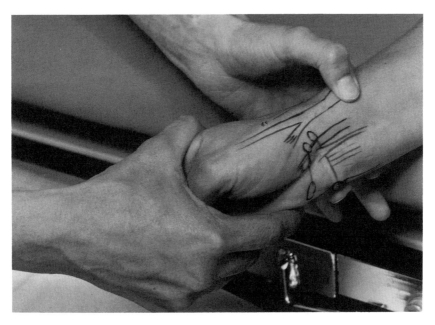

Figure 20–35 Transverse friction of the common tendon sheath of the abductor pollicis longus and extensor pollicis brevis.

nation. The needle is inserted directly proximal to the styloid process of the radius.

INSERTION TENDOPATHY OF THE ABDUCTOR POLLICIS LONGUS

Functional Examination
- Resisted thumb palmar abduction is painful.
- Resisted radial abduction of the thumb can be painful.

Transverse Friction

An insertion tendopathy of the abductor pollicis longus is rarely seen. Sometimes it occurs from overuse, but more often it is the result of trauma incurred while playing sports such as volleyball, handball, and water polo. It is seen most often in conjunction with traumatic arthritis of the trapeziometacarpal joint or a lesion of the medial collateral ligament of the metacarpophalangeal joint.

Position of the Patient

The patient sits next to the short end of the treatment table. The forearm rests in maximal supination, and the wrist and hand hang over the edge of the table.

Position of the Therapist

The therapist sits next to the long side of the treatment table, diagonally facing the patient.

If the right side is being treated, the therapist uses the right hand to support the patient's hand, holding the thumb in ulnar adduction and the wrist in slight extension.

The tip of the thumb of the therapist's other hand is placed directly ulnar to the lesion. The insertion is located on the radiovolar side of the base of the first metacarpal.

Performance

The transverse friction is performed in an ulnar to a radial direction by means of radial deviation of the wrist and slight adduction of the arm (Figure 20–36).

Duration of Treatment

Usually four to six treatments are necessary to achieve complete relief of pain. The patient should be seen three times weekly, and the transverse friction should be performed for 10 to 15 minutes per session.

An injection of triamcinolone acetonide, 10 mg/mL, is also a very effective treatment.

Injection

Generally, transverse friction treatments provide excellent results for this problem. Occasionally, however, an injection is required.

Position of the Patient

The patient sits next to the short end of the treatment table. The maximally supinated forearm rests on the table with the wrist and hand hanging over the edge of the table. A small towel or pillow can also be placed under the forearm in order to allow for extension in the hand.

Position of the Physician

With one hand, the physician grasps the patient's hand, maintaining the position of wrist extension and ulnar adduction in the thumb. With the other hand, the physician locates the insertion of the abductor pollicis longus at the radiovolar aspect of the base of metacarpal I.

Performance

A syringe is filled with 0.5 mL of triamcinolone acetonide, 10 mg/mL. A 2-cm long needle is inserted vertically—because of the patient's hand position, the insertion lies in

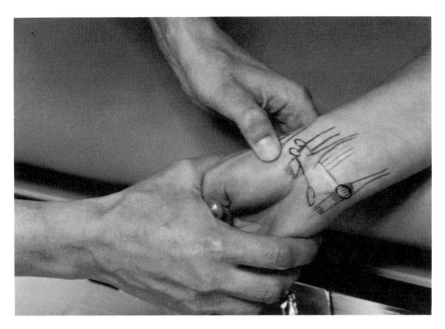

Figure 20–36 Transverse friction of the insertion of the abductor pollicis longus at the radiovolar aspect of the base of the first metacarpal.

the horizontal plane (Figure 20–37). The lesion is injected in a dropwise fashion, guided by the patient's feelings of pain. The amount of solution that can be injected varies from 0.2 to 0.5 mL, depending on the resistance.

Follow-Up

The hand and wrist are partially immobilized in a sling for 3 days, and activities that could affect the afflicted area negatively should be reduced significantly for the next 3 to 4 days. After approximately 1 week, activities can be increased gradually. The patient's condition should be reassessed in 2 weeks.

One injection is usually sufficient to achieve full recovery.

TENOSYNOVITIS OF THE FLEXOR POLLICIS LONGUS

Functional Examination

- Passive retroposition of the thumb is painful because of stretching.

- In severe cases, resisted ulnar adduction and opposition of the thumb can be painful.

Transverse Friction

Transverse friction for a tenosynovitis of the flexor pollicis longus is a very effective treatment, whether the lesion is located in the carpal region or at the level of the thenar eminence. Patience is required in both instances because the lesion lies so deep.

An injection of triamcinolone acetonide, 10 mg/mL, between the tendon and its sheath is also an effective treatment. However, the tendon is difficult to find, and searching with the needle in this richly vascularized area is not recommended.

Position of the Patient

The patient sits next to the short end of the treatment table. The forearm rests in maxi-

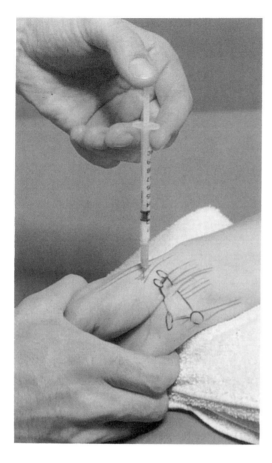

Figure 20–37 Injection of the insertion of the abductor pollicis longus at its insertion on the radiovolar aspect of the base of the first metacarpal.

The tips of the index and middle fingers of the other hand are placed directly ulnar to the site of the lesion. This positioning is suitable for a problem at the level of the thenar eminence as well as in the carpal region.

Performance

The transverse friction is performed by means of wrist extension with slight arm adduction, during which the fingertips are moved in an ulnar to a radial direction over the lesion (Figure 20–38).

Duration of Treatment

The patient should be seen three times per week for 15- to 20-minute sessions of transverse friction. Generally, 4 to 5 weeks of treatment are necessary to achieve full recovery.

TRAUMATIC ARTHRITIS OF THE TRAPEZIOMETACARPAL JOINT

Functional Examination

- Passive retroposition of the thumb is limited and painful.
- Sometimes resisted radial abduction of the thumb is painful.

mal supination on the table with the wrist and hand hanging over the edge.

Position of the Therapist

The therapist sits next to the long side of the treatment table, diagonally facing the patient.

If the right side is being treated, the therapist grasps the patient's hand from the volar aspect with the fingers of the right hand, fixing it in slight extension. The therapist's right thumb holds the patient's thumb in retroposition.

Transverse Friction of the Volar Aspect of the Joint Capsule

The trapeziometacarpal joint is one of the few joints that, posttraumatically, respond very well to transverse friction.

Transverse friction is also indicated for the first stages of osteoarthrosis.

Position of the Patient

The patient sits next to the short side of the treatment table with the forearm resting in maximal supination on the table.

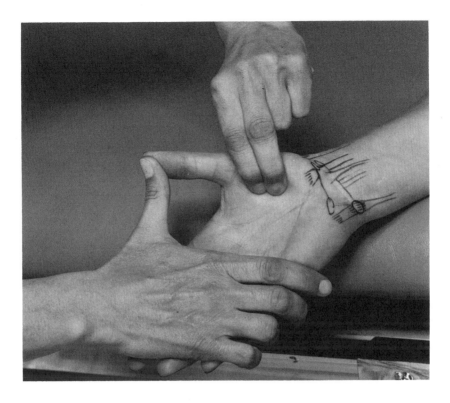

Figure 20–38 Transverse friction for a tenosynovitis of the flexor pollicis longus at the level of the thenar eminence.

Position of the Therapist

The therapist sits next to the long side of the treatment table, diagonally facing the patient.

If the right thumb is being treated, the therapist's right hand is placed on the table; the dorsum of the patient's hand lies on the dorsum of the therapist's hand. The therapist's thumb grasps the patient's thumb from the volar aspect and brings it into retroposition. In so doing, the volar aspect of the joint capsule is stretched (Figure 20–39).

The thumb of the therapist's other hand is then placed on the ulnar side of the lesion.

Performance

The transverse friction is performed in an ulnar to a radial direction by means of thumb adduction (Figures 20–40A and 20–40B).

Transverse Friction of the Lateral (Radial) Aspect of the Joint Capsule

Position of the Patient

The position of the patient is the same as that for transverse friction of the volar part of the joint capsule, except that the patient's forearm is in slight supination and the wrist

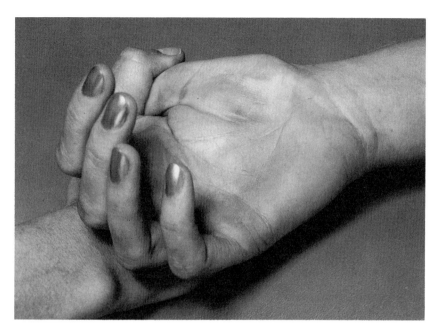

Figure 20–39 Hand position for transverse friction of the volar aspect of the capsule of the trapeziometacarpal joint.

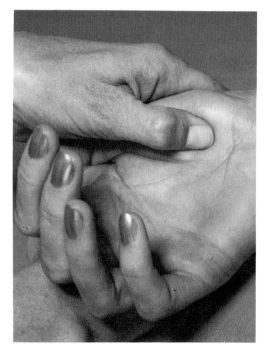

Figure 20–40A Initial position in transverse friction of the volar aspect of the joint capsule.

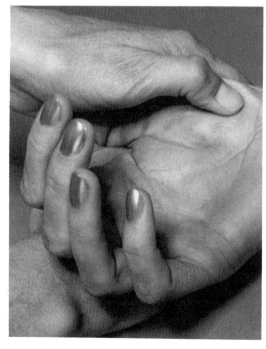

Figure 20–40B End position in transverse friction of the volar aspect of the joint capsule.

rests in ulnar deviation over the edge of the table.

Position of the Therapist

The position of the therapist is similar to that described for the volar part, except that the therapist supports the patient's hand from the radial aspect, holding the thumb in opposition and the wrist in ulnar deviation (Figure 20–41A).

The tip of the therapist's index finger is placed on the ulnar-volar side of the lesion.

Performance

The index finger is reinforced by the middle finger. The active phase of the transverse friction occurs through wrist extension. In so doing, the fingers are moved in an ulnar-volar to a radial-dorsal direction over the lesion (Figure 20–41B).

Duration of Treatment

The transverse friction should be performed for 7 to 10 minutes at the volar as well as the lateral aspects of the joint capsule. The patient should be seen two or three times per week. Generally 2 to 3 weeks of treatment are needed to reach full recovery.

If a limitation of motion in retroposition exists, the joint is also treated with joint-specific mobilization techniques. In addition, it may be necessary to support the joint with tape or a splint during the recovery period.

Stabilization by Means of Taping

Sometimes in the treatment of traumatic arthritis, whether there are ligamentous lesions or not, it is beneficial to supplement the transverse friction treatment with taping. However, in instances of severe instability,

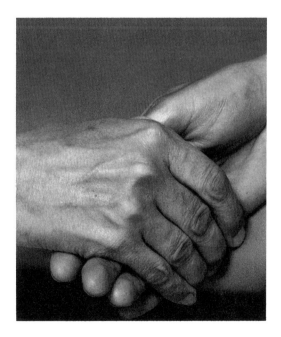

Figure 20–41A Positioning for transverse friction of the lateral part of the capsule of the trapezio-metacarpal joint.

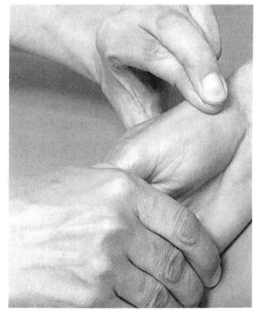

Figure 20–41B Transverse friction of the lateral part of the capsule of the trapeziometacarpal joint.

surgical treatment is indicated. In other forms of arthritis, it may also be necessary to tape the joint to prevent the particularly painful motion of retroposition.

Position of the Patient

The patient sits next to the treatment table. The elbow, which is flexed approximately 90°, is supported on the treatment table.

Position of the Therapist

The therapist sits or stands next to the treatment table.

Performance

To limit the retroposition motion, the thumb is immobilized in the resting (or maximal loose-packed) position. A 2-cm wide adhesive tape is placed on the dorsal aspect of the wrist at the level of the styloid process of the ulna. Via the dorsum of the wrist, the tape runs over the trapeziometacarpal joint, over the thenar eminence, and between the thumb and index finger (Figure 20–42). The tape again runs over the joint, and then extends further to the styloid process of the ulna, where it ends at the volar aspect of the wrist (Figure 20–43).

The entire construction is then repeated in reverse, whereby the second tape slightly overlaps the first tape (Figure 20–42). Thus the tapes cross over the joint to be immobilized.

In the same way, the metacarpophalangeal joint can be immobilized, except that the tape crosses directly over this joint (Figure 20–44).

OSTEOARTHROSIS OR TRAUMATIC ARTHRITIS OF THE TRAPEZIOMETACARPAL JOINT

Functional Examination

- Passive retroposition of the thumb is painful and limited (capsular pattern).

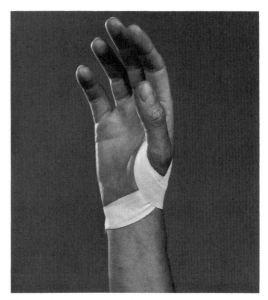

Figure 20–42 Taping of the trapeziometacarpal joint.

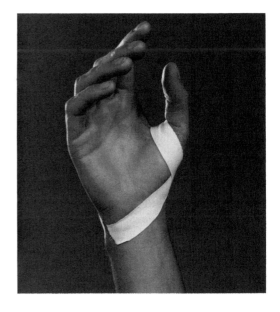

Figure 20–43 Tape construction of the trapeziometacarpal joint, volar view.

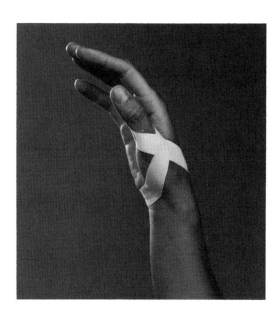

Figure 20–44 Tape construction for the immobilization of the metacarpophalangeal joint.

- Sometimes resisted radial abduction is painful.

Intra-articular Injection

An intra-articular injection is indicated in some cases of traumatic arthritis, for arthritides of a rheumatic nature, and for osteoarthrosis in the second and sometimes third stages.

Position of the Patient

The patient sits next to the treatment table with the forearm resting in slight supination. The hand hangs over the edge of the table with the wrist positioned in slight ulnar deviation.

Position of the Physician

The physician sits next to the treatment table, diagonally facing the patient.

With one hand the physician grasps the patient's thumb and exerts a pull so that the joint space is easier to palpate.

Performance

A syringe containing 1 mL of triamcinolone acetonide, 10 mg/mL, with a 2-cm long needle is inserted at an angle of 60° into the forearm (Figure 20–45). After only approximately 1.5 cm of the needle has been inserted is the needle intra-articular. Therefore, if the needle contacts bone before it is inserted 1.5 cm, it has to be maneuvered to a slightly different angle until it has been inserted for a distance of 1.5 cm or until resistance is no longer encountered. At this point the solution is injected. Depending on the resistance, the amount that can be injected varies from 0.6 to 1 mL.

Follow-Up

For 3 days after the injection, the affected part should be taped or the arm placed in a sling. During the next several days, impinging activities should be kept to a minimum. Over the next 2 weeks, the patient should continue at a reduced level of activities. The patient is seen for reassessment 2 weeks after the intra-articular injection.

In most cases of traumatic arthritis, only one injection is necessary for full recovery. In instances of rheumatoid and other arthritides of a rheumatic nature, additional injections depend on the reaction to the first injection. If the first injection resulted in a long period of pain relief, the treatment can be repeated several times.

In osteoarthrosis, the results are variable. After receiving an injection, patients sometimes remain without symptoms for years.

TRAUMATIC ARTHRITIS OF THE METACARPOPHALANGEAL AND INTERPHALANGEAL JOINTS OF THE THUMB

Functional Examination

- Passive flexion and extension are painful and limited; flexion is more limited than extension (capsular pattern).

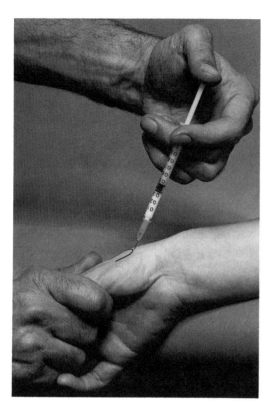

Figure 20–45 Intra-articular injection of the trapeziometacarpal joint.

Stabilization by Means of Taping

Taping is a very easy way to immobilize not only flexion but also extension in the metacarpophalangeal and interphalangeal joints of the thumb.

Position of the Patient

The patient sits next to the treatment table. The elbow is flexed approximately 90° and is supported on the table.

Position of the Therapist

The therapist stands next to the treatment table.

Performance

A 2-cm wide adhesive tape is placed in a circular manner between the metacarpophalangeal and interphalangeal joints of the thumb when immobilizing the metacarpophalangeal joint. The tape is placed in a circular manner around the distal phalanx when immobilizing the interphalangeal joint.

To restrict flexion, a piece of tape approximately 25 cm long, with the adhesive side facing away from the thumb, is placed between the thumb and the circular tape (Figure 20–46A). This piece is then folded over and laid along the forearm over the course of the wrist extensors (Figure 20–46B).

To restrict extension, almost the same construction is used. In this instance, the long strip of tape runs over the thenar eminence to the distal-volar aspect of the forearm (Figure 20–47).

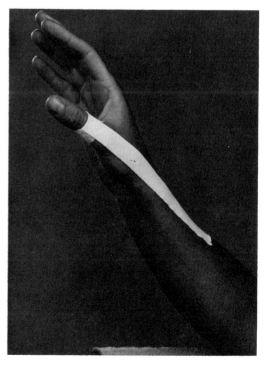

Figure 20–46A Tape construction to immobilize flexion in the metacarpophalangeal joint.

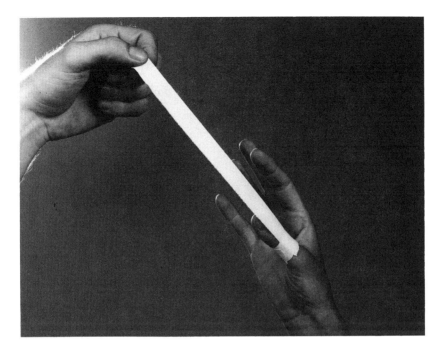

Figure 20–46B The long strip is folded back.

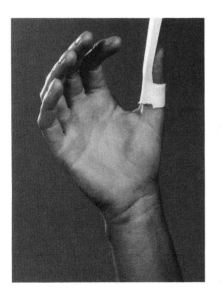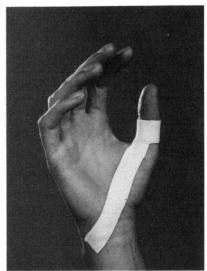

Figure 20–47 Tape construction to immobilize the extension of the first metacarpophalangeal joint.

TRAUMATIC ARTHRITIS OF THE METACARPOPHALANGEAL AND INTERPHALANGEAL JOINTS OF THE FINGERS

Functional Examination

- Passive flexion and extension are painful and limited. Flexion elicits these symptoms to a greater extent than extension (capsular pattern).

Intra-articular Injection

Arthritides of the finger joints generally react very well to intra-articular injections of corticosteroid (Figures 20–48 and 20–49).

Position of the Patient

The patient sits next to the treatment table. The forearm rests in pronation on the table with the hand placed on a small pillow or a towel roll. The joint to be injected is positioned in approximately 90° flexion.

Position of the Physician

With the thumb and index finger, the physician exerts slight traction on the finger to be injected.

Performance

A syringe containing 0.5 mL of triamcinolone acetonide, 10 mg/mL, with a 1-cm long needle is inserted horizontally at either the radial or ulnar side of the joint. In 90° flexion, the metacarpophalangeal joint line is approximately 1 cm from the knuckle.

Follow-Up

For 3 days the joint is immobilized either with the arm in a sling or by taping.

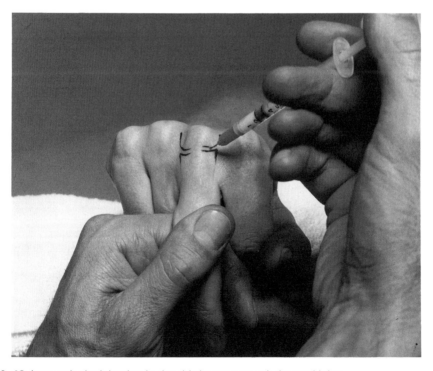

Figure 20–48 Intra-articular injection in the third metacarpophalangeal joint.

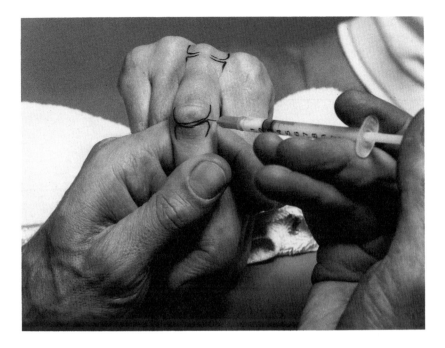

Figure 20–49 Intra-articular injection in the third proximal interphalangeal joint.

Generally, the results are good. One or two injections usually achieve complete relief of pain. If a second injection is necessary, it is administered 2 weeks after the first one. Usually the joint remains sensitive for a long time, however, particularly when bumping it against something or when given a firm handshake. In these instances, taping the joint is indicated, particularly for athletes participating in sports such as soccer, handball, and water polo.

Stabilization by Means of Taping

The method of taping described in this section also can be applied in lesions of the finger extensors or flexors.

Position of the Patient

The patient sits next to the treatment table. The elbow is flexed approximately 90° and is supported on the table.

Position of the Therapist

The therapist stands next to the treatment table, diagonally facing the patient.

Performance

An anchor tape is placed, circularly, both proximal and distal to the joint being immobilized (Figure 20–50A), which in this instance is the second proximal interphalangeal joint of the index finger. Care is taken to ensure that the circulation in the finger is not inadvertently stopped.

In instances of a traumatic arthritis, both the flexion and extension motions are restricted. Therefore, a 10- to 12-cm strip of tape is placed on both the dorsal and palmar aspects of the distal anchor—the dorsal strip is attached with its adhesive side up, and the palmar strip is attached with the adhesive side pointing down (Figure 20–50B).

Both strips are then folded over proximally and attached to the finger (Figure 20–50C).

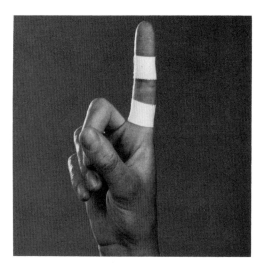

Figure 20–50A First the two anchors are placed, one proximal and one distal to the joint.

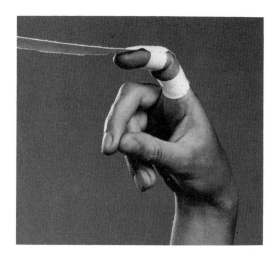

Figure 20–50B The long strip is folded over and taped to the dorsal side of the finger. The same is applied to the volar side of the finger.

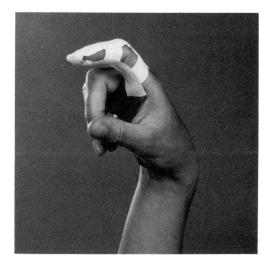

Figure 20–50C Tape construction to immobilize the proximal interphalangeal joint of the index finger.

TENDOVAGINITIS STENOSANS OF THE FINGER FLEXORS (TRIGGER FINGER)

Functional Examination

- Locking occurs during active finger flexion or extension.

Injection

Trigger finger denotes the condition of stenosing tendovaginitis or a nodule in the flexor tendon. It is characterized by momentary spasmodic locking of the finger in either flexion or extension, followed by a snapping whereby movement is again possible.

Although it is not always successful, injection for a trigger finger is worth trying. The patient can get at least temporary relief and sometimes the results are permanent.

Position of the Patient

The patient sits next to the treatment table. The forearm rests in maximal supination on the table and the other hand fixes the forearm.

Position of the Physician

The physician sits next to the treatment table, diagonally facing the patient.

Using thumb and index finger, the physician grasps the patient's finger from the dorsal aspect.

Performance

A syringe is filled with 0.5 mL of triamcinolone acetonide, 10 mg/mL. After locating the thickening in the tendon just proximal to the metacarpophalangeal joint, a 2-cm long needle is inserted at an angle of approximately 30° into the finger (Figure 20–51). Approximately 0.2 to 0.4 mL of solution is injected between the tendon and its sheath, as well as into the thickened tendon.

Follow-Up

For 3 days the finger is immobilized by means of taping or putting the arm in a sling. After that, the patient returns to normal activities.

Results vary widely. If the patient continues to have significant complaints, surgery may be indicated.

STRAIN OF THE ADDUCTOR POLLICIS, OBLIQUE HEAD

Functional Examination

- Resisted ulnar adduction and opposition of the thumb are painful.
- Passive retroposition of the thumb can be painful because of stretching.

Transverse Friction

Lesions of the adductor pollicis, oblique head, usually occur as the result of a hyperextension (retroposition) trauma of the thumb. Such trauma commonly results from falls or, for example, in sports, when a ball hits the thumb during volleyball or handball. It is often seen in conjunction with a traumatic ar-

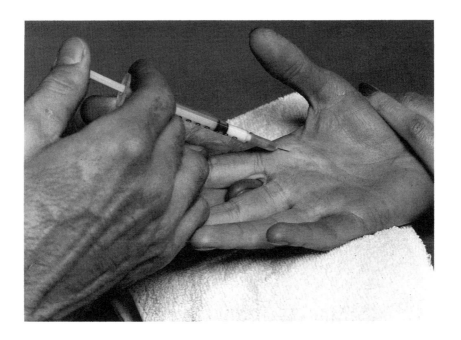

Figure 20–51 Injection for a trigger finger.

thritis of the trapeziometacarpal I or metacarpophalangeal I joint.

Position of the Patient

The patient sits next to the short end of the treatment table. The forearm rests in maximal supination on the table, and the hand lies in slight extension at the edge of the table.

Position of the Therapist

The therapist sits next to the long side of the treatment table, diagonally facing the patient.

If the right side is being treated, the therapist grasps the patient's fingers with the right hand, holding the wrist in slight extension. With the thumb, the therapist exerts pressure against the volar aspect of the patient's inter-phalangeal I joint in order to position the patient's thumb in retroposition.

The therapist's thumb is placed just ulnar to the site of the lesion, which is located at the base of the thenar eminence, in line with the third metacarpal. The fingers of this hand exert counterpressure against the dorsal aspect of the patient's hand (Figure 20–52).

Performance

Transverse friction is performed in an ulnar to a radial direction by means of thumb adduction and slight wrist extension.

Duration of Treatment

The patient should be seen three times per week for 15-minute sessions of transverse friction. Usually, three to six treatments are necessary to achieve complete recovery.

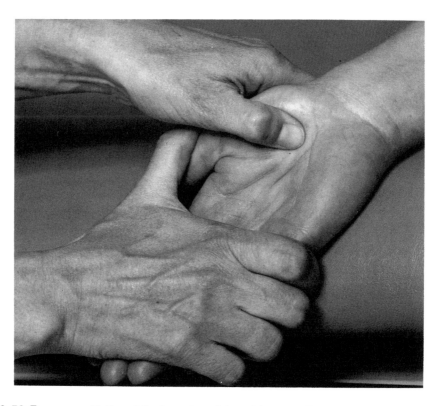

Figure 20–52 Transverse friction of the insertion of the adductor pollicis, oblique head.

STRAIN/OVERUSE OF THE DORSAL INTEROSSEI

Functional Examination

- Resisted abduction of the fingers is painful.
- Sometimes passive flexion or extension of the metacarpophalangeal joint is painful at end-range.

Transverse Friction of the Muscle Belly

We have not yet seen patients with lesions of the palmar interosseous muscles. Thus, the following discussion is limited to lesions of the dorsal interossei. Most often, lesions of the dorsal interossei either occur traumatically (eg, the result of a metacarpal fracture) or are due to overuse—seen particularly in musicians who play string instruments.

Position of the Patient

The patient sits next to the short end of the treatment table with the forearm resting in pronation on the table.

Position of the Therapist

The therapist sits next to the long side of the treatment table, diagonally facing the patient.

If the right side is being treated, the therapist places the tip of the right middle finger at the site of the lesion. (The dorsal interosseus II, between the middle and index fingers, is used here as an example.)

The thumb and index finger of the other hand grasp the head of metacarpal III from dorsal and palmar aspects, respectively, bringing it in a dorsal direction. This position of the hand is adapted in the treatment of each dorsal interosseous muscle lesion.

Performance

The middle finger is reinforced by the index finger. The transverse friction is performed through forearm supination during which the tip of the middle finger is moved from radial to ulnar over the lesion (Figures 20–53A and 20–53B).

Transverse Friction of the Tendon or Insertion

Sometimes the tendon or the insertion is affected. In this case, a different initial position and transverse friction technique are necessary. In the following example, the dorsal interosseous II tendon is affected at the radial aspect of the middle finger directly distal to the metacarpophalangeal III joint of the right hand.

Position of the Patient

The patient is in the same position as for transverse friction of the muscle belly.

Position of the Therapist

With the distal phalanx of the right index finger, the therapist grasps the patient's metacarpal III from the volar aspect, pushing it dorsally. At the same time, the right thumb pushes the metacarpal II volarly. The therapist's other fingers grasp the patient's index finger. In this way, the tendon can be reached for treatment.

With the other hand, the therapist grasps the patient's middle finger between thumb and index finger, in which the thumb lies just volar to the site of the lesion.

Performance

Transverse friction is performed through slight thumb adduction, which moves the thumb in a volar to dorsal direction, transversely over the fibers of the affected tendon (Figure 20–54).

Duration of Treatment

Regardless of the duration of symptoms, even if the symptoms have existed for several years, only two or three treatments are necessary if the muscle belly is affected. At the most, six treatments are needed for a lesion of the tendon or insertion.

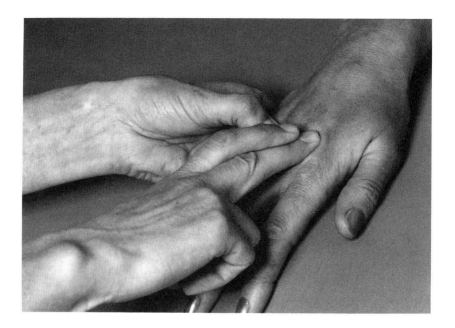

Figure 20–53A Transverse friction of the muscle belly of the dorsal interosseous II muscle, initial position.

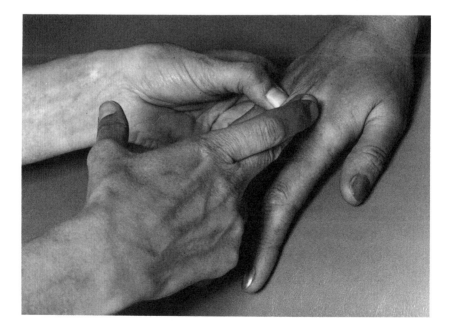

Figure 20–53B End position of transverse friction of the muscle belly.

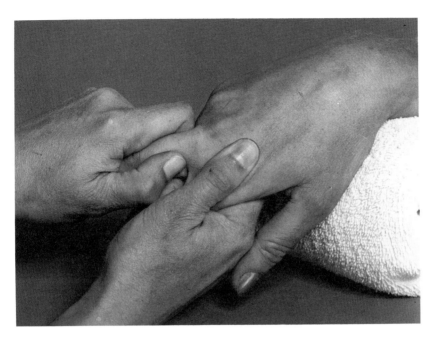

Figure 20–54 Transverse friction of the dorsal interosseous II tendon.

CARPAL TUNNEL SYNDROME— COMPRESSION NEUROPATHY OF THE MEDIAN NERVE

Functional Examination

- The Phalen test provokes pain.
- The Tinel test provokes pain.

Treatment of the carpal tunnel syndrome is partially dependent on the cause. For instance, a tenosynovitis of the flexor digitorum profundus can lead to narrowing of the carpal tunnel. This tenosynovitis is often the result of overuse. For example, after a vigorous period of training, a motocross rider can develop a carpal tunnel syndrome. In this case, the treatment consists of 3 weeks of rest (no training), during which the symptoms should disappear.

Night Splint

As long as there are no neurological deficits, the initial treatment should always be conservative. Particularly in patients who complain of symptoms at night, good results can be achieved by wearing a well-cushioned splint that fixes the wrist in a neutral position and leaves the fingers free to move. This splint is worn until the symptoms have resolved. This can be tested after 2 to 3 weeks of wearing the splint, by leaving it off occasionally at night. If symptoms do not return, the splint can be left off more and more often.

Injection

If improvement with rest or splinting is insufficient, an injection of the carpal tunnel with 1 mL of local anesthetic is indicated. The intention during this injection is to remain *perineural*. If paresthesia occurs while the needle is being inserted, the needle has contacted the nerve. At this point, the needle should be partially withdrawn immediately. *An accidental injection into the nerve can cause permanent nerve damage.* The use of a short-beveled needle in perineural injections is safer, because there is less danger that damage will occur if the nerve is accidentally hit by the needle. During injection of the solution, however, tingling symptoms from the median nerve usually arise. This is an indication that the needle is correctly located, and the rest of the corticosteroid should be deposited.

Position of the Patient

The patient sits next to the short side of the treatment table. The forearm is positioned in maximal supination and the hand hangs slightly in extension over the edge of the table.

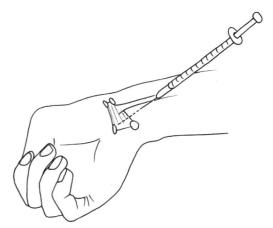

Figure 20–55 Injection into the carpal tunnel.

Position of the Physician

The physician sits next to the long side of the treatment table, diagonally in front of the patient.

Performance

A 4-cm needle is inserted approximately 2 cm proximal to a line connecting the pisiform and tubercle of the scaphoid, directly ulnar to the palmaris longus tendon (Figure 20–55). If this tendon is not present (in 20% of all cases), the needle is inserted directly ulnar from the midline. The needle is pushed dis-

tally, bringing the tip 1½ to 2 cm further into the carpal tunnel.

Surgery

Good to excellent results are usually achieved with injection therapy. However, sometimes the symptoms recur too quickly. If symptoms continue to recur after three injections, surgery may be indicated. Immediate operative treatment is indicated in cases of objective sensory or motor deficits.

General considerations when giving injections

Before injecting the solution, aspiration should always be performed. Aspiration is important to ensure that the injection is not accidentally given into a blood vessel. If this occurs, there is risk of toxic side effects and false-negative results.

When giving an intra-articular injection, the first drop of solution always should be injected into the subcutaneous tissue. In this way, the danger of a bacterial arthritis is diminished—the possibly nonsterile plug of skin, which may be in the opening of the needle, is not brought into the joint.

21

Peripheral Compression Neuropathies in the Wrist and Hand Region

FUNCTIONAL ANATOMY

Although motor deficits do not occur in every compression syndrome of the upper extremity, an overview of the normal innervation of the muscles should be kept on hand. Of course, these innervations are subject to significant variance, particularly distal in the extremity. In various anatomy books, descriptions of branching patterns and topography differ. Even the distribution of the segments is subject to interindividual differences. Therefore, the overview presented in Table 21–1 should be used only as a rough guide.

Regarding sensory innervation, there is even greater variance among individuals. Therefore, the examiner who is making a diagnosis should not hold rigidly to one diagram. Regarding innervation of the hand, however, the following rules generally apply:

- The fifth finger and the ulnar aspect of the fourth finger are supplied entirely by the ulnar nerve.
- The other parts of the fingers are supplied dorsally by the radial nerve and palmarly by the median nerve.

RADIAL NERVE

For anatomy of the radial nerve and proximal compression neuropathies, refer to Chapter 14, Peripheral Compression Neuropathies in the Elbow Region.

ULNAR NERVE

For anatomy of the ulnar nerve and proximal compression neuropathies, refer to Chapter 14, Peripheral Compression Neuropathies in the Elbow Region.

Distal Compression of the Ulnar Nerve

Functional Anatomy

Compression of the ulnar nerve in the wrist area can occur in three different sites: (1) before the nerve bifurcates into a superficial and a deep branch, (2) both branches after the bifurcation, or (3) one of the branches after the bifurcation.

Compression can occur in the region of Guyon's tunnel, particularly against the pisiform or against the hook of the hamate bone. This is often seen in motocross racers.

Causes are generally direct trauma or microtrauma (using a screwdriver, a cane, or a crutch; playing Olympic handball). A tenoosseous tendinitis of the flexor carpi ulnaris can also cause compression of the nerve. Tumors rarely cause compression in this area.

Clinical Findings

- Sensory (superficial branch): There is burning pain in the fifth finger and ulnar half of the fourth finger, only palmar. First the patient complains of hyperesthesia and later of anesthesia.

Table 21–1 Normal Innervation of the Muscles

Muscle	Nerve	Segments
Abductor pollicis longus	Radial	C7, C8
Extensor pollicis longus	Radial	C7, C8
Extensor pollicis brevis	Radial	C7, C8
Extensor indicis	Radial	C7, C8
Abductor pollicis brevis	Median	C8, T1
Opponens pollicis	Median	C8, T1
Flexor pollicis brevis	Median	C8, T1
	Ulnar	
Adductor pollicis	Ulnar	C8, T1
Palmaris brevis	Ulnar	C8, T1
Abductor digiti minimi	Ulnar	C8, T1
Flexor digiti minimi brevis	Ulnar	C8, T1
Opponens digiti minimi	Ulnar	C8, T1
Lumbricals I and II	Median	C8, T1
Lumbricals III and IV	Ulnar	C8, T1
Palmar interossei	Ulnar	C8, T1
Dorsal interossei	Ulnar	C8, T1

- Motor (deep branch): There is loss of strength of the flexor pollicis brevis and adductor pollicis. In a later stage, there is also weakness of the interossei with noticeable atrophy.

Treatment

If there are only sensory disturbances, a perineural injection of a corticosteroid at the site of the compression is administered. If there are motor deficits, surgical decompression should be performed as quickly as possible.

Metacarpal Tunnel Syndrome

Functional Anatomy

The metacarpal tunnel syndrome involves compression of the common palmar digital nerves in the metacarpal tunnels. These nerves are the sensory terminal branches of the median and ulnar nerves.

Possible Causes

- Trauma, usually involving hyperextension and lateral deviation of one or more fingers
- Space-occupying lesion, such as tenosynovitis of the finger flexors
- Lesions of the lumbricals (extremely rare)
- Arthritis of a metacarpophalangeal joint
- Trigger finger (tendovaginitis stenosans of the finger flexors)
- Chronic irritation, for instance, caused by use of a cane

Differential Diagnosis

- Tenosynovitis of the finger flexors
- Arthritis of a metacarpophalangeal joint
- Carpal tunnel syndrome

Clinical Findings

- The patient complains of pain in one or two fingers. Sensory disturbances may be present, ranging from hyperesthesia to anesthesia.

- Hyperextension of the finger's metacarpophalangeal joint is very painful.
- There is pain on palpation between the heads of the involved metacarpals.

Treatment

The treatment of choice is local perineural injection of a corticosteroid. Several injections may be necessary, performed at intervals of 2 weeks between the injections. This therapy is particularly successful after a one-time trauma or in a tenosynovitis. If the problem recurs, surgery is indicated.

MEDIAN NERVE

For anatomy of the median nerve and proximal compression neuropathies, refer to Chapter 14, Peripheral Compression Neuropathies in the Elbow Region.

Carpal Tunnel Syndrome

Functional Anatomy

The median nerve can become compressed in the carpal tunnel. This is the tunnel formed underneath the flexor retinaculum proper through which the tendons of the flexor pollicis longus and the flexors digitorum profundus and superficialis run together with the median nerve (Figure 21–1).

Note: At its *ulnar* end, the flexor retinaculum has a deep and superficial layer that attaches to the hook of the hamate and pisiform, respectively. These two ulnar layers form a tunnel for the ulnar nerve and artery (Guyon's tunnel) (see Distal Compression of the Ulnar Nerve). At its *radial* end, the flexor retinaculum has a superficial layer that attaches to the tubercles of the scaphoid and trapezium, as well as a deep layer attaching to the deep ulnar edge of the trapezium. These

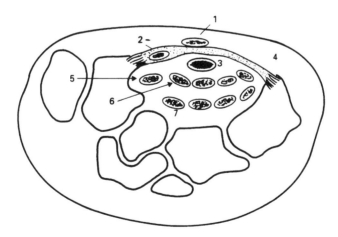

Figure 21–1 Left carpal tunnel. **1**, Tendon of the palmaris longus; **2**, tendon of the flexor carpi radialis; **3**, median nerve; **4**, flexor retinaculum; **5**, tendon of the flexor pollicis longus; **6**, tendons of the flexor digitorum superficialis; **7**, tendons of the flexor digitorum profundus.

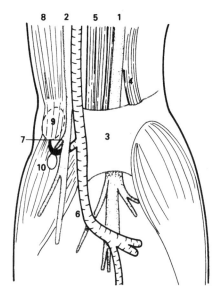

Figure 21–2 Volar aspect of the left wrist. **1**, Median nerve; **2**, ulnar nerve; **3**, flexor retinaculum; **4**, tendon of the flexor carpi radialis; **5**, tendons of the flexor digitorum superficialis; **6**, ulnar artery; **7**, deep ramus of the ulnar nerve; **8**, flexor carpi ulnaris; **9**, pisiform; **10**, hook of the hamate.

two radial layers of the retinaculum form a tunnel for the tendon of the flexor carpi radialis (Figure 21–2).

Possible Causes

- Tenosynovitis, particularly of the tendons of the flexor digitorum profundus
- Trauma, as the result of a Colles' fracture, fracture of the scaphoid, or a carpal dislocation (particularly of the lunate)
- Tumor
- Ganglion
- Tophi in gout
- Rheumatoid arthritis (in 30% of the cases, even before symptoms of rheumatoid arthritis are manifested)

Differential Diagnosis

Because pain from a carpal tunnel syndrome often radiates upward to the neck, the following should be ruled out:

- thoracic outlet syndrome
- cervical (disc-related) problems
- pronator teres syndrome

Clinical Findings

- Carpal tunnel syndrome is seen, particularly in women between the ages of 40 and 50 years.
- The patient often complains of paresthesia in the arm and hand (particularly the palmar aspect of the first three fingers). The symptoms are usually worse at night than during the day (brachialgia paresthetica nocturna).
- Sometimes there is atrophy of the opponens pollicis.
- In instances of tenosynovitis of the finger flexors, local swelling is often visible and palpable.
- Phalen's test usually produces symptoms. This test consists of holding the wrist passively in maximal palmar flexion. Within 60 seconds tingling and numbness arise. If the wrist is held passively in extension and pressure is exerted with the thumb at the level of the carpal tunnel, or the examiner taps the fingers at this site (Tinel's test), pain and paresthesia usually arise in the hand.

Treatment

Treatment depends on the cause. Therapeutic measures include the use of a night splint, positioning the wrist in the neutral position and allowing movement of the fingers, and injection of a corticosteroid into the carpal tunnel; the needle is inserted approximately 4 cm proximal to the carpal tunnel, directly ulnar to the palmaris longus. An injection is particularly effective in instances of a flexor digitorum profundus tenosynovitis. If the problem recurs, surgery may be indicated.

Metacarpal Tunnel Syndrome

See Ulnar Nerve for detailed information on this syndrome.

PART III—WRIST AND HAND REVIEW QUESTIONS

1. What repeatedly performed movement can cause a lesion of the articular disc in the wrist? Give two sports examples.

2. In which carpal joints are arthrotic changes most commonly seen?

3. When a patient, after an accident, has a painful circumferential swelling of the wrist along with a significant loss of function, one thinks in the first instances of _____

4. What is a carpal boss?

5. Which tendons run through the second dorsal tunnel of the wrist?

6. Name the 10 most important structures that run through the carpal tunnel.

7. What is a ganglion?

8. Which test is most important in determining a carpal instability?

9. Which passive test is frequently positive with a tenosynovitis of the extensor carpi ulnaris when the lesion lies just proximal to the styloid process of the ulna?

10. Which test is always positive with a de Quervain syndrome?

11. Which muscles bring the index finger and the middle finger together?

12. Where is a tendovaginitis stenosis of the flexor pollicis longus usually localized? Name the synonym for this lesion.

13. Which ligament is the most important for stability between the capitate and the lunate?

14. Define the space of Poirier.

15. Which function is generally disturbed with a carpal instability?

16. A traumatic arthritis of the trapeziometacarpal joint occurs generally as a result of a _____ trauma.

17. What is the capsular pattern of the trapeziometacarpal joint?

18. The so-called skier's thumb is the second most frequent injury (after knee injuries) from skiing accidents. Which structure is affected?

19. What is the capsular pattern of the metacarpophalangeal joints?

20. Where are the so-called Heberden's nodes localized? With which disease are they associated?

21. Describe briefly the etiology of a buttonhole deformity.

22. Describe briefly the etiology of a swan neck deformity.

23. A Dupuytren's contracture is a disorder of the palmar aponeurosis. It is chiefly localized in what area?

24. Name the juvenile osteochondroses of the wrist/hand and give the localization of each.

25. Which structures run through Guyon's tunnel?

26. Give the localization and the etiology of the metacarpal tunnel syndrome.

27. Name five causes of the carpal tunnel syndrome.

28. Name a common metacarpal localization for a ganglion.

29. Which part of the capsulo ligamentous structures of the distal radioulnar joint stop pronation of the forearm?

30. How can one best locate the distal radioulnar joint?

PART III—WRIST AND HAND REVIEW ANSWERS

1. By repeatedly performed ulnar deviation, such as in baseball/softball and batting in cricket.

2. In the joints of the radial row, especially between the radius and scaphoid and between the trapezium and metacarpal I.

3. A carpal fracture, typically of the scaphoid.

4. Irritation of the soft tissue structures at the bases of metacarpals II and/or III and the trapezoid and capitate. The irritation occurs as a result of repeatedly performed forceful extension of the wrist or as a result of a single traumatic wrist extension.

5. The tendons of the extensors carpi radialis longus and brevis.

6. —Four tendons of the flexor digitorum profundus.

   —Four tendons of the flexor digitorum superficialis.

   —The tendon of the flexor pollicis longus.

   —Median nerve.

7. A ganglion is the result of mucine degeneration of the joint capsule or of a tendon sheath whereby a cyst develops.

8. The apprehension test.

9. Passive supination of the forearm.

10. Finkelstein's test.

11. Palmar interosseus I and dorsal interosseus II.

12. —At the level of the head of metacarpal I.

    —Trigger thumb.

13. The palmar radiocapitate ligament.

14. Poirier's space is the triangle that is formed by the palmar ligaments between the radius and the capitate, between the radius and the lunate and triquetrum, and between the capitate and the triquetrum.

15. The ability to grip forcefully.

16. Hyper-retroposition.

17. Retroposition is limited; other motions are not limited or are minimally limited.

18. The ulnar collateral ligament of the metacarpophalangeal I joint.

19. Flexion is slightly more limited than extension.

20. —At the level of the distal interphalangeal finger joints.

    —Arthrosis of the finger joints.

21. Forceful flexion of the proximal interphalangeal joint with, as a result, a rupture of the middle part of the extensor digitorum communis tendon. The head of the proximal phalanx is positioned dorsally between the two parts of the stretched tendon, as through a buttonhole.

22. Traumatic hyperextension of the proximal interphalangeal joint with rupture of the palmar fibrocartilaginous plate of the joint, thus allowing the tendon of the extensor digitorum communis to pull this joint into hyperextension.

23. The fourth and fifth rays.

24. —Kienböck's disease—lunate.

    —Burns' disease—head of one of the metacarpals.

—Thiemann's disease—proximal interphalangeal joints.

25. A branch from the ulnar nerve and a branch from the ulnar artery.

26. It concerns the common palmar digital nerves in the intermetacarpal tunnels; this is the passage between the deep and the superficial transverse metacarpal ligaments between the heads of the metacarpals. It usually concerns a traumatic lesion such as hyperextension and ulnar or radial deviation of one or more fingers. Less frequent causes include tenosynovitis of the finger flexors, arthritis or arthrosis of a metacarpophalangeal joint, a trigger finger, or chronic irritation, for instance, from use of a cane.

27. —Tenosynovitis of the finger flexors, especially from the flexor digitorum profundus.

   —Carpal instability.

   —Carpal fracture.

   —Colles' fracture.

   —Rheumatoid arthritis of the carpus.

28. Between the heads of metacarpals II and III.

29. The dorsal part.

30. In the zero position of the wrist, hand, and finger joints, palpate the tendon of the extensor digiti minimi (raise little finger), just radial from the head of the ulna. In this position, the distal radioulnar joint lies below the tendon of the extensor digiti minimi.

REFERENCES

1. Takechi H, Kono M. The osseous structure of the carpal groove. *J Bone Joint Surg [Br]*. 1983;67:130–132.

2. Gelberman RH, Hergenroeder PT, Hargens AR, Lundborg GN, Akeson WH. The carpal tunnel syndrome: a study of carpal canal pressure. *J Bone Joint Surg [Am]*. 1981;63:380–383.

3. Kapandji IA. *Bewegingsleer*. Part 1: *De Bovenste Extremiteit*. Utrecht: Bohn, Scheltema & Holkema; 1983.

4. De Lange A, Kauer JMG, Huiskes R. Kinematic behaviour of the human wrist joint: a rontgenstereophotogrammetric analysis. *J Orthop Res*. 1985;3:56–64.

5. Kauer JMG. Functional anatomy of the wrist. *Clin Orthop*. 1980;149:9–20.

6. Kauer JMG. The interdependence of carpal articular chains. *Acta Anat Scand*. 1974; 88:481–501.

7. Berger RA, Crownshield RD, Flatt AE. The three dimensional rotational behaviors of the carpal bones. *Clin Orthop*. 1982;167:303–310.

8. Legrand JJ. The lunate bone: a weak link in the articular column of the wrist. *Anat Clin*. 1983;5:57–64.

9. Delattre JF, Ducasse A, Flament JB, Kenesi C. The mechanical role of the digital fibrous sheath: application to reconstructive surgery of the flexor tendons. *Anat Clin*. 1983;5:187–197.

10. Taleisnik J. The ligaments of the wrist. *J Hand Surg*. 1976;1-2:110–118.

11. Dobyns JG, Linscheid RI, Chao E, et al. Traumatic Instability of the Wrist. *American Academy of Orthopaedic Surgeons Instructional Course Lectures*. Chicago: American Academy of Orthopaedic Surgeons; 1975;24:182–199.

12. Taleisnik J. *The Wrist*. New York: Churchill Livingstone; 1985.

13. Panting AL. Dislocations of the lunate with and without fracture of the scaphoid. *J Bone Joint Surg*. 1984; 66B:391-395.

14. Johnson RP, Carrera GF. Chronic capitolunate instability. *J Bone Joint Surg [Am]*. 1986;68:1164–1175.

PART III—SUGGESTED READING

Addison A. Knuckle pads causing extensor tendon tethering. *J Bone Joint Surg [Br]*. 1984;66:128–130.

Allen PR. Idiopathic avascular necrosis of the scaphoid: a report of two cases. *J Bone Joint Surg [Br]*. 1983;65:333–335.

Allender E. Prevalences, incidences, and remission rates of some common rheumatic diseases or syndromes. *Scand J Rheumatol*. 1974;3:145–153.

Allieu Y. *Instabilité du carpe et sport*. Presented at the Five Sports Medicine Days of St Jan Hospital. Brugge, Belgium: 1986.

Amis AA, Jones MM. The interior of the flexor tendon sheath of the finger. *J Bone Joint Surg [Br]*. 1988;70:583–587.

Ansink BJJ, Meerwijk GM van, et al. *Neurologie voor Paramedische Beroepen*. Utrecht: Bunge; 1982.

Araki S, Ohtani T, Tanaka T. Acute dislocation of the extensor digitorum communis tendon at the metacarpophalangeal joint: a report of five cases. *J Bone Joint Surg [Am]*. 1987;69:616–619.

Bell MJ, Hill RJ, McMurtry RY. Ulnar impingement syndrome. *J Bone Joint Surg [Br]*. 1985;67:126–129.

Bellinghausen HW, Gilula LA, Young LV, Weeks PM. Post-traumatic palmar carpal subluxation: report of two cases. *J Bone Joint Surg [Am]*. 1983;65:998–1006.

Benini A. *Das Karpaltunnelsyndrom und die übrigen Kompressionssyndrome des Nervus Medianus*. Stuttgart: Georg Thieme Verlag; 1974.

Berger A. Weichteilverletzungen im Handbereich. *Orthopaedie*. 1988;17:74–81.

Bergfeld JA, Leach RE, Longmire WT, et al. Diagnostiek en behandeling van letsel van hand en pls. *Patient Care*. 1982:41–48.

Bolton-Maggs BG, Helal BH, Revell PA. Bilateral avascular necrosis of the capitate: a case report and a review of the literature. *J Bone Joint Surg [Br]*. 1984; 66:557–559.

Bradish CF. Carpal tunnel syndrome in patients on haemodialysis. *Anat Clin*. 1985;5:153–157.

Buck-Gramcko D. Verletzungen der Beuge- und Strecksehnen an Hand und Unterarm und ihre Behandlung. *Orthopaedie*. 1988;17:82–88.

Carpentier Alting MP. Ziekte van De Quervain, een vergeten diagnose? *Ned Tijdschr Geneeskd*. 1982;126:1433–1435.

Carter SR, Aldridge MJ. Stress injury of the distal radial growth plate. *J Bone Joint Surg [Br]*. 1988;70:834–836.

Chow SP, So YC, Pun WK, Luk KDK, Leong JCY. Thenar crush injuries. *J Bone Joint Surg [Br]*. 1988;70:135–139.

Clain A, ed. *Hamilton Bailey's Demonstrations of Physical Signs in Clinical Surgery*. Bristol: John Wright & Sons; 1965.

Conway WF, Destouet JM, Gilula LA, Bellinghausen HW, Weeks PM. The carpal boss: an overview of radiographic evaluation. *Radiology*. 1985;156:29–31.

Crawford Adams J. *Outline of Orthopaedics*. 6th ed. London: Churchill Livingstone; 1967.

Cuono CB, Watson HK. The carpal boss: surgical treatment and etiological considerations. *Plast Reconstr Surg*. 1979:88–93.

Cyriax J. *Textbook of Orthopaedic Medicine*. Vol. 1. 7th ed. London: Baillière Tindall; 1978.

Darrow JC, Linscheid RL, Dobyns JH, Mann III JM, Wood MB, Beckenbaugh RD. Distal ulnar recession for disorders of the distal radioulnar joint. *J Hand Surg [AM]*. 1985;10:482–490.

Dias JJ, Taylor M, Thompson J, Brenkel IJ, Gregg PJ. Radiographic signs of union of scaphoid fractures. *J Bone Joint Surg [Br]*. 1988;70:299–301.

Din KM, Meggitt BF. Mallet thumb. *J Bone Joint Surg [Br]*. 1983;65:606–607.

Ecke H, Faupel L. Verletzungen der Handwurzel. *Muench Med Wochenschr*. 1984;126:789–794.

Elias N. *Über den Prozeß der Zivilisation*. Two Vol. 5th ed. Baden-Baden: Suhrkamp; 1978.

Fehring TK, Milek MA. Isolated volar dislocation of the radiocarpal joint: a case report. *J Bone Joint Surg [Am]*. 1984;66:464–467.

Feindel W, Stratford J. The role of the cubital tunnel in tardy ulnar palsy. *Can J Surg*. 1985;1:287–300.

Feldmeier C. *Verletzungen und Schäden der Hand*. Munich: W. Zuckschwerdt Verlag; 1988.

Fisk GR. The wrist. *J Bone Joint Surg [Br]*. 1984;66:396–407.

Ford DJ, Ali MS. Acute carpal tunnel syndrome: complications of delayed decompression. *J Bone Joint Surg [Br]*. 1986;68:759.

Fowler JL. Dislocation of the triquetrum and lunate: brief report. *J Bone Joint Surg [Br]*. 1988;70:665.

Garcia-Elias M, Abanco J, Salvador E, Sanchez R. Crush injury of the carpus. *J Bone Joint Surg [Br]*. 1985;67:286–289.

Gardner E, Gray DJ, O'Rahilly R. *Anatomy*. Philadelphia: Saunders; 1975.

Gelberman RH, Pfeffer GB, Galbraith RT, Szabo RM, Rydevik B, Dimick M. Results of treatment of severe carpal-tunnel syndrome without internal neurolysis of the median nerve. *J Bone Joint Surg [Am]*. 1987;69:896–903.

Graham HK, McCoy GF, Mollan RAB. A new injury of the distal radio-ulnar joint. *J Bone Joint Surg [Br]*. 1985;67:302–304.

Gray H, Williams PL, Warwick R. *Gray's Anatomy*. 36th ed. London: Churchill Livingstone; 1980.

Haak A, Steendijk R, de Wijn IF. *De samenstelling van het menselijk lichaam*. Assen: Van Gorcum; 1968.

Hafferl A. *Lehrbuch der topographischen Anatomie des Menschen*. Berlin: Springer Verlag; 1957.

Hamilton WJ, Simon G, Hamilton SGI. *Surface and Radiological Anatomy*. 5th ed. London: Macmillan Press Ltd; 1976.

Hauser H, Rheiner P. Computed tomography of the hand, part II: pathological conditions. *Medicamundi*. 1983;28:129–134.

Hauser H, Rheiner P, Gajisin S. Computed tomography of the hand, part I: normal anatomy. *Medicamundi*. 1983;28:90–94.

Haymaker W, Woodhall B. *Peripheral Nerve Injuries*. 2nd ed. Philadephia: Saunders; 1956.

Healy EJ, Seybold WD. *A Synopsis of Clinical Anatomy*. Philadelphia: Saunders; 1969.

Heerkens YF, Meijer OG. *Tractus-anatomie*. Amsterdam: Interfaculty Physical Education; 1980.

Henderson JJ, Arafa MAM. Carpometacarpal dislocation: an easily missed diagnosis. *J Bone Joint Surg [Br]*. 1987;69:212–214.

Hoppenfeld S. *Physical Examination of the Spine and Extremities*. New York: Appleton-Century-Crofts; 1976.

Iftikhar TB, Hallmann BW, Kaminski RS, Ray AK. Spontaneous rupture of the extensor mechanism causing ulnar dislocation of the long extensor tendon of the long finger: two case reports. *J Bone Joint Surg [Am]*. 1984;66:1108–1109.

Janis JL, Mahl GF, Kagan J, Holt RR. *Personality, Dynamics, Development, and Assessment*. New York: Harcourt, Brace and World, Inc; 1969.

Jones WA. Beware the sprained wrist. *J Bone Joint Surg [Br]*. 1988;70:293–296.

Kauer JMG. Bewegungsanalyse des Handgelenkes. *Extracta Orthopaedica*. 1987; 10:25–33.

Kawai H, Yamamoto K, Yamamoto T, Tada K, Kaga K. Excision of the lunate in Kienböck's disease. *J Bone Joint Surg [Br]*. 1988;70:287–292.

Kinnen L. Polsletsels en Sport. Presented at the Five Sports Medicine Days at the St Jan Hospital. Brugge, Belgium: 1986.

Klein Rensink GJ, Smits M. Entrapment neuropathieën. *Tijdschr Ned Belg Orthop Geneeskd*. 1983;3,2:33–48.

Koebke J, Tischendorf F. Die Hand: eine funktionelle und biomechanische Analyse. Teil 1: Knochen, Bänder und Gelenke. *Physikal Ther*. 1984;5:242–248.

Koebke J, Tischendorf F. Die Hand: eine funktionelle und biomechanische Analyse. Teil 2: Muskeln, Sehnen und Sehnenscheiden. *Physikal Ther*. 1984;5:540–545.

Kopell HP. Carpal tunnel compression median neuropathy treated non-surgically. *N Engl J Med*. 1958;58:744.

Krause R, Reif G, Feldmeier C. Überlastungssyndrome und Verletzungen der Hand und des Unterarmes beim Sportklettern. *Praktische Sport-Trumatologie und Sportmedizin*. 1987;2:10–14.

Lohman AGM. *Vorm en beweging. Leerboek van het bewegingsapparaat van de mens*. Two Vol. 4th ed. Utrecht: Bohn, Scheltema & Holkema; 1977.

McMinn RMH, Hutching RT. *A Color Atlas of Human Anatomy*. London: Wolfe Medical Publications Ltd; 1977.

Meerwijk GM van. *Syllabus Onderzoeken en Behandelen*. Amsterdam: Stichting Akademie voor Fysiotherapie Amsterdam; 1979: chap 16.

Mumenthaler M. *Der Schulter-Arm-Schmerz*. Bern: Hans Huber; 1982.

Mumenthaler M, Schliack H. *Läsionen peripherer Nerven*. Stuttgart: Georg Thieme Verlag; 1977.

Ono K, Ebara S, Fuji T, et al. Myelopathy hand: new clinical signs of cervical cord damage. *J Bone Joint Surg [Br]*. 1987;69:215–219.

Phalen GS. The carpal-tunnel syndrome. *Clin Orthop*. 1972;83:29–40.

Rhoades CE, Mowery CA, Gelberman RH. Results of internal neurolysis of the median nerve for severe carpal-tunnel syndrome. *J Bone Joint Surg [Am]*. 1985; 67:253–256.

Russe O, Gerhardt JJ, King PS. *An Atlas of Examination, Standard Measurements and Diagnosis in Orthopaedics and Traumatology*. Bern: Hans Huber Verlag; 1972.

Shea JD, McClain EJ. Ulnar nerve compression syndrome at and below the wrist. *J Bone Joint Surg [Am]*. 1969;51:1095.

Sobotta J, Becher PH. *Atlas of Human Anatomy*. Vols 1, 2, 3. 9th English ed. Berlin: Urban & Schwarzenberg; 1975.

Szabo RM, Gelberman RH, Dimick MP. Sensibility testing in patients with carpal tunnel syndrome. *J Bone Joint Surg [Am]*. 1984;66:60–64.

Thompson WAL, Kopell HP. Peripheral entrapment neuropathies of the upper extremity. *N Engl J Med*. 1959;260:1261–1265.

Wainapel SF. Elektrodiagnostisch onderzoek van het carpale-tunnelsyndroom na een Colles-fractuur (distale radiusfractuur). *Am J Phys Med*. 1981;60:126–131.

Wilhelm A. Unklare Schmerzzustände an der oberen Extremität. *Orthopaedie*. 1987;16:458–464.

Wilhelm A. Kompressionssyndrome des Nervus ulnaris und Nervus medianus im Handbereich. *Orthopaedie*. 1987;16:465–471.

Williams PL, Warwick R, eds. *Gray's Anatomy*. 36th ed. Edinburgh: Longman; 1980.

Winkel D, Fisher S. *Schematisch handboek voor onderzoek en behandeling van weke delen aandoeningen van het bewegingsapparaat*. 6th ed. Delft: Nederlandse Akademie voor Orthopedische Geneeskunde; 1982.

Schematic Topography of Upper Extremity Nerves and Blood Vessels

BRACHIAL PLEXUS

The nerves supplying the shoulder and the arm originate from a relatively small section of the spinal cord; they consist of the ventral rami of the four lower cervical segments (C5, C6, C7, and C8), as well as part of the upper thoracic segments (T1). Occasionally, C4 and T2 also contribute to innervation of the arm. In this section only the *ventral* rami of the nerve roots are discussed. The dorsal rami supply the neck muscles and do not play a role in innervation of the arm.

The ventral rami from C5 to T1 run through the posterior scalenic triangle, which is formed by the middle and anterior scalene muscles. The first rib lies at the floor of this triangular passageway. Upon leaving the posterior scalenic triangle, the rami form the easily visible and palpable *brachial plexus*. To avoid unnecessary discomfort, extreme care should be used during palpation in this region.

The brachial plexus runs from the posterior scalenic triangle, in a straight line, to the neurovascular bundle in the axilla. Palpation of the plexus, after it leaves the posterior scalenic triangle, can be more easily conducted by drawing a line from the dorsal border of the sternocleidomastoid muscle (at the level of the cricoid cartilage) to the middle of the clavicle. Palpate along this line with the subject's head laterally flexed to the opposite side.

The nerves lie on top of the subclavian artery in the scalenic triangle, but in the axilla they surround the artery from all sides. Before entering the axilla, they pass underneath the clavicle, and run dorsally to the pectoralis minor muscle. In its supraclavicular part, the brachial plexus consists of three *trunks*, lying one on top of the other. In the axilla, they reorganize into cords. This is where the large nerves running to the arm originate (Figures A–1 and A–2):

Lateral Cord

- Lateral pectoral nerve
- Musculocutaneous nerve
- Median nerve, lateral part

Posterior Cord

- Subscapular nerve
- Thoracodorsal nerve
- Radial nerve
- Axillary nerve

Medial Cord

- Medial pectoral nerve
- Medial cutaneous nerve of the arm
- Medial cutaneous nerve of the forearm
- Ulnar nerve
- Median nerve, medial part

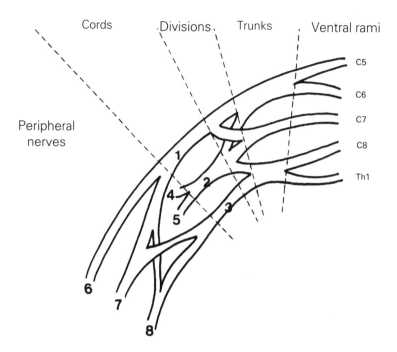

Figure A–1 Schematic representation of the right brachial plexus. **1**, Lateral cord; **2**, posterior cord; **3**, medial cord; **4**, axillary nerve; **5**, radial nerve; **6**, musculocutaneous nerve; **7**, median nerve; **8**, ulnar nerve.

Most nerves for the shoulder region originate even before the brachial plexus runs underneath the clavicle (pars supraclavicularis). These nerves are as follows:

- dorsal scapular nerve
  —innervates the levator scapula and rhomboid muscles
  —sometimes palpable directly behind the brachial plexus
  —runs in the direction of the levator muscle
- subclavian nerve
  —innervates the subclavius muscle and sternoclavicular joint
  —usually not palpable
- suprascapular nerve
  —at the level of the scapular notch, runs dorsolateral to the supraspinatus

muscle and further to the acromioclavicular joint, glenohumeral joint, and infraspinatus muscle
  —occasionally palpable just before it reaches the scapular notch
- subscapular nerve
  —runs from the brachial plexus in a dorsocaudal direction
  —innervates the subscapularis and teres major muscles
  —not palpable
- long thoracic nerve
  —from the start, runs steeply downward, then caudally over the thoracic wall to the serratus anterior
  —palpable as a vertical cord on the thorax, behind the ventral axillary wall (pectoralis major)

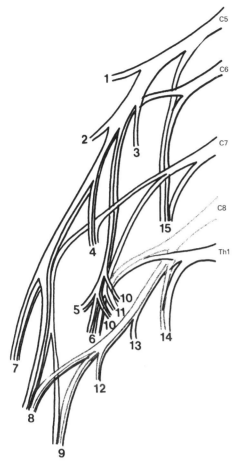

Figure A–2 Simplified illustration of the right brachial plexus. **1**, Dorsal scapular nerve; **2**, suprascapular nerve; **3**, subclavian nerve; **4**, lateral pectoral nerve; **5**, axillary nerve; **6**, radial nerve; **7**, musculocutaneous nerve; **8**, median nerve; **9**, ulnar nerve; **10**, subscapular nerve; **11**, thoracodorsal nerve; **12**, medial cutaneous nerve of the forearm; **13**, medial cutaneous nerve of the arm; **14**, medial pectoral nerve; **15**, long thoracic nerve.

- thoracodorsal nerve
  —travels on a course similar to that of the long thoracic nerve, but slightly more dorsal
  —innervates the latissimus dorsi muscle
  —palpable as a vertical cord on the thorax, in front of the dorsal axillary wall

(latissimus dorsi, teres major) and dorsal to the long thoracic nerve

All of the above-mentioned branches from the supraclavicular part of the brachial plexus arise from trunks. Further distally, the brachial plexus reorganizes into cords, which accompany the axillary artery through the axilla. In this region, the nerves to the arm arise.

- axillary nerve
  —arises from the posterior cord, runs dorsally in the axilla, then through the lateral axillary space (quadrangular space) with the posterior humeral circumflex artery
  —innervates the deltoid and teres minor muscles
  —palpable deep within the axilla with the arm hanging in a relaxed position (Moving dorsally to the neurovascular bundle, the palpating index finger slides upward. The axillary nerve is located just underneath the infraglenoid tubercle.)
- radial nerve (Figure A–3)
- median nerve (Figure A–5)
- musculocutaneous nerve (Figure A–6)
- ulnar nerve (Figure A–7)
- medial cutaneous nerves of the arm and forearm
  —originate at the medial cord and run distally along the ulnar side of the arm (The medial cutaneous nerve of the arm travels from the ventral wall of the axilla to approximately midarm, and the medial cutaneous nerve of the forearm courses from midarm to just beyond the elbow.)

Radial Nerve

Derivation

The radial nerve derives from the posterior cord. Its roots are C5 to T1 (Figures A–1 and A–2).

Course

The radial nerve passes between the distal third of the axillary artery and the subscapularis muscle, then distally through the tendons of the latissimus dorsi and teres major. Together with the deep brachial artery, it leaves the proximal part of the medial bicipital sulcus. Behind the humerus, the radial nerve takes a spiral course anteriorly. After giving off motor and sensory branches, it penetrates the lateral intermuscular septum. From there it runs through a groove formed by the medial brachialis and lateral brachioradialis muscles.

Between the biceps tendon and the lateral epicondyle, the nerve divides into a superficial branch and a deep branch. The deep branch (posterior interosseous nerve) runs dorsally between both heads of the supinator muscle. The superficial branch runs distally along the ulnar aspect of the brachioradialis. Approximately 7 cm before reaching the wrist, the superficial branch turns dorsally and ends in four or five dorsal digital nerves (Figure A–3).

Palpation

Draw a straight line from the deltoid tuberosity to the lateral humeral epicondyle, and divide this line into three equal parts. The radial nerve can be palpated at the point where the upper and middle thirds meet. Approximately 1 cm lateral to the biceps tendon, the nerve is accessible for electrical stimulation. Palpation of the superficial ramus is possible in the region of the anatomical snuffbox. It crosses, superficially, over the extensor pollicis longus tendon (Figure A–4).

Lesions

Injuries to the radial nerve especially occur as a result of proximal humerus fractures, as well as the improper use of axillary crutches. Severe injuries can lead to the so-called drop hand.

After the nerve splits, at the level of the elbow, the deep branch runs under a tendinous arch, which is part of the extensor carpi radia-

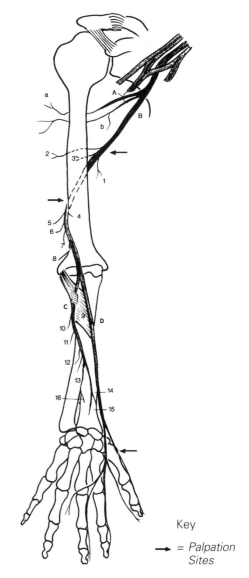

Key

→ = Palpation Sites

Figure A–3 Radial nerve and axillary nerve, right arm. **A**, axillary nerve; **B**, radial nerve; **C**, radial nerve, deep branch (posterior interosseous nerve); **D**, radial nerve, superficial branch. *Innervated by the axillary nerve:* **a**, deltoid; **b**, teres minor. *Innervated by the radial nerve:* **1**, triceps, medial head; **2**, triceps, lateral head; **3**, triceps, long head; **4**, brachialis (partially innervated); **5**, extensor carpi radialis longus; **6**, brachioradialis; **7**, extensor carpi radialis brevis; **8**, anconeus; **9**, supinator; **10**, extensor digitorum communis; **11**, extensor carpi ulnaris; **12**, extensor digiti minimi; **13**, extensor pollicis longus; **14**, abductor pollicis longus; **15**, extensor pollicis brevis; **16**, extensor indicis proprius.

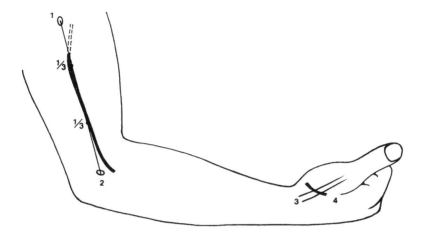

Figure A–4 Palpation of a cutaneous nerve. Localize the deltoid tuberosity **(1)**, and the lateral humeral epicondyle **(2)**. The radial nerve crosses an imaginary line connecting the two points, at a point where the upper and middle thirds of the line meet. **3**, Extensor pollicis longus tendon; **4**, palpable part of the superficial branch of the radial nerve.

lis brevis tendon. This tendinous arch is not present in everyone. If it does exist, the nerve can get compressed at this site and cause signs and symptoms similar to those of tennis elbow. This can happen when forcefully repeated supination or wrist extension with radial deviation leads to irritation of the deep radial branch (posterior interosseous nerve) or superficial branch (somewhat further distally). An injury such as this could be incurred, for example, while playing tennis when a backhand stroke is made with a maximally extended elbow.

Median Nerve

Derivation

The median nerve derives from the lateral and medial cords. Its roots are C5 to T1 (Figures A–1 and A–2).

Course

The median nerve runs lateral to the brachial artery in the medial bicipital sulcus. Further distally, it can be found at the medial side of the coracobrachialis insertion. In the cubital fossa, it runs medial to the biceps ten-

don, then courses between the heads of the pronator teres. At the level of the wrist, the median nerve runs between the palmaris longus and flexor carpi radialis muscles, then underneath the flexor retinaculum through the carpal tunnel. After leaving the carpal tunnel, it divides into branches (Figures A–5 and A–8).

Palpation

The median nerve can be palpated over a relatively long distance in the medial bicipital sulcus. A second site of palpation is at the wrist, where the nerve runs between the palmaris longus and flexor carpi radialis tendons. Flexing and extending the wrist facilitates this palpation (Figure A–5).

Lesions

The most significant lesion of the median nerve is summarily termed carpal tunnel syndrome. This syndrome is described as a compression of the median nerve in the carpal tunnel, most frequently caused by arthritides, tenovaginitides, and luxations. The patient's chief complaints are tingling in the arm and

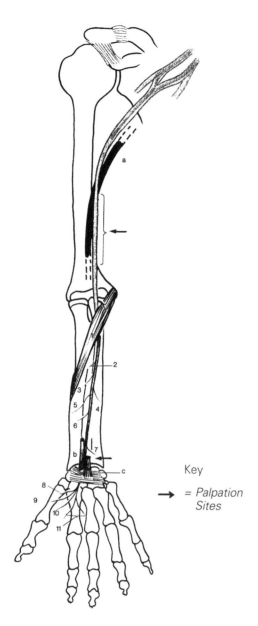

Key

→ = Palpation
      Sites

Figure A–5 Median nerve (C5 to T1), right arm.
a, brachial artery; **b**, flexor carpi radialis tendon;
c, palmaris longus tendon. *Innervated by the
median nerve:* **1**, pronator teres; **2**, palmaris longus; **3**, flexor carpi radialis; **4**, flexor digitorum
profundus (II and III); **5**, flexor digitorum
superficialis; **6**, flexor pollicis longus; **7**, pronator
quadratus; **8**, abductor pollicis brevis; **9**, opponens pollicis; **10**, flexor pollicis brevis, superficial
head; **11**, lumbricals (I and II).

hand—which occurs particularly at night—
and later, the inability to perform forceful
thumb opposition.

The median nerve also can be compressed
between both heads of the pronator teres
muscle, resulting in a pronator teres syndrome. This condition is difficult to differentiate from a carpal tunnel syndrome. Assessing
sensory loss in the thenar eminence helps to
make the diagnosis. Just proximal to the
transverse carpal ligament (flexor retinaculum), the nerve gives off a sensory branch
(palmar cutaneous branch) to the thenar
eminence. Thus, if the nerve is affected at the
level of the pronator teres, there should be
evidence of a sensory disturbance in the thenar region, which would not be present with a
carpal tunnel syndrome.

Musculocutaneous Nerve

Derivation

The musculocutaneous nerve derives from
the lateral cord. Its roots are C5 to C7 (Figures A–1 and A–2).

Course

The musculocutaneous nerve penetrates
the coracobrachialis muscle, then runs distally between the biceps and brachialis,
where it courses along the lateral side of the
biceps. From here it enters the humeral fascia, where it becomes superficial. In its superficial course, it is called the lateral cutaneous
nerve of the forearm and has two branches
that run along the radial aspect of the forearm
(Figure A–6).

Palpation

Occasionally, the nerve can be palpated
where it enters the coracobrachialis muscle.
In order to do so, the palpating finger slides
along the medial bicipital sulcus until reaching the caudal part of the axilla, where the
entrance site is sought (Figure A–6).

Lesions

Lesions of the musculocutaneous nerve are
rare.

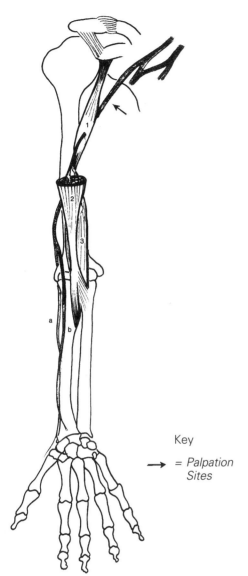

Key

➜ = *Palpation Sites*

Figure A–6 Musculocutaneous nerve (C5 to C7), right arm. **a**, pars posterior; **b**, pars anterior. *Innervated by the musculocutaneous nerve:* **1**, coracobrachialis; **2**, biceps; **3**, brachialis.

Ulnar Nerve

Derivation

The ulnar nerve derives from the medial cord. Its roots are C8 and T1, sometimes C7 (Figures A–1 and A–2).

Course

The ulnar nerve accompanies the axillary and brachial arteries medially to midarm level. It penetrates the medial intermuscular septum and then runs with the superior ulnar collateral artery through the medial epicondylar groove (sulcus nervi ulnaris), which is formed by the olecranon and the medial humeral epicondyle.

After leaving the groove, the ulnar nerve first runs between both heads of the flexor carpi ulnaris and then travels radially to this muscle as it courses distally. At midforearm, the nerve courses along the ulnar side of the ulnar artery, eventually becoming more superficial in its course (Figures A–7 and A–8).

In the wrist region, the ulnar nerve runs on the radial side of the pisiform, through Guyon's tunnel. An imaginary line connecting the medial humeral epicondyle to the radial side of the pisiform provides a rough impression of the ulnar nerve's course.

Palpation

It is possible to palpate the ulnar nerve proximally in the medial bicipital sulcus and behind the medial epicondyle. Occasionally, it is also palpable just proximal to the wrist (Figure A–7).

Lesions

The ulnar nerve is most frequently injured in the region of the cubital tunnel (epicondylar groove). If the groove is too shallow or if the fascia that fixes the nerve is too lax, repeated subluxations lead to irritation of the nerve. Fractures of the medial epicondyle are often complicated by accompanying damage to the ulnar nerve. Hypertonia of the flexor carpi ulnaris muscle (eg, overuse) can also lead to compression of the nerve.

In the hand region, painful tingling, especially in the little finger, sometimes occurs as a result of constant pressure (eg, in bicyclists).

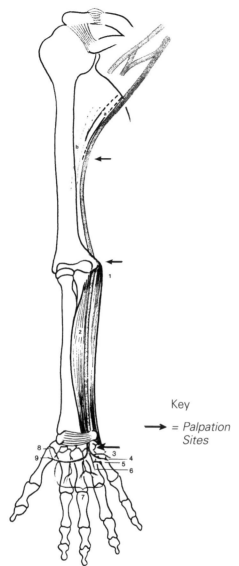

Key

→ = *Palpation Sites*

Figure A–7 Ulnar nerve (C8-T1), right arm. **a**, brachial artery; **b**, median nerve. *Innervated by the median nerve:* **1**, flexor carpi ulnaris; **2**, flexor digitorum profundus (IV and V); **3**, palmaris brevis; **4**, abductor digiti minimi; **5**, opponens digiti minimi; **6**, flexor digiti minimi; **7**, lumbricals (III and IV) interossei; **8**, abductor pollicis; **9**, flexor pollicis brevis, deep head.

ARTERIES OF THE UPPER EXTREMITIES

On the left side, the subclavian artery originates directly from the aorta, and on the right side it arises from the brachiocephalic trunk. As it leaves the thorax, it runs over the first rib and between the insertions of the middle and anterior scalenes (lying on the floor of the posterior scalenic triangle), just caudal to the brachial plexus. Just before the scalenic triangle, it gives off a number of branches to the thorax, neck, shoulder, and back of the head. Topographically, the course of the vertebral artery is of the greatest significance (artery for neck and back of the head).

Taking essentially the shortest route, the subclavian artery runs from the posterior scalenic triangle, underneath the clavicle, behind the pectoralis minor (after which it is called the axillary artery), to the neurovascular bundle of the axilla. Along this route, the artery again gives off numerous branches, particularly dorsally to the scapular region. In the axilla, a ring of humeral arteries is given off, of which the posterior humeral circumflex artery is the most clinically significant. The posterior humeral circumflex artery runs together with the axillary nerve through the lateral axillary space (quadrangular space) and is susceptible to injury in instances of humeral head dislocations.

On leaving the axilla, the axillary artery is called the brachial artery. It runs distally in the medial bicipital sulcus without giving off any branches. Underneath the biceps aponeurosis, the radial artery arises from the brachial artery; somewhat later, the ulnar artery arises (Figure A–8).

Brachial Artery

Derivation

The brachial artery derives from the axillary artery.

Course

The brachial artery runs in the medial bicipital sulcus, underneath the teres major tendon. Further distally, it turns ventrally and divides into the radial and ulnar arteries in the cubital fossa (Figure A–8).

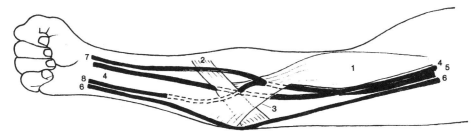

Figure A–8 Right arm, relationship of the most important arteries and nerves (volar). **1**, Biceps; **2**, pronator teres; **3**, biceps aponeurosis; **4**, median nerve; **5**, brachial artery; **6**, ulnar nerve; **7**, radial artery; **8**, ulnar artery.

Palpation

Obvious pulsation can be felt in the medial bicipital sulcus.

Lesions

Because of its superficial course in the arm, the brachial artery is susceptible to compression and injuries.

Radial Artery

Derivation

The radial artery derives from the brachial artery.

Course

The radial artery runs from the cubital fossa along the ulnar aspect of the radius to the radial styloid process (Figure A–8). Its proximal part is covered by the brachioradialis muscle. Further distally, the artery lies just underneath the skin and fascia. In the region of the wrist, the radial artery divides into a superficial artery and a deep artery. The deep branch is the main branch, which runs underneath the extensor pollicis brevis tendon, over the floor of the anatomical snuffbox, and under the extensor pollicis longus tendon. It then penetrates the dorsal interosseous I muscle to meet the deep branch of the ulnar artery (coming from the other side), in the palm of the hand. Together, the two arteries form the deep palmar arch.

The smaller superficial branch of the radial artery crosses over the carpal tunnel and hypothenar eminence (or penetrates the hypothenar eminence) and forms the superficial palmar arch along with the superficial branch of the ulnar artery.

Palpation

The radial artery is easy to palpate just radial to the flexor carpi radialis tendon. From here, it runs underneath the abductor pollicis longus and extensor pollicis brevis tendons through the first extensor tunnel. After that, it is palpable in the anatomical snuffbox, just where it penetrates the first dorsal interosseous muscle.

Lesions

Lesions of the radial artery are rare.

Ulnar Artery

Derivation

The ulnar artery derives from the brachial artery.

Course

The proximal third of the ulnar artery is hidden under the wrist flexors. After that, the artery runs under an imaginary line connecting the medial humeral epicondyle to the ulnar side of the pisiform (Figure A–8).

In the palm, the ulnar artery gives off a deep branch and a superficial branch, both of which anastomose with the corresponding branches of the radial artery. The superficial branch of the ulnar artery is the main branch. It runs over the carpal tunnel and radially to the hypothenar eminence, and is the main contributor to the superficial palmar carpal arch. The smaller deep branch crosses over the carpal tunnel as well, penetrates the hypothenar eminence, and joins together with the deep radial branch to supply the deep palmar carpal arch.

The superficial palmar carpal arch is located in the palm between the palmar aponeurosis and the tendons of the finger flexors. The deep palmar carpal arch lies between the tendons of the finger flexors and the interossei and metacarpals.

Palpation

The ulnar artery can be palpated between the flexor carpi ulnaris and the flexor digitorum superficialis. The superficial branch of the ulnar artery is palpable radial to the hypothenar eminence.

Lesions

There may be compression in Guyon's tunnel.

VEINS OF THE UPPER EXTREMITIES

Each of the smaller arteries is accompanied by two veins of similar names. However, proximal to the axilla, there are only the axillary and subclavian veins (bilaterally). Besides these deep veins, there are also several important superficial veins:

- cephalic vein, which arises on the radial side, runs proximally along the lateral bicipital sulcus, and flows into the axillary vein in Mohrenheim's groove
- basilic vein, which arises on the ulnar side and flows into the brachial vein in the medial bicipital sulcus
- median cubital vein, which flows into the cephalic and basilic veins (in varying patterns) in the cubital fossa

Further proximally, the veins generally run ventral to the arteries of the same name. For instance, the subclavian vein runs through the anterior scalenic triangle (the subclavian artery runs through the posterior scalenic triangle), taking the internal jugular vein with it. Afterward, they are called the brachiocephalic veins. Both brachiocephalic veins join to form the superior vena cava.

Cephalic Vein

Derivation

The cephalic vein derives from the venous plexus at the dorsum of the hand and the venous branches from the forearm and arm.

Course

The course of the cephalic vein varies among individuals. It originates at the dorsum of the hand and runs proximally along the volar aspect of the radial side of the forearm. In the cubital fossa, the cephalic vein gives a branch to the median cubital vein. It then runs along the lateral aspect of the arm in the groove between the brachialis and biceps muscles, and later in Mohrenheim's groove (between the deltoid and pectoralis major muscles) in order to reach the infraclavicular fossa. Here it penetrates the fascia and empties into the axillary vein.

Palpation

The cephalic vein can be palpated lateral to the biceps tendon. In this area, it also has a constant flow.

Lesions

Lesions of the cephalic vein are rare.

Basilic Vein

Derivation

The basilic vein derives from the ulnar part of the venous plexus at the dorsum of the hand and venous branches in the forearm and arm.

Course

The basilic vein runs along the dorsoulnar aspect of the forearm, then courses in a volar direction just distal to the cubital fossa. After passing the cubital fossa, it runs medial to the biceps, where it pierces the fascia (basilic hiatus) at the point between the lower and middle thirds of the arm.

Finally, the basilic vein runs on the medial side of the brachial artery, where its name changes to axillary vein after crossing the teres major. Along its course, the basilic vein often anastomoses with the cephalic vein.

Palpation

Palpation of the basilic vein is difficult. Sometimes it can be seen and palpated just proximal to the cubital fossa and in the forearm in the region where it courses from dorsal to volar. Palpation can be simplified by following the easily identified median cubital vein.

Lesions

Lesions of the basilic vein are rare.

Median Cubital Vein

Derivation

The medial cubital vein derives from the cephalic vein.

Course

The median cubital vein connects the cephalic vein (laterodistally) to the basilic vein (medioproximally) at the level of the elbow.

Palpation

Despite its variable course, the median cubital vein is easy to find. The vein can be identified more clearly by making a firm fist with a taut elastic tourniquet on the upper arm.

Lesions

Lesions of the median cubital vein are rare.

Appendix B

Algorithms for the Diagnosis and Treatment of the Upper Extremities

LEGEND

Pain

    ○ = Sometimes painful
    ● = Painful
  ●● = Most painful test
  ( ) = eg, ● (●) Signifies pain, and sometimes is the most painful test

Limitation of Motion

    ○ = Sometimes (minimal) limitation of motion
    ● = Minimal limitation of motion
  ●● = Moderate limitation of motion
●●● = Severe limitation of motion
  ( ) = eg, ●● (●) Signifies moderate to severe limitation of motion

Muscle Weakness

    ○ = Sometimes (minimal) weakness
    ● = Moderate weakness
  ●● = Severe weakness

    □ = Hypermobility or instability
    ! = Test not performed
    + = Positive, but without pain, limitation of motion, weakness, or hypermobility
    ★ = Muscle tightness
  ( ) = Sometimes, eg, (+) signifies sometimes positive; (★) signifies sometimes muscle tightness

Symbols and Indications

$\equiv$ Possibilities mentioned are of equal rank; one can make a choice from the available data

1
2 Graded order of ranking; information is listed in order of importance or preference
3

$\downarrow\equiv$ Listed according to the passage of time

$\triangleright$ Indicates the sequence

$\longrightarrow$ In all probability, the following occurs

$---\rightarrow$ It could possibly lead to the following

$\pm$ Approximately

DIAGRAM FOR BASIC ORTHOPAEDIC EXAMINATION

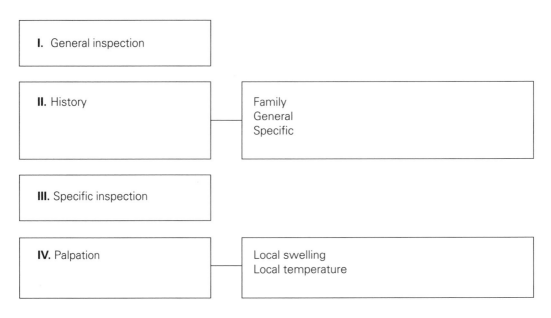

I. General inspection

II. History — Family / General / Specific

III. Specific inspection

IV. Palpation — Local swelling / Local temperature

Before beginning the functional examination, ask the patient what he or she feels "at this moment" (at rest). During the functional examination, note whether the patient reports any change with each movement or test.

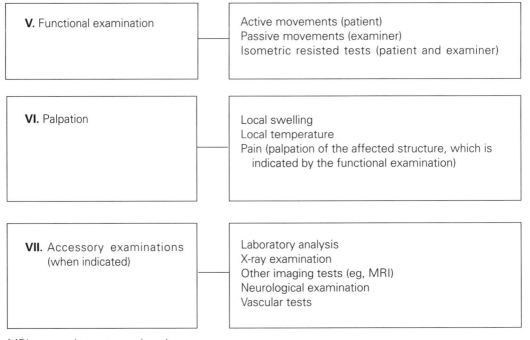

V. Functional examination — Active movements (patient) / Passive movements (examiner) / Isometric resisted tests (patient and examiner)

VI. Palpation — Local swelling / Local temperature / Pain (palpation of the affected structure, which is indicated by the functional examination)

VII. Accessory examinations (when indicated) — Laboratory analysis / X-ray examination / Other imaging tests (eg, MRI) / Neurological examination / Vascular tests

MRI, magnetic resonance imaging.

General Inspection and History

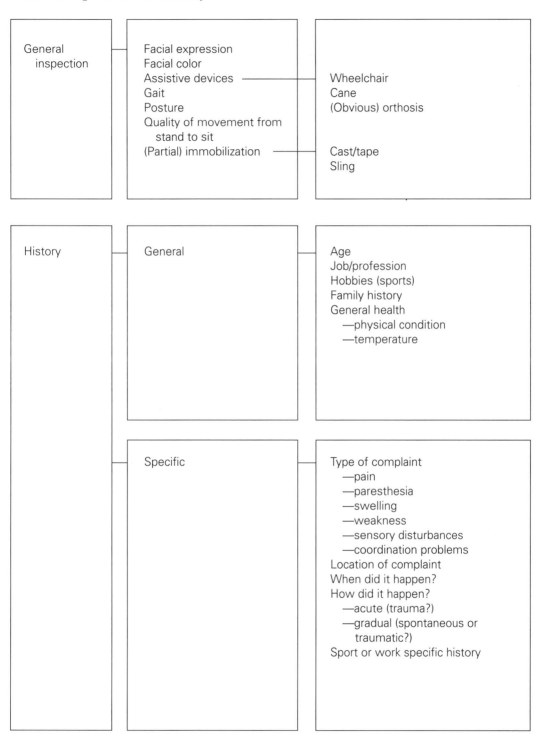

Specific Inspection

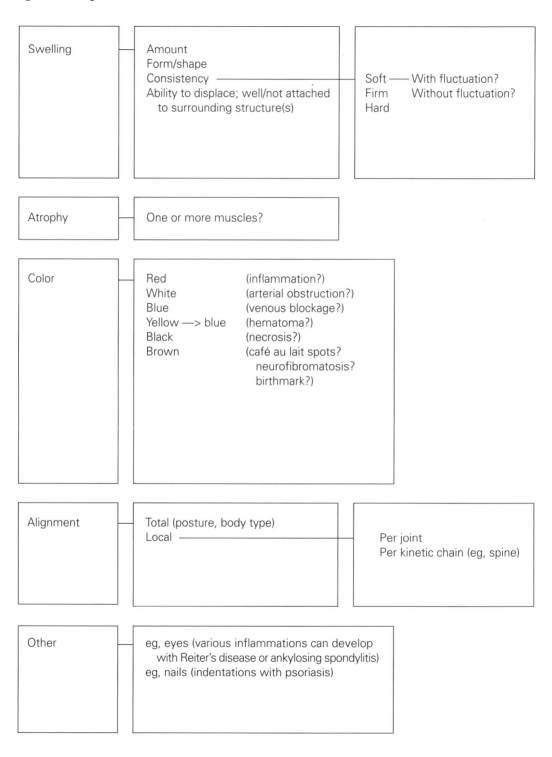

| Swelling | Amount
Form/shape
Consistency ———————
Ability to displace; well/not attached
    to surrounding structure(s) | Soft —— With fluctuation?
Firm   Without fluctuation?
Hard |

| Atrophy | One or more muscles? |

| Color | Red   (inflammation?)
White   (arterial obstruction?)
Blue   (venous blockage?)
Yellow —> blue   (hematoma?)
Black   (necrosis?)
Brown   (café au lait spots?
                        neurofibromatosis?
                        birthmark?) |

| Alignment | Total (posture, body type)
Local ———————— | Per joint
Per kinetic chain (eg, spine) |

| Other | eg, eyes (various inflammations can develop
    with Reiter's disease or ankylosing spondylitis)
eg, nails (indentations with psoriasis) |

Functional Examination

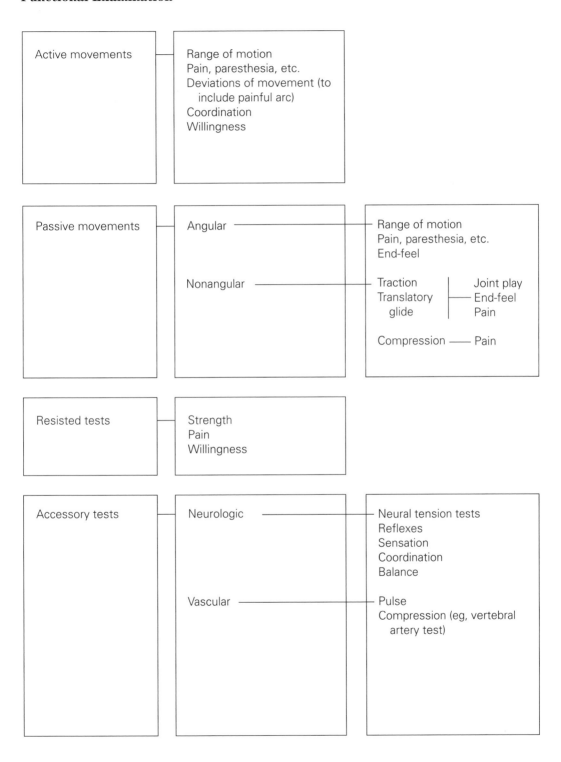

DIAGRAM FOR BASIC FUNCTIONAL EXAMINATION FINDINGS 1

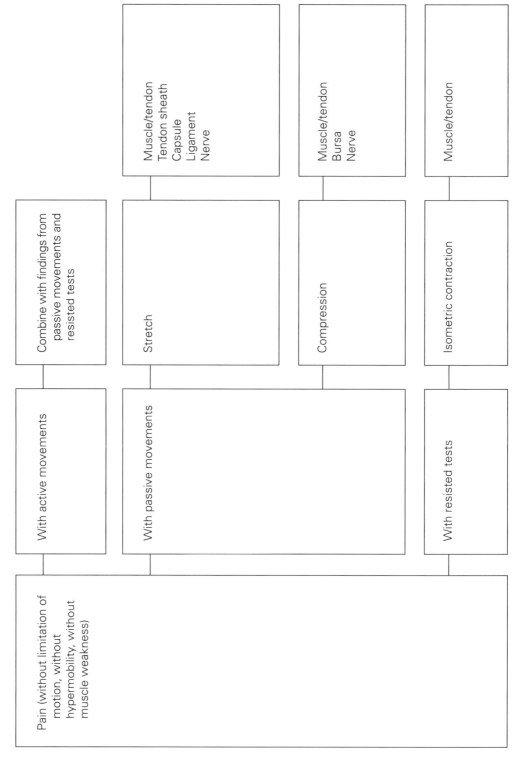

Pain (without limitation of motion, without hypermobility, without muscle weakness)

With active movements — Combine with findings from passive movements and resisted tests

With passive movements — Stretch — Muscle/tendon, Tendon sheath, Capsule, Ligament, Nerve

Compression — Muscle/tendon, Bursa, Nerve

With resisted tests — Isometric contraction — Muscle/tendon

DIAGRAM FOR BASIC FUNCTIONAL EXAMINATION FINDINGS 2

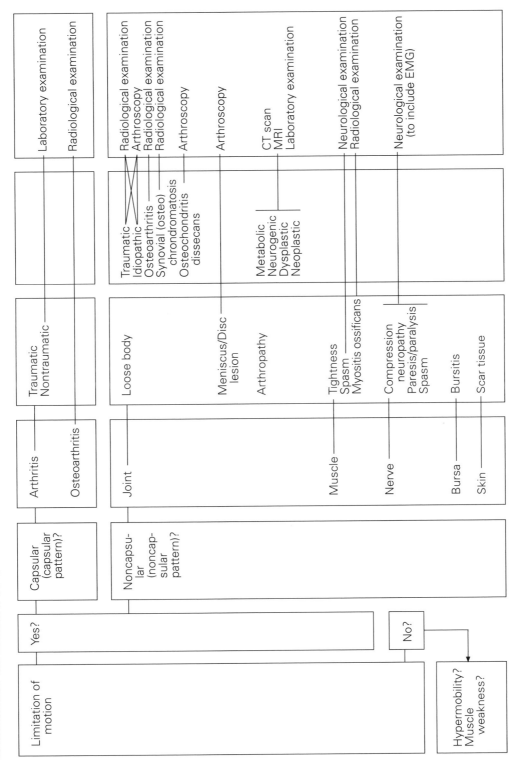

DIAGRAM FOR BASIC FUNCTIONAL EXAMINATION FINDINGS 3

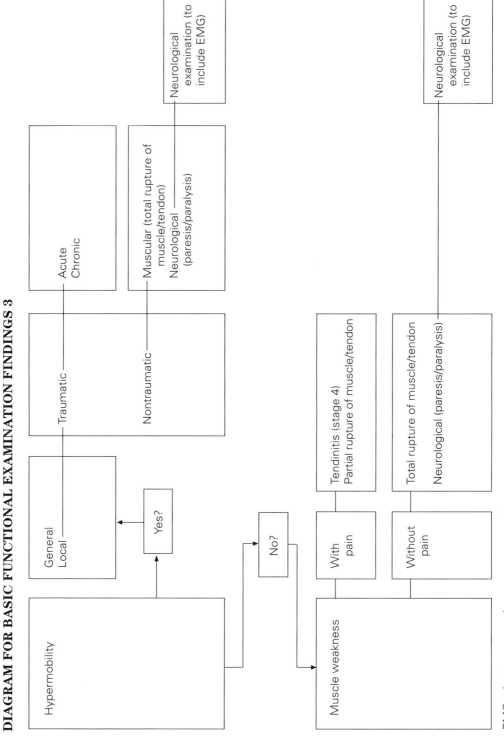

EMG, electromyography

DIAGRAM FOR BASIC TREATMENT

Primary prevention	1 Information
	    • General
	        —posture
	        —body mechanics
	        —nutrition
	    • Work specific
	    • Sport specific
	2 Working conditions adapted to the working activities (ergonomics)
	3 Sport conditions
	    • Surface
	    • Equipment
	        —eg, shoes, racquet, etc.
	    • Clothes
	    • Warm up/cool down
	    • Taping

Secondary prevention (= treatment)	1 Causal treatment
	    • See primary prevention, 1, 2, 3
	2 Local treatment
	    • eg, transverse friction, ultrasound, cryotherapy
	    • Mobilization (manipulation)
	    • Stretching
	    • Muscle strengthening
	    • Injection
	    • Taping
	    • Stabilization
	3 General treatment
	    • Limitation of activities
	    • General conditioning
	    • Medication

Tertiary prevention	Prevent progression of the lesion by means of the measures listed under secondary prevention

LOCAL TREATMENT

Lesion	Physical therapist	Physician	Patient
Joint and ligamentous lesions	Specific mobilization and/or manipulation of movement limitations Stabilization exercise program and taping or bracing of hypermobilities or instabilities Transverse friction massage for ligament sprains and small partial ruptures Modalities	Aspiration Intra-articular injection Injection (of ligament insertions)	Active exercises after mobilization/manipulation Possibly transverse friction massage Muscle-strengthening exercises
Musculotendinous lesions	Transverse friction massage Stretching Muscle-strengthening exercises Modalities	Injection (tendon insertion, musculotendinous junction, muscle belly) Injection (tenosynovitis, tenovaginitis)	Stretching exercises Muscle-stretching exercises When possible, transverse friction massage
Bursitis	Correction of local articular and/or muscular disturbances Modalities	Aspiration Injection	Maintain mobility after joint mobilization/manipulation and/or muscle stretching
Compression neuropathy	Correction of possible muscle tightness by means of muscle stretching Modalities	Perineural injection	Stretching exercises

DIAGRAM FOR BASIC TREATMENT OF TENDINITIS

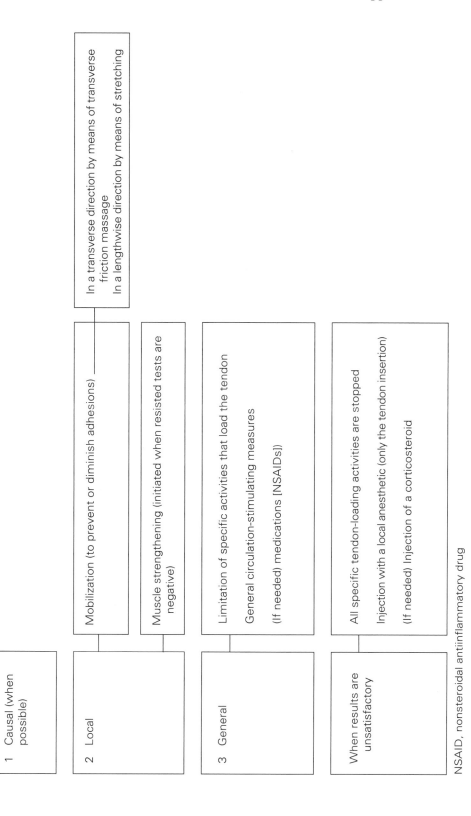

1 Causal (when possible)

2 Local

Mobilization (to prevent or diminish adhesions)

In a transverse direction by means of transverse friction massage
In a lengthwise direction by means of stretching

Muscle strengthening (initiated when resisted tests are negative)

3 General

Limitation of specific activities that load the tendon

General circulation-stimulating measures

(If needed) medications [NSAIDs])

When results are unsatisfactory

All specific tendon-loading activities are stopped

Injection with a local anesthetic (only the tendon insertion)

(If needed) Injection of a corticosteroid

NSAID, nonsteroidal antiinflammatory drug

END-FEEL

The quality of the resistance that the examiner feels at the end of a joint range of motion is determined by:
1. the structure restricting the movement
2. the particular lesion of the joint
3. gender
4. age
5. general flexibility
6. how the examiner performs the test

There are as many kinds of end-feel as there are motions. Furthermore, there is a difference both interindividually and intraindividually.

The end-feel is best specified by using a visual analogue scale: |——————| The left end of the scale indicates the softest possible end-feel; the right end indicates the hardest possible end-feel.

Normal end-feel is specified here with a black line above the scale.

Pathological end-feel is specified with a gray line above the scale.

Types of end-feel	Restricting structure	Example
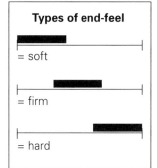 = soft	Soft tissue between long bones or between extremity and trunk	Elbow flexion Hip flexion
= firm	Capsuloligamentous structures Musculature	Shoulder external rotation Hip abduction
= hard	Capsuloligamentous structures	Elbow extension Knee extension

Pathological end-feel	Description	Example
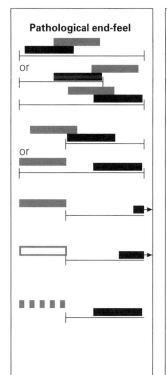	"Too hard" for what is expected	Elbow flexion with arthritis Elbow extension with arthritis
	"Too soft" for what is expected	Knee hyperextension, post-traumatically
	"Springing back" when either a soft or a hard end-feel is expected	Hip adduction (in 90° flexion) with a loose body Elbow extension with a loose body
	"Bounces back" more severe stage than springing back	Blocked knee extension by a meniscus
	"Empty"; not able to test end-feel due to a willful limitation of motion because of pain	Shoulder abduction with an acute subacromiodeltoid bursitis
	"Spasm"; an unconscious limitation of motion as a result of severe pathology	Fracture Tumor Severe inflammation

ARTHROLOGY (THE SCIENCE OF JOINTS)

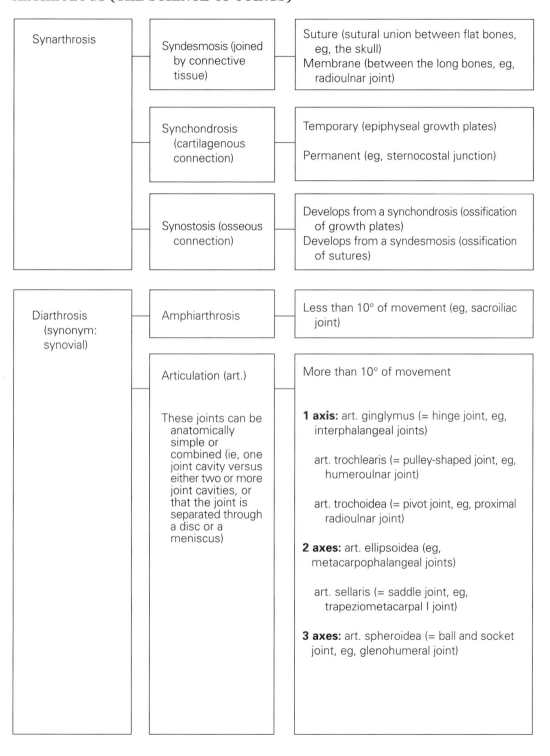

Synarthrosis	Syndesmosis (joined by connective tissue)	Suture (sutural union between flat bones, eg, the skull) Membrane (between the long bones, eg, radioulnar joint)
	Synchondrosis (cartilagenous connection)	Temporary (epiphyseal growth plates) Permanent (eg, sternocostal junction)
	Synostosis (osseous connection)	Develops from a synchondrosis (ossification of growth plates) Develops from a syndesmosis (ossification of sutures)

Diarthrosis (synonym: synovial)	Amphiarthrosis	Less than 10° of movement (eg, sacroiliac joint)
	Articulation (art.) These joints can be anatomically simple or combined (ie, one joint cavity versus either two or more joint cavities, or that the joint is separated through a disc or a meniscus)	More than 10° of movement **1 axis:** art. ginglymus (= hinge joint, eg, interphalangeal joints) art. trochlearis (= pulley-shaped joint, eg, humeroulnar joint) art. trochoidea (= pivot joint, eg, proximal radioulnar joint) **2 axes:** art. ellipsoidea (eg, metacarpophalangeal joints) art. sellaris (= saddle joint, eg, trapeziometacarpal I joint) **3 axes:** art. spheroidea (= ball and socket joint, eg, glenohumeral joint)

ANALYSIS OF MOVEMENT: GENERAL

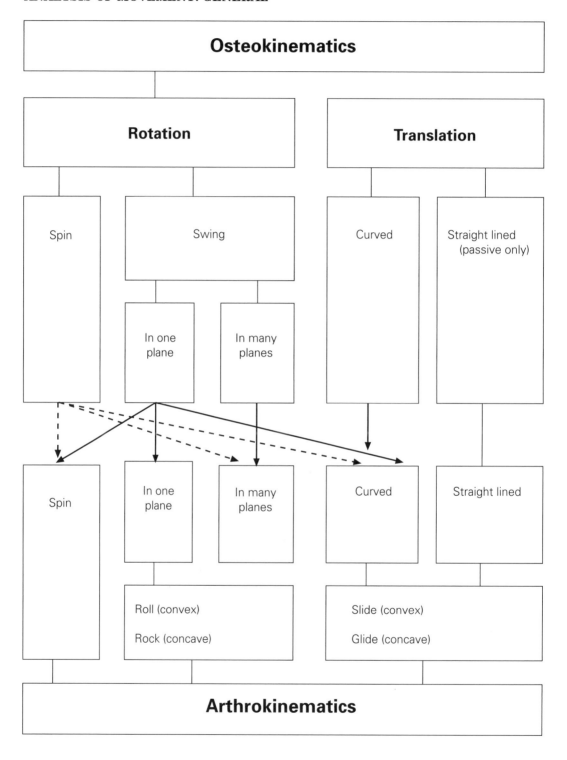

ASSESSMENT OF THE MOBILITY OF THE PERIPHERAL JOINTS

Normal mobility	From the anatomical zero position, normal mobility is the average amount of movement possible per joint per motion. It is determined according to the SFTR method (sagittal, frontal, transverse, and rotation), and was unanimously accepted by the orthopaedic associations of all English-speaking countries, in Vancouver, BC, in 1964. Gender and age play a very important role, and there can be significant individual differences. Therefore, it is essential to compare findings with those of the other side.
Hypomobility	Less than normal mobility is present without necessary pathology. There are no clinical signs and/or symptoms.
Limitation of motion	Less than normal mobility is present, as well as less range of motion than on the other side. There is pathology, and there are clinical signs from the affected joint or its surrounding structures.
Hypermobility	More than normal mobility is present without necessary pathology. There are no clinical signs and/or symptoms. Through overuse or trauma, a hypermobile joint can lead to problems earlier than a joint with normal mobility. Hypermobile joints can dislocate earlier than joints with normal mobility.
Hypermobility syndrome	General hypermobility is present, which can be hereditary, incidental, or due to a pathological connective tissue syndrome such as Ehlers-Danlos syndrome, Marfan syndrome, or osteogenesis imperfecta. General hypermobility can also be present with other disorders, for instance, with Down syndrome.

Instability
    Subluxation
    Dislocation
	There is incomplete dislocation of a joint.
	There is complete loss of contact between the joint surfaces of the two joint partners.
	The amount of instability is determined by use of passive tests in the functional examination. For certain joints, radiological criteria are also utilized.
	One differentiates between functional stability and functional instability.

Functional stability	The patient does not have a feeling of instability in the joint during activities. There can be other complaints, such as pain and swelling.
Functional instability	During activities, the patient has an unstable feeling in the joint or a "giving way" such as in the knee; or the patient experiences a shooting pain followed by a short moment of inability to move (or a "paralyzed" feeling in) the joint (eg, shoulder, wrist).

PROGRESSION OF GENERAL JOINT-SPECIFIC TREATMENT FOR A LIMITATION OF MOTION

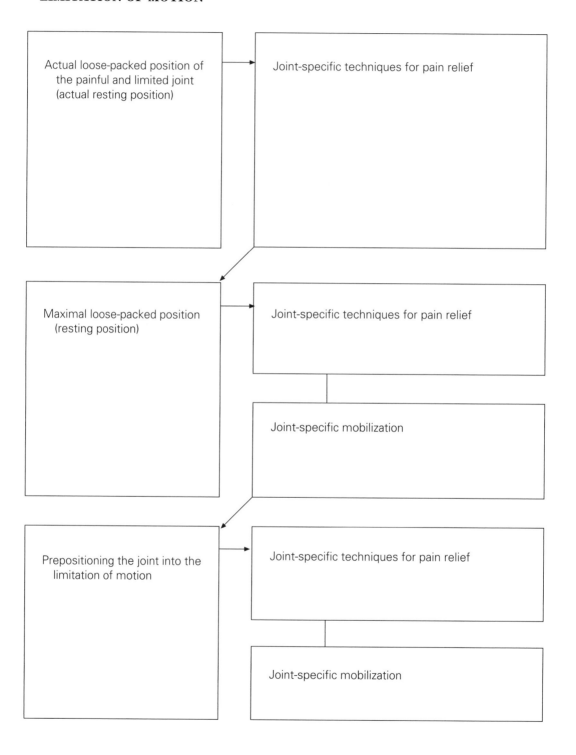

GENERAL JOINT MOBILIZATION DIAGRAM

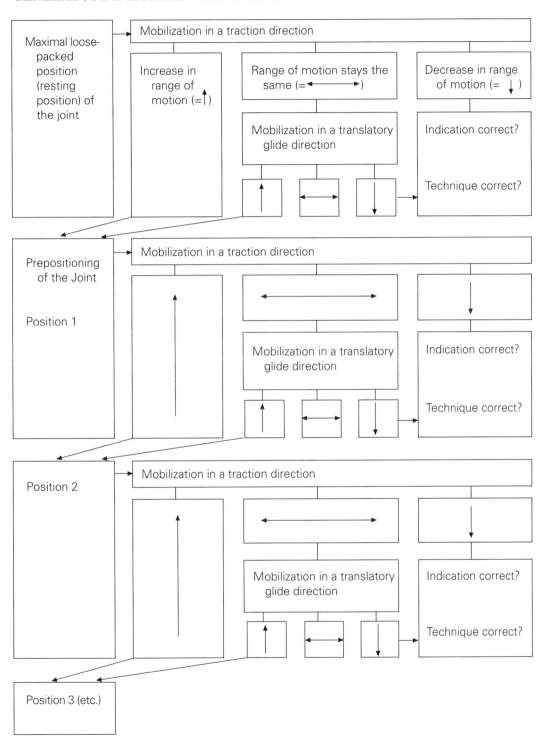

Appendix C

Algorithms for the Diagnosis and Treatment of the Upper Extremities—General

ZERO POSITION, MAXIMAL LOOSE-PACKED POSITION, MAXIMAL CLOSE-PACKED POSITION—UPPER EXTREMITIES

Joint	Zero position	Maximal loose-packed position	Maximal close-packed position
Shoulder Glenohumeral Joint	The best way to assume this position is with 90° elbow flexion; the forearm makes an angle of 90° (in the horizontal plane) to the spine of the scapula	± 55° abduction from the zero position	Maximal glenohumeral abduction, external rotation, and extension
Acromioclavicular joint	The physiological posture of the shoulder girdle; strong inter- and intra-individual differences	Same as the zero position	Maximal glenohumeral abduction without rotation
Sternoclavicular joint	See acromioclavicular joint	See acromioclavicular joint	Maximal elevation of the arm
Elbow Humeroulnar joint	Forearm and upper arm in the frontal plane, the elbow in 0° flexion, the forearm in 90° supination	± 70° elbow flexion and 10° forearm supination	Maximal elbow extension and forearm supination (for the anterior part of the joint: maximal flexion)
Humeroradial joint		Maximal elbow extension and forearm supination	± 90° elbow flexion and 5° forearm supination
Proximal radioulnar joint	The elbow flexed 90°, forearm in the middle between pro- and supination, the wrist in the zero position and the hand in the sagittal plane	± 70° elbow flexion and 35° forearm supination	± 5° forearm supination
Distal radioulnar joint		±10° supination	
Wrist (carpus) Consists of: Radiocarpal joints Intercarpal joints	The longitudinal axis through the radius and the longitudinal axis through metacarpal III are in line with each other	From the zero position, slight palmar flexion and ulnar deviation	Wrist in maximal extension

ZERO POSITION, MAXIMAL LOOSE-PACKED POSITION, MAXIMAL CLOSE-PACKED POSITION—UPPER EXTREMITIES

Joint	Zero position	Maximal loose-packed position	Maximal close-packed position
Midhand (metacarpus)			
Consists of:			
Intermetacarpal joint			
Carpometacarpal joint of the thumb	The middle position between maximal palmar abduction and dorsal adduction	The middle position between maximal palmar abduction and dorsal adduction as well as radial abduction and ulnar adduction	Maximal opposition
Carpometacarpal joints II–V	See zero position of the wrist	See zero position of the wrist	Wrist in maximal extension
Fingers			
Consist of:			
Distal and proximal interphalangeal joints	The longitudinal axis through the metacarpal bone and its articulating phalanx are in line with each other	Slight flexion	Maximal extension
Metacarpophalangeal joints II–V		Slight flexion and slight ulnar deviation	Maximal flexion
Metacarpophalangeal joint of the thumb		Slight flexion	Maximal extension

CAPSULAR PATTERN—UPPER EXTREMITIES

Joint	Limitation of Motion (passive angular movements)
Glenohumeral joint	External rotation > abduction > internal rotation (± 3:2:1)
Acromioclavicular joint	No true capsular pattern; pain (and sometimes slight limitation) at the end-range of each motion, particularly with horizontal adduction of the arm
Sternoclavicular joint	See above: acromioclavicular joint
Humeroulnar joint	Flexion > extension (± 4:1)
Humeroradial joint	No true capsular pattern
Proximal radioulnar joint	No true capsular pattern; pronation and supination painful at end-range of motion
Distal radioulnar joint	See above: proximal radioulnar joint
Wrist (carpus)	Flexion ± = extension
Radiocarpal joint Midcarpal joint Carpometacarpal joint	See above: carpus
Carpometacarpal I joint (art. carpometacarpea pollicis/art. trapeziometacarpal joint)	Retroposition
Metacarpophalangeal joints	Flexion > extension (± = 2:1)
Interphalangeal joints: proximal (PIP) distal (DIP)	Flexion > extension (± 2:1)

END-FEEL AND STRUCTURES THAT CAUSE THE END-FEEL 1

The end-feel is specified on the visual analogue scale: ———— The left end of the scale indicates
the softest possible end-feel: the right end indicates the hardest possible end-feel. Given here are
the average normal "end-feels" for normal joints.

Movement	End-feel	Structures
Shoulder		
Elevation	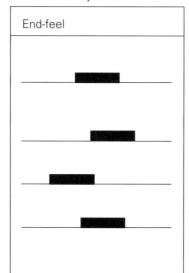	Capsuloligamentous structures from all of the joints in the shoulder girdle
Abduction		Axillary recess of the glenohumeral joint
Internal rotation		Posterior capsule of the glenohumeral joint
External rotation		Anterior capsuloligamentous structures of the glenohumeral joint

Elbow		
Extension	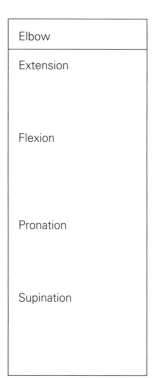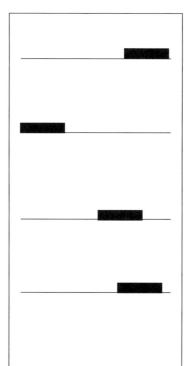	Anteromedial capsuloligamentous complex, particularly the pars anterior of the ulnar collateral ligament
Flexion		Usually soft tissue between humerus and radius-ulna Sometimes the posterior capsule
Pronation		In particular, the dorsal capsuloligamentous complex of the distal radioulnar joint
Supination		In particular, the volar capsuloligamentous complex of the distal radioulnar joint

END-FEEL AND STRUCTURES THAT CAUSE THE END-FEEL 2

The end-feel is specified on the visual analogue scale: —————— The left end of the scale indicates the softest possible end-feel; the right end indicates the hardest possible end-feel. Given here are the average normal "end-feels" for normal joints.

Movement	End-feel	Structures
Distal radioulnar joint See elbow pronation and supination Wrist Extension		Volar tendons and capsuloligamentous complex
Flexion		Dorsal tendons and capsuloligamentous complex
Radial deviation		In particular, ulnar carpal collateral ligament
Ulnar deviation		In particular, radial carpal collateral ligament

Carpometacarpal I joint Retroposition		Volar capsuloligamentous complex

Fingers (art. metacarpophalangeal and interphalangeal Extension		Volar tendons and capsuloligamentous complex
Flexion		Dorsal tendons and capsuloligamentous complex

Appendix D

Algorithms for the Diagnosis and Treatment of the Shoulder

LIMITATION OF MOTION IN THE SHOULDER

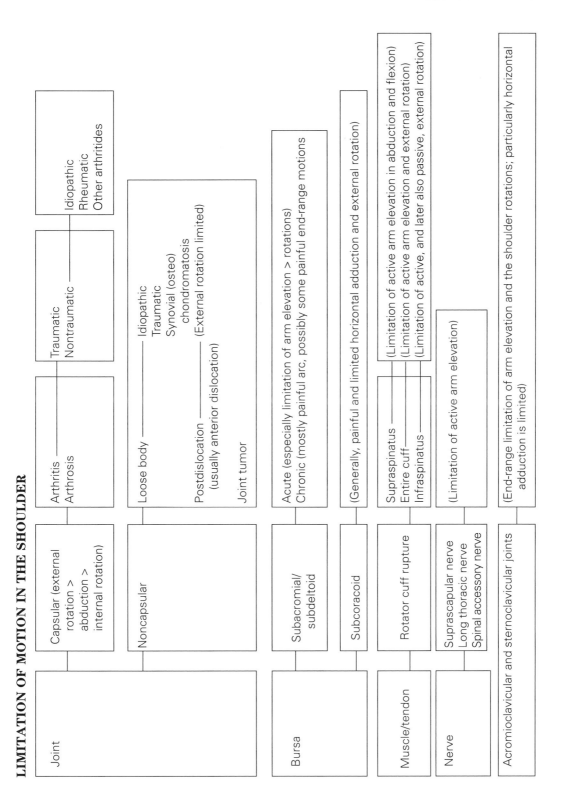

LIMITATIONS OF MOTIONS IN THE SHOULDER—ARTICULAR CAUSES

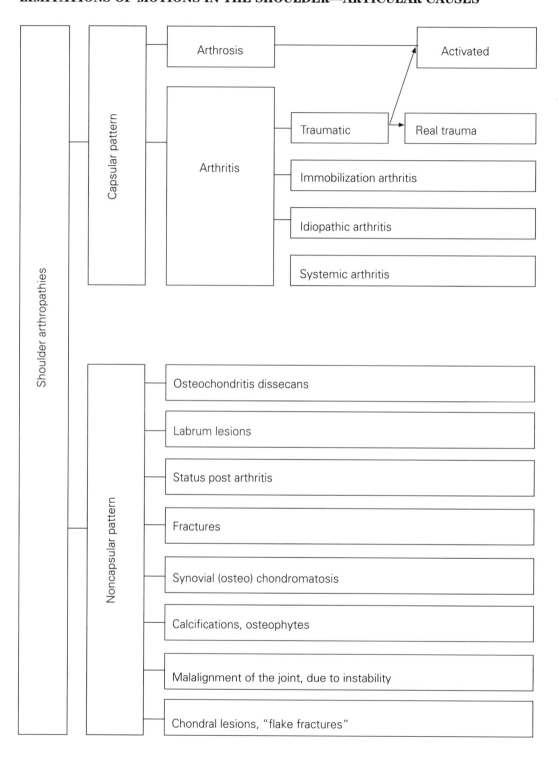

INTERPRETATION OF FINDINGS FOR ARM ELEVATION

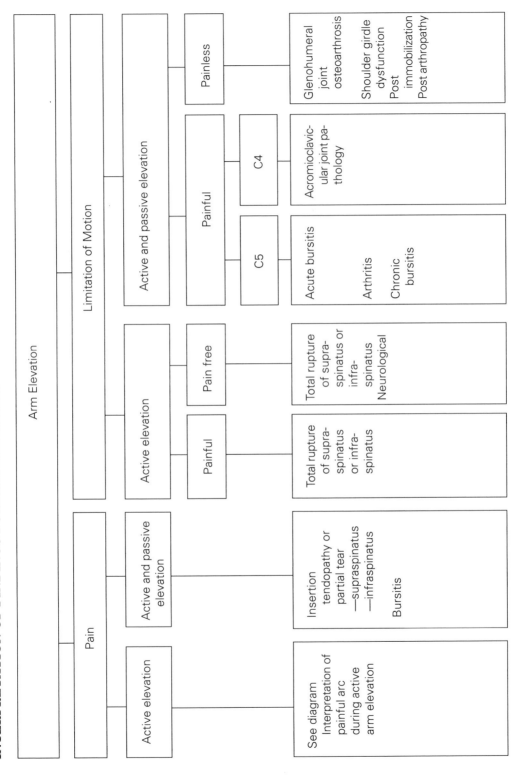

INTERPRETATION OF PAINFUL ARC DURING ACTIVE ARM ELEVATION

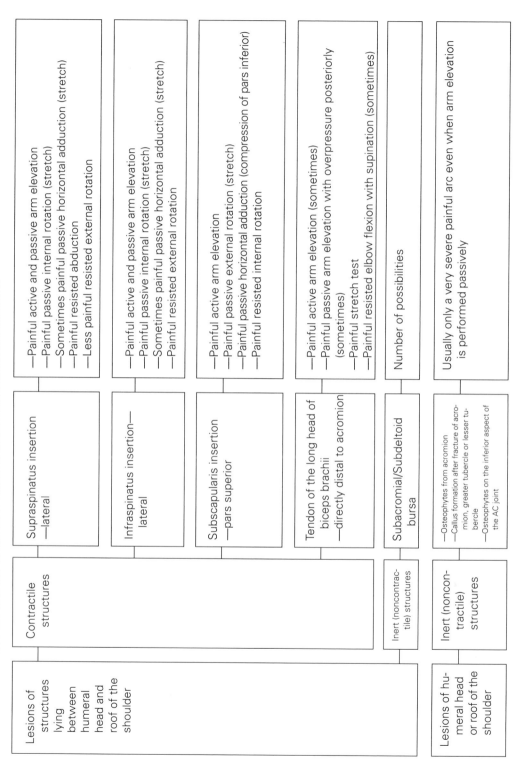

Lesions of structures lying between humeral head and roof of the shoulder

Contractile structures

Supraspinatus insertion
—lateral
—Painful active and passive arm elevation
—Painful passive internal rotation (stretch)
—Sometimes painful passive horizontal adduction (stretch)
—Painful resisted abduction
—Less painful resisted external rotation

Infraspinatus insertion—
lateral
—Painful active and passive arm elevation
—Painful passive internal rotation (stretch)
—Sometimes painful passive horizontal adduction (stretch)
—Painful resisted external rotation

Subscapularis insertion
—pars superior
—Painful active arm elevation
—Painful passive external rotation (stretch)
—Painful passive horizontal adduction (compression of pars inferior)
—Painful resisted internal rotation

Tendon of the long head of biceps brachii
—directly distal to acromion
—Painful active arm elevation (sometimes)
—Painful passive arm elevation with overpressure posteriorly (sometimes)
—Painful stretch test
—Painful resisted elbow flexion with supination (sometimes)

Inert (noncontractile) structures

Subacromial/Subdeltoid bursa
Number of possibilities

Lesions of humeral head or roof of the shoulder

Inert (noncontractile) structures
—Osteophytes from acromion
—Callus formation after fracture of acromion, greater tubercle or lesser tubercle
—Osteophytes on the inferior aspect of the AC joint

Usually only a very severe painful arc even when arm elevation is performed passively

SUBACROMIAL/SUBDELTOID

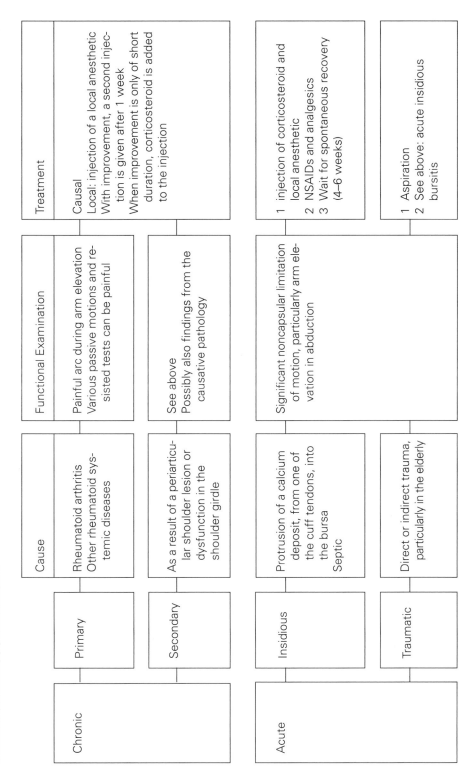

		Cause	Functional Examination	Treatment
Chronic	Primary	Rheumatoid arthritis Other rheumatoid systemic diseases	Painful arc during arm elevation Various passive motions and resisted tests can be painful	Causal Local: injection of a local anesthetic With improvement, a second injection is given after 1 week When improvement is only of short duration, corticosteroid is added to the injection
	Secondary	As a result of a periarticular shoulder lesion or dysfunction in the shoulder girdle	See above Possibly also findings from the causative pathology	
Acute	Insidious	Protrusion of a calcium deposit, from one of the cuff tendons, into the bursa Septic	Significant noncapsular limitation of motion, particularly arm elevation in abduction	1 injection of corticosteroid and local anesthetic 2 NSAIDs and analgesics 3 Wait for spontaneous recovery (4–6 weeks)
	Traumatic	Direct or indirect trauma, particularly in the elderly		1 Aspiration 2 See above: acute insidious bursitis

INTERPRETATION OF PAINFUL PASSIVE HORIZONTAL ADDUCTION OF THE ARM

	Affected structure	Other positive findings in the functional examination*
Pain occurring as a result of stretch	Suprascapular nerve	—Limitation of active arm elevation —Weak abduction —Weak external rotation
	Supraspinatus muscle	—Painful active and passive arm elevation —Painful arc —Painful resisted abduction —Less painful resisted external rotation —Painful passive internal rotation
	Infraspinatus muscle	—Painful active and passive arm elevation —Painful arc —Painful resisted external rotation —Painful passive internal rotation
Pain occurring as a result of compression	Subscapularis muscle (pars inferior)	—Painful active arm elevation —Painful arc (when the pars superior is also affected) —Painful resisted internal rotation —Painful passive external rotation
	Subacromial/Subdeltoid bursa	—Number of possibilities —Painful arc almost always present
	Subcoracoid bursa	—Painful passive external rotation in 0° abduction —Negative (pain free) passive external rotation in 90° abduction
	Acromioclavicular joint	—Painful end-range arm elevation, external rotation, and internal rotation —Sometimes resisted adduction is painful
	Sternoclavicular joint	—Painful end-range arm elevation, external rotation, and internal rotation

*Not all the tests mentioned here are always positive.

CAUSES OF SHOULDER INSTABILITY 1a

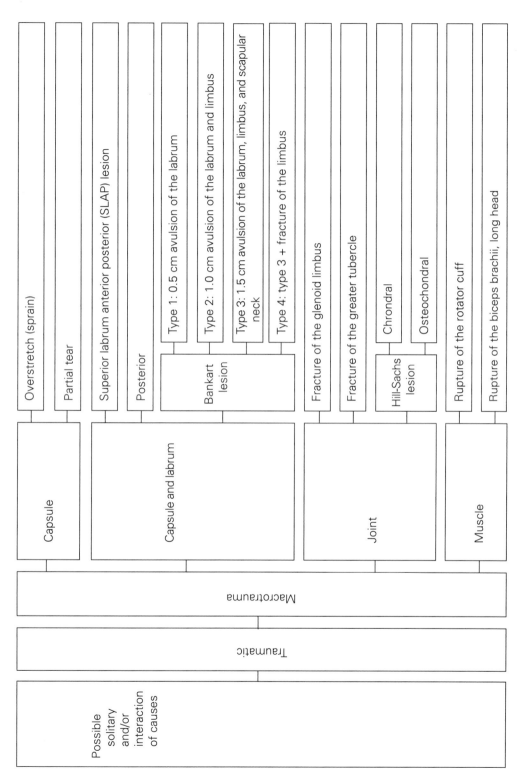

CAUSES OF SHOULDER INSTABILITY 1b

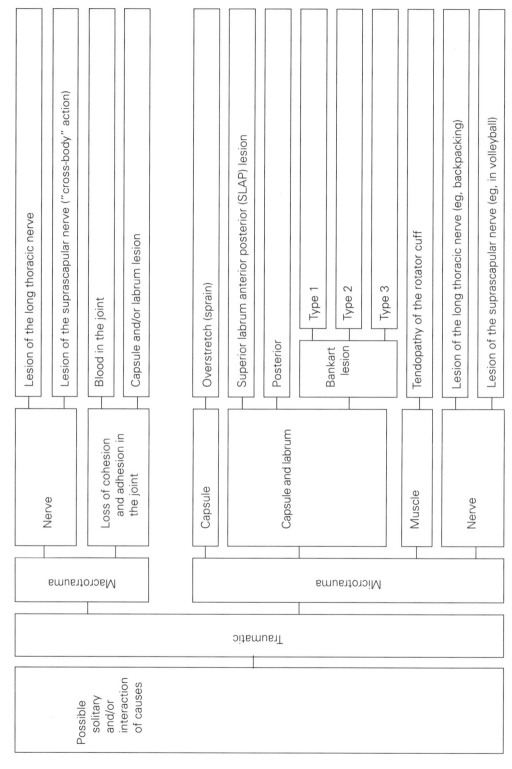

CAUSES OF SHOULDER INSTABILITY 2

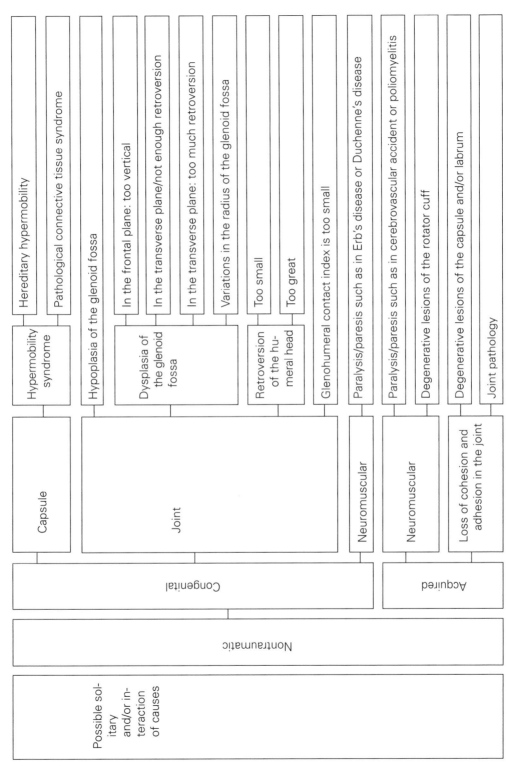

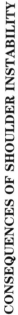

CONSEQUENCES OF SHOULDER INSTABILITY

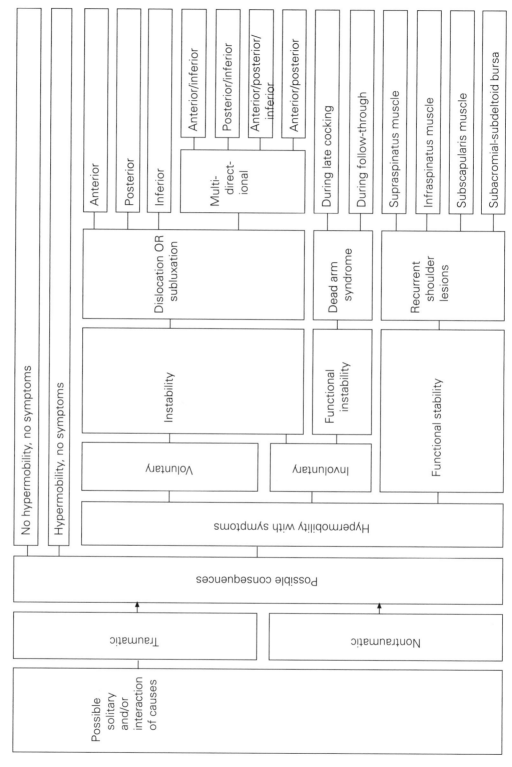

TEST SEQUENCE IN SHOULDER INSTABILITY a

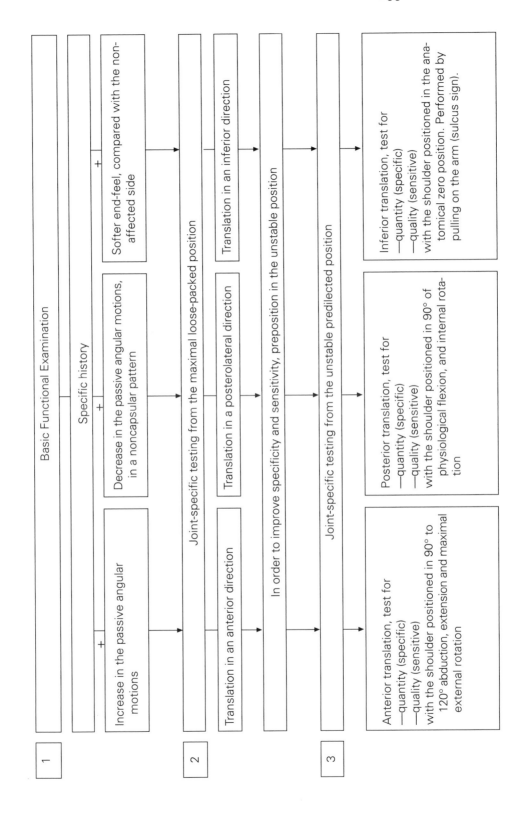

1 Basic Functional Examination

Specific history

Increase in the passive angular motions
+
Decrease in the passive angular motions, in a noncapsular pattern
+
Softer end-feel, compared with the non-affected side

2 Joint-specific testing from the maximal loose-packed position

Translation in an anterior direction
Translation in a posterolateral direction
Translation in an inferior direction

In order to improve specificity and sensitivity, preposition in the unstable position

3 Joint-specific testing from the unstable predilected position

Anterior translation, test for
—quantity (specific)
—quality (sensitive)
with the shoulder positioned in 90° to 120° abduction, extension and maximal external rotation

Posterior translation, test for
—quantity (specific)
—quality (sensitive)
with the shoulder positioned in 90° of physiological flexion, and internal rotation

Inferior translation, test for
—quantity (specific)
—quality (sensitive)
with the shoulder positioned in the anatomical zero position. Performed by pulling on the arm (sulcus sign).

TEST SEQUENCE IN SHOULDER INSTABILITY b

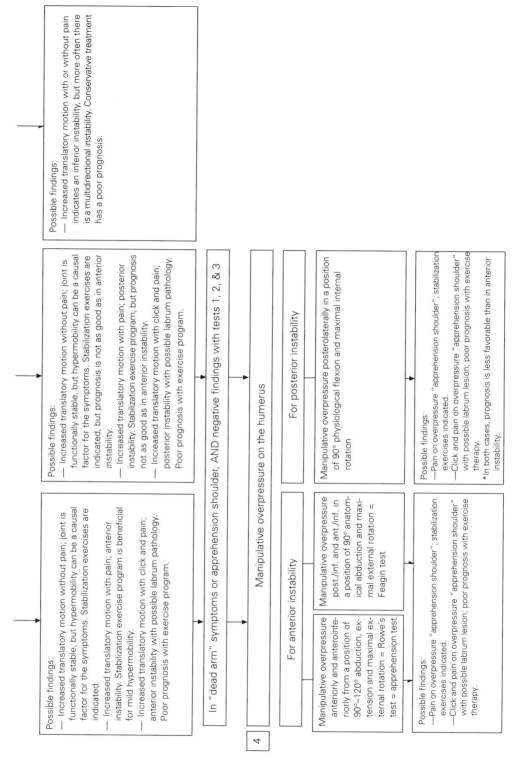

Possible findings:
— Increased translatory motion without pain; joint is functionally stable, but hypermobility can be a causal factor for the symptoms. Stabilization exercises are indicated.
— Increased translatory motion with pain; anterior instability. Stabilization exercise program is beneficial for mild hypermobility.
— Increased translatory motion with click and pain; anterior instability with possible labrum pathology. Poor prognosis with exercise program.

Possible findings:
— Increased translatory motion without pain; joint is functionally stable, but hypermobility can be a causal factor for the symptoms. Stabilization exercises are indicated, but prognosis is not as good as in anterior instability.
— Increased translatory motion with pain; posterior instability. Stabilization exercise program, but prognosis not as good as in anterior instability.
— Increased translatory motion with click and pain; posterior instability with possible labrum pathology. Poor prognosis with exercise program.

Possible findings:
— Increased translatory motion with or without pain indicates an inferior instability, but more often there is a multidirectional instability. Conservative treatment has a poor prognosis.

In "dead arm" symptoms or apprehension shoulder, AND negative findings with tests 1, 2, & 3

Manipulative overpressure on the humerus

4

For anterior instability

Manipulative overpressure anteriorly and anteroinferiorly from a position of 90°–120° abduction, extension and maximal external rotation = Rowe's test = apprehension test

Manipulative overpressure post./inf. and ant./inf. in a position of 90° anatomical abduction and maximal external rotation = Feagin test

For posterior instability

Manipulative overpressure posterolaterally in a position of 90° physiological flexion and maximal internal rotation

Possible findings:
—Pain on overpressure "apprehension shoulder"; stabilization exercises indicated.
—Click and pain on overpressure "apprehension shoulder" with possible labrum lesion; poor prognosis with exercise therapy.

Possible findings:
—Pain on overpressure "apprehension shoulder"; stabilization exercises indicated.
—Click and pain on overpressure "apprehension shoulder" with possible labrum lesion; poor prognosis with exercise therapy.
*In both cases, prognosis is less favorable than in anterior instability.

DIAGNOSIS AND TREATMENT OF STERNOCLAVICULAR JOINT LESIONS

Category	Subtype	Description	Treatment
Arthritis	Capsular pattern (all motions are painful and slightly limited at end-range)	Traumatic	With severe pain, intra-articular injection Spontaneous recovery With residual dysfunction: mobilization
		Nontraumatic (most common: rheumatoid arthritis, acute septic arthritis) Subacute degeneration (swelling in the joint without trauma; usually benign swelling at the medial end of the clavicle)	Dependent on the cause With residual dysfunction: mobilization Seldom necessary due to minimal symptoms Spontaneous recovery
Arthritis (usually seen in middle-aged women)		Primary (occurs without previous trauma or pathology in the joint)	Seldom necessary due to minimal symptoms Mobilization
Instability	Noncapsular pattern	Subluxation (can occur spontaneously or as a result of a trauma)	Intra-articular injection in cases with severe pain Symptoms gradually resolve, although subluxation remains
		Dislocation presternal retrosternal suprasternal	In the presence of severe symptoms: surgery

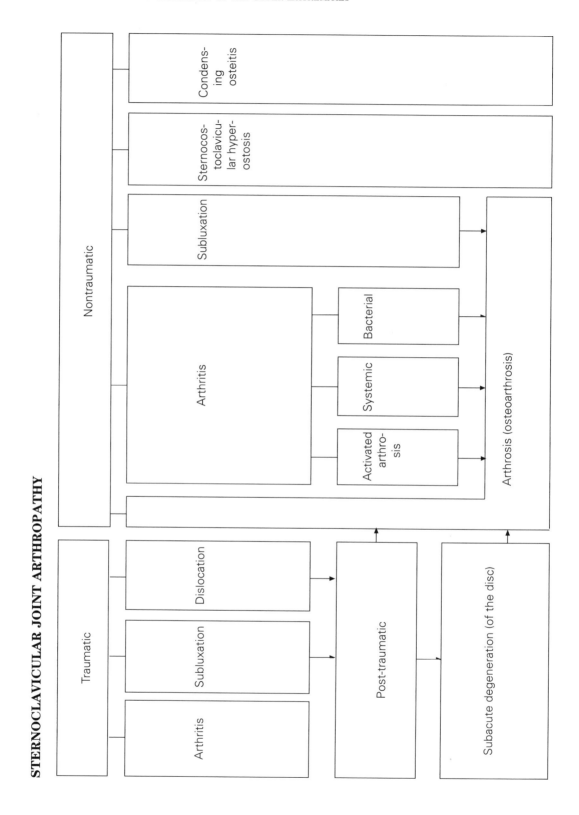

DIAGNOSIS AND TREATMENT OF ACROMIOCLAVICULAR JOINT LESIONS

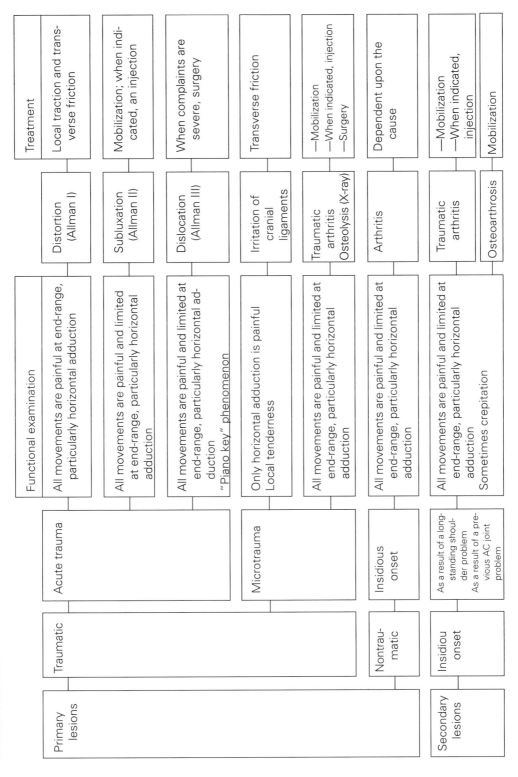

DIAGNOSIS DIAGRAM FOR THE SHOULDER 1a

Functional examination of the shoulder

Pathology	Glenohumeral joint	Traumatic arthritis	Immobilization arthritis	Idiopathic arthritis	Shoulder-hand syndrome	Osteoarthrosis
1 Active elevation of both arms		● ● (●)	● ● (●)	● ● (●)		○
2 Active elevation of one arm		● ()	● ()	()		○
3 Painful arc test						
4 With the arm elevated, overpressure medially		()	()	()		○
5 With the arm elevated, overpressure posteriorly		()	()	()	Burning pain in the shoulder area, diffuse swelling on the dorsal aspect of the hand and fingers	○
6 Active extension-internal rotation						○ (○)
7 Passive internal rotation		()	()			○ (○)
8 Passive glenohumeral abduction: mobility						●
9 Passive glenohumeral abduction: end-feel						●
10 Passive adduction from an extended-internally rotated position						(○)
11 Passive horizontal adduction		!	!	!		
12 Active external rotation						● (●)
13 Passive external rotation						● (●)
14 Biceps brachii stretch test						
15 Resisted adduction						

Note: See Appendix B for legend

Loose body	Anterior instability	Posterior instability	Inferior instability	Complex instability	**Acromioclavicular joint** Arthritis	Subluxation	Dislocation	Osteolysis of the lateral end of the clavicle	**Sternoclavicular joint** Subluxation	Osteoarthrosis	Subacute degeneration
					○				●		○
					○				●		○
					○						
					●○	○	●	●	●		●
					●○	○	●	●	●		●
					●				●● ○		
○○					●● ●●	●	●	● (●)	●● ○	*Usually no pain or local swelling*	●●
	○		○	○	●○	○	●	●	●		●
					○	○	○				

DIAGNOSIS DIAGRAM FOR THE SHOULDER 1b

Functional examination of the shoulder	**Pathology**	**Glenohumeral joint**	Traumatic arthritis	Immobilization arthritis	Idiopathic arthritis	Shoulder-hand syndrome	Osteoarthrosis
16 Resisted abduction			○	○	○		
17 Resisted external rotation			○	○	○		
18 Resisted internal rotation			○	○	○		
19 Resisted elbow flexion							
20 Resisted elbow extension							
21 Throwing test			!	!	!		
22 External rotation test			!	!	!	Functional examination of the shoulder is often negative	
23 Anterior subluxation test			!	!	!		
24 Anterior drawer test			!	!	!		
25 Posterior drawer test			!	!	!		
26 Resisted abduction with pull							
27 Resisted external rotation with pull							
28 Resisted internal rotation with pull							

	Loose body	Anterior instability	Posterior instability	Inferior instability	Complex instability	**Acromioclavicular joint**	Arthritis	Subluxation	Dislocation	Osteolysis of the lateral end of the clavicle	**Sternoclavicular joint**	Subluxation	Osteoarthrosis	Subacute degeneration
Sudden blocking of the joint and limitation of one or more motions	○ ●● (□) □○	○ ○ □○	○ ○ □○○ □○	○ ○ □○○ □○										
"Piano key" phenomenon									✓					
Functional examination is usually negative												✓		

DIAGNOSIS DIAGRAM FOR THE SHOULDER 2a

Functional examination of the shoulder

Pathology	Acute subacromial/Subdeltoid bursitis	Chronic subacromial/Subdeltoid bursitis	Subcoracoid bursitis	Supraspinatus tendopathy	Supraspinatus tendopathy with calcification	Rupture of supraspinatus tendon
1 Active elevation of both arms	● ● ●					● ● ●
2 Active elevation of one arm	● ● ●					● ● ●
3 Painful arc test		● (●)		○		
4 With the arm elevated, overpressure medially	● ● ●	○		○		
5 With the arm elevated, overpressure posteriorly	!	○				
6 Active extension-internal rotation		○		○		
7 Passive internal rotation	● ● ●	○		○		
8 Passive glenohumeral abduction: mobility	● ● ●					
9 Passive glenohumeral abduction: end-feel	!	○			See supraspinatus tendopathy	
10 Passive adduction from an extended-internally rotated position	!	○		○		
11 Passive horizontal adduction	!	○	○			
12 Active external rotation	● ● ●					
13 Passive external rotation	● ● ●	○	● ●			
14 Biceps brachii stretch test						
15 Resisted adduction						

Note: See Appendix B for legend.

Infraspinatus tendopathy	Subscapularis tendopathy	Tenosynovitis of the long head of the biceps brachii	Dislocation of the long head of the biceps brachii tendon	Rupture of the long head of the biceps brachii tendon	Suprascapular nerve compression neuropathy	Long thoracic nerve lesion	Accessory nerve lesion	Rheumatic polymyalgia
						●●	●	
○	○	○						
○								
		○						
○		○						
○								
○								
○	○							
○	○							
	○							
		●●						

DIAGNOSIS DIAGRAM FOR THE SHOULDER 2b

Functional examination of the shoulder

Pathology	Acute subacromial/Subdeltoid bursitis	Chronic subacromial/Subdeltoid bursitis	Subcoracoid bursitis	Supraspinatus tendopathy	Supraspinatus tendopathy with calcification	Rupture of supraspinatus tendon
16 Resisted abduction				● (●)		●
17 Resisted external rotation				○		
18 Resisted internal rotation						
19 Resisted elbow flexion						
20 Resisted elbow extension				○		
21 Throwing test		Various resisted tests can be painful				
22 External rotation test						
23 Anterior subluxation test						
24 Anterior drawer test						
25 Posterior drawer test						
26 Resisted abduction with pull				●●		
27 Resisted external rotation with pull						
28 Resisted internal rotation with pull						

Condition	Findings / Notes
Infraspinatus tendopathy	● (●) ○ ● ●
Subscapularis tendopathy	● (●) ● (●)
Tenosynovitis of the long head of the biceps brachii	○ ○
Dislocation of the long head of the biceps brachii tendon	Functional examination is usually negative; with an external rotation-abduction movement an (uncomfortable) click can be felt.
Rupture of the long head of the biceps brachii tendon	Functional examination is usually negative; with contraction of the biceps brachii "swelling" of the muscle belly can be seen directly proximal to the elbow
Suprascapular nerve compression neuropathy	○ ○
Long thoracic nerve lesion	
Accessory nerve lesion	
Rheumatic polymyalgia	Constant pain in both shoulders and hips. In 30%, temporal arteritis

Appendix E

Algorithms for the Diagnosis and Treatment of the Elbow

DIFFERENTIAL DIAGNOSIS OF ANTERIOR ELBOW PAIN

Pathology	Functional examination
Biceps brachii muscle: —Insertion tendopathy —Tendinitis —Musculotendinous junction strain or overuse	Painful resisted elbow flexion and forearm supination Passive forearm pronation can be painful with an insertion tendopathy
Bicipitoradial bursitis	Painful passive forearm pronation Resisted elbow flexion from a position of maximal forearm pronation is very painful Resisted elbow flexion from a position of maximal forearm supination is not painful
Brachialis muscle strain or overuse	Painful resisted elbow flexion
Brachialis myositis ossificans	Limitation of elbow flexion and extension in a noncapsular pattern Resisted flexion can be weak and painful
Articular pathology of the elbow:	
—Capsular	Flexion limitation > > extension limitation
—Noncapsular, eg, anterior loose body	Elbow flexion limited
Pronator teres syndrome (Compression neuropathy of median nerve)	Repeatedly performed resistance of forearm pronation produces the symptoms (pain and/or paresthesia) Tenderness on palpation at the level of the bicipital aponeurosis
Referred pain from:	
—Cervical spine, C6 —Thoracic outlet compression syndrome —Shoulder —Possibly wrist/hand	Functional examination of the elbow (also after provocation of the complaints) is negative

DIFFERENTIAL DIAGNOSIS OF LATERAL ELBOW PAIN

Pathology	Functional examination
Tennis elbow Type I: extensor carpi radialis longus insertion tendopathy Type II: extensor carpi radialis brevis insertion tendopathy Type III: extensor carpi radialis brevis tendinitis Type IV: overuse of extensor carpi radialis brevis musculotendinous junction and/or proximal muscle belly Type V: extensor digitorum insertion tendopathy	Painful resisted wrist extension Painful resisted wrist radial deviation Usually, painful resisted extension of 2nd and 3rd fingers When resisted extension of 4th and 5th fingers is also painful: tennis elbow, type V Sometimes: painful passive elbow extension painful resisted elbow flexion painful resisted forearm supination Palpation further differentiates the location of the lesion
Radial nerve compression neuropathy	All positive findings with the tennis elbow can also be positive here! The local tenderness is in a different place than the predilection sites for the tennis elbow Sometimes only resisted extension of the middle finger is painful
Humeroradial joint lesion	Painful passive forearm supination and/or pronation Local tenderness
Radial head subluxation (in children 3–8 years)	Painfully limited elbow flexion and extension
Radial collateral ligament lesion	Painful passive varus test in slight elbow flexion Sometimes slight limitation of motion in a capsular pattern
Loose body in the elbow joint (in the lateral compartment)	Painful flexion or extension limitation of motion in the elbow Sometimes painful resisted wrist extension
Panner's disease (humeral capitulum osteochondrosis in children 8–14 years)	Painless limitation of elbow extension Sometimes local swelling
Supinator muscle strain	Painful resisted forearm supination Sometimes painful passive forearm pronation
Referred pain from: —Cervical spine —Thoracic outlet compression syndrome —Shoulder —Wrist/hand	Functional examination of the elbow (also after provocation of the complaints) is negative

DIFFERENTIAL DIAGNOSIS OF MEDIAL ELBOW PAIN

Pathology	Functional examination
Golfer's elbow Type I: insertion tendopathy of the wrist flexors on the medial humeral epicondyle Type II: musculotendinous junction of the wrist flexors, about 1 cm distal to the medial humeral epicondyle	Painful resisted wrist flexion Painful resisted forearm pronation Sometimes: slight limitation of motion in a capsular pattern slightly painful resisted radial and/or ulnar deviation of the wrist slightly painful resisted finger flexion
Medial humeral epicondyle periostitis (as a result of direct trauma)	Functional examination negative Local tenderness
Traumatic arthritis of the humeroulnar joint (as a result of a hyperextension and/or valgus trauma)	Limitation of motion in a capsular pattern Sometimes painful valgus test (in slight flexion)
Ulnar collateral ligament lesion	Painful passive valgus test in slight elbow flexion Sometimes (slight) limitation of motion in a capsular pattern
Pronator teres insertion tendopathy	Painful resisted forearm pronation
Ulnar nerve (compression) neuropathy	Functional examination of the elbow is negative It may be possible to see anterior dislocation of the nerve during elbow flexion Symptoms are reproduced by palpation of the ulnar nerve
Referred pain, from: —Cervical spine —Thoracic outlet compression syndrome —Shoulder —Hand/wrist	Functional examination of the elbow (also after provocation of the complaints) is negative

LIMITATION OF MOTION IN THE ELBOW

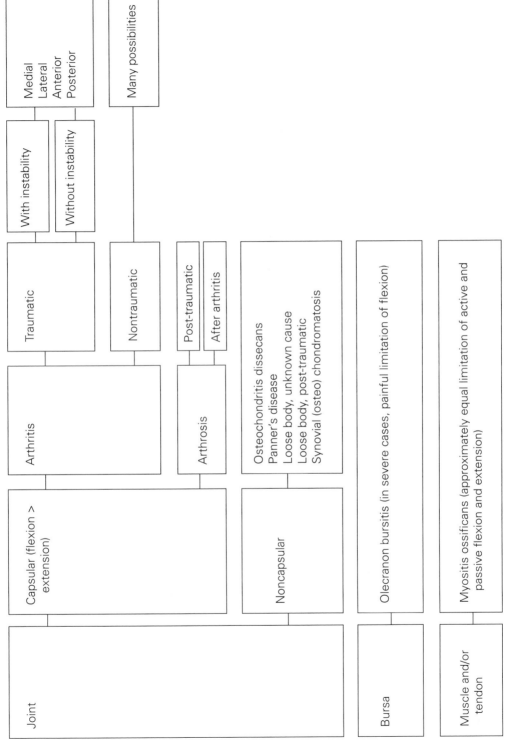

INTERPRETATION OF A LIMITATION OF MOTION IN THE ELBOW

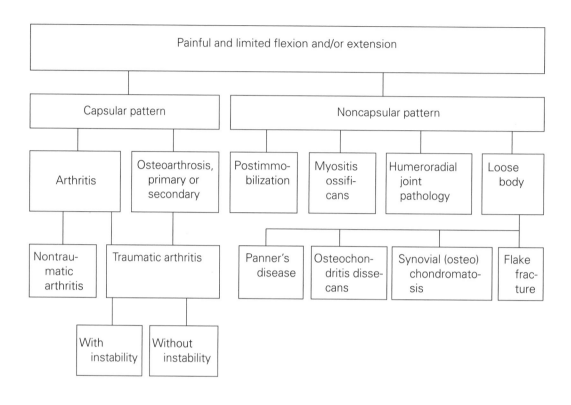

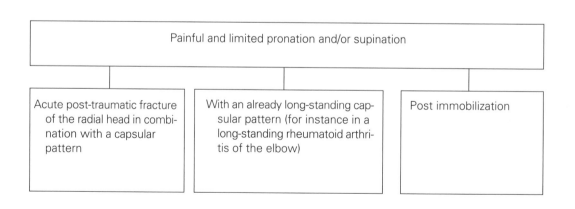

INTERPRETATION OF PAIN WITHOUT A LIMITATION OF MOTION IN THE ELBOW

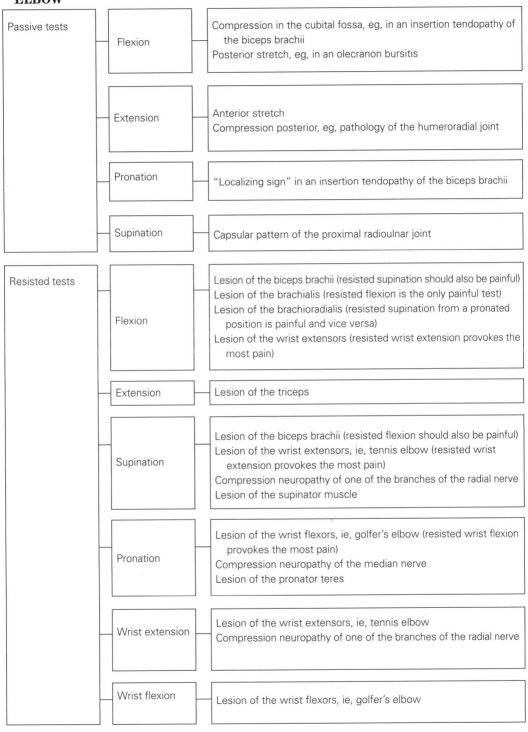

Passive tests	Flexion	Compression in the cubital fossa, eg, in an insertion tendopathy of the biceps brachii Posterior stretch, eg, in an olecranon bursitis
	Extension	Anterior stretch Compression posterior, eg, pathology of the humeroradial joint
	Pronation	"Localizing sign" in an insertion tendopathy of the biceps brachii
	Supination	Capsular pattern of the proximal radioulnar joint
Resisted tests	Flexion	Lesion of the biceps brachii (resisted supination should also be painful) Lesion of the brachialis (resisted flexion is the only painful test) Lesion of the brachioradialis (resisted supination from a pronated position is painful and vice versa) Lesion of the wrist extensors (resisted wrist extension provokes the most pain)
	Extension	Lesion of the triceps
	Supination	Lesion of the biceps brachii (resisted flexion should also be painful) Lesion of the wrist extensors, ie, tennis elbow (resisted wrist extension provokes the most pain) Compression neuropathy of one of the branches of the radial nerve Lesion of the supinator muscle
	Pronation	Lesion of the wrist flexors, ie, golfer's elbow (resisted wrist flexion provokes the most pain) Compression neuropathy of the median nerve Lesion of the pronator teres
	Wrist extension	Lesion of the wrist extensors, ie, tennis elbow Compression neuropathy of one of the branches of the radial nerve
	Wrist flexion	Lesion of the wrist flexors, ie, golfer's elbow

TENNIS ELBOW

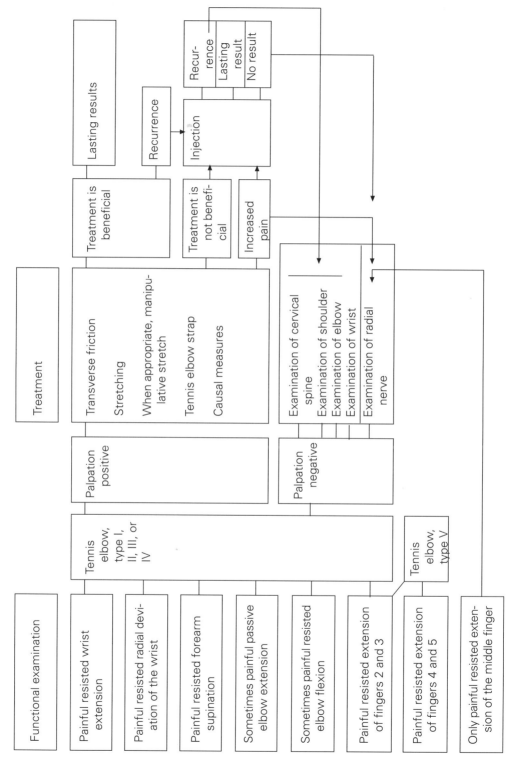
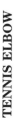

ASEPTIC NECROSES OF THE ELBOW JOINT

	Osteochondritis dissecans	Panner's disease
Age	15–20 years	± 10 years (age span 4–16 years)
Gender	Male:female = 9:1	Male
Localization	Usually on the dominant side —humeral capitulum —humeral trochlea —radial head (often osteochondritis dissecans processes are also occurring in other joints)	Most often humeral capitulum
Clinical stages and functional examination	1. Early stage: no pain slight recurrent swelling slight limitation of extension 2. Middle stage: activity-related pain locking of the elbow limitation of flexion and extension joint crepitation 3. Late stage: constant pain disturbance of ADLs also limitation of pronation and supination	Minimal findings: —Painless limitation of extension —Seldom activity-related pain —Seldom swelling —Spontaneous recovery in 3–4 months (more pain and limitation when the radial head or the humeral trochlea is affected)
X-ray examination	All stages have typical findings on X-ray	Typical findings on X-ray These changes remain visible about 3 years
Treatment	Surgery	Reassure the parents Participation in sports limited or stopped

INSTABILITY OF THE ELBOW A

	Medial instability	Lateral instability	Posterior instability	Anterior instability
Frequency	Most frequent form of elbow instability	Seldom occurring elbow instability; radial head (sub) dislocation, as a form of lateral instability occurs more often: children (up to 8 years) > adults	Occurring second most frequently after medial instability: posterolateral > posteromedial > posterior	Least occurring instability: an anterior (sub) dislocation of the radius or ulna
Cause	Hyperextension and/or valgus trauma	Varus trauma Radial head dislocation in children: sudden traction on the radius	Traumatic force from anterior against the forearm with a fixed upper arm, or from posterior against the upper arm with a fixed forearm	Traumatic force from posterior against a flexed elbow
Chief complaints	With a nonreduced dislocation: severe pain, and movement is impossible After reduction: pain anteromedial and lateral (as a result of compression) Chronic instability: quickly fatiguing arm muscles, and clicking or shifting in the joint	Acute: Severe pain and limitation of motion Radial head subluxation in adults: minimal complaints Radial head dislocation in adults: pain and limitation of motion Radial head dislocation in children: elbow held in about 90° flexion Pain in the elbow and in the wrist (distal radioulnar joint)	Acute: diffuse pain and inability to move Chronic: avoids maximal extension out of fear for redislocating	Acute: diffuse pain and severe limitation of motion After reduction: diffuse pain
Functional examination (after reduction)	Limited flexion > extension (traumatic arthritis) Positive valgus test: abnormal mobility and painful	Radial head subluxation in adults: occasional audible click with pronation and supination Radial head dislocation in adults: limitation of flexion Radial head dislocation in children: severe limitation of flexion	Limited flexion > > extension (traumatic arthritis) Positive varus test: abnormal mobility and pain	Limited flexion > > extension (traumatic arthritis)

INSTABILITY OF THE ELBOW B

	Medial instability	Lateral instability	Posterior instability	Anterior instability
Complications	In adolescents: apophyseal avulsion fracture of the humeral medial epicondyle In adults: strain of the common tendon insertion of the wrist flexors Fracture Compression fracture, lateral ulnar nerve entrapment	Seldom: radial head fracture	In about 2% of the cases, a chronic instability occurs	Olecranon fracture or other fractures
Treatment	Surgery	Surgery Radial head dislocation in children: manual reduction	Surgery In young patients: 4–6 weeks immobilization in a cast Patients with minimal complaints: specific muscle strengthening	Surgery

DIAGNOSIS DIAGRAM FOR THE ELBOW 1a

Lesions **Functional examination of the elbow**	Traumatic arthritis	Nontraumatic arthritis (eg, rheumatoid arthritides)		Osteoarthrosis	Subluxation/dislocation of the head of the radius: in children
1 Active extension of both elbows	○ (●)	○ (●)		○	
2 Active flexion of both elbows	● ●● (●)	● ●● (●)		●●	
3 Active pronation of both forearms					
4 Active supination of both elbows					
5 Passive elbow extension	● (●)	● (●)		○	● ●●●
6 Passive elbow flexion	● ●● (●)	● ●● (●)		●●	
7 Passive forearm pronation					It is often impossible to perform the functional examination
8 Passive forearm supination					
9a Passive valgus test	○				
9b Passive varus test					

Note: See Appendix B for legend.

Panner's disease	Osteochondritis dissecans	Surgical Osteochondromatosis	Loose body: in adults	Fracture of the radial head	Sprain of the radioulnar joint		Subcutaneous olecranon bursitis	Bicipitoradial bursitis
○ ●	○	● ●●(●)	● ●(●)	○ (●)				
	○	○ ●●(●)	● ●(●)	● ●●(●)			○	
	○			○				●
	○			○	○			
○ ●	○	● ●●(●)	● ●(●)	● (●)				
	○	● ●●(●)	● ●(●)	● ●●(●)			○	
	○			●				●●
	○			●	●●			

DIAGNOSIS DIAGRAM FOR THE ELBOW 1b

Functional examination of the elbow	Traumatic arthritis	Nontraumatic arthritis (eg, rheumatoid arthritides)		Osteoarthrosis	Subluxation/dislocation of the head of the radius: in children
10 Resisted elbow flexion	O	O			
11 Resisted elbow extension					
12 Resisted forearm pronation					
13 Resisted forearm supination					
14 Resisted dorsal extension of the wrist					
15 Resisted palmar flexion of the wrist					
16 Resisted radial deviation of the wrist					
17 Resisted ulnar deviation of the wrist					
18 Resisted extension of the 2nd and 3rd fingers					
19 Resisted extension of the 4th and 5th fingers					

Panner's disease	Osteochondritis dissecans	Surgical Osteochondromatosis	Loose body: in adults	Fracture of the radial head	Sprain of the radioulnar joint		Subcutaneous olecranon bursitis	Bicipitoradial bursitis

DIAGNOSIS DIAGRAM FOR THE ELBOW 2a

Functional examination of the elbow	**Lesions** Lesion of the brachialis muscle	Myositis ossificans (in the brachialis muscle)	Lesions of the biceps brachii muscle	Muscle or musculotendinous junction	Insertion tendopathy
1 Active extension of both elbows	○	○ ● ● (◉)		○	○
2 Active flexion of both elbows	○	○ ● ● (◉)		○	○
3 Active pronation of both forearms					○
4 Active supination of both elbows				○	○
5 Passive elbow extension	○	○ ● ● (◉)		○	○
6 Passive elbow flexion		○ ● ● (◉)			
7 Passive forearm pronation					●
8 Passive forearm supination					
9a Passive valgus test					
9b Passive varus test					

Lesion of the triceps brachii muscle	Golfer's elbow	Tennis elbow, Types I to IV	Tennis elbow, Type V	Lesion of the supinator muscle	Lesion of the pronator teres muscle	Compression neuropathy: superficial radial nerve	Compression neuropathy: posterior interosseous nerve	Compression neuropathy: recurrent radial nerve	Compression neuropathy: ulnar nerve	Compression neuropathy: median nerve
○										
○									○	
					○					
				○						
	○	○	○		○					○
○									○	
				○						
					○					
	○				○				○	
		○								

DIAGNOSIS DIAGRAM FOR THE ELBOW 2b

Functional examination of the elbow	**Lesions** Lesion of the brachialis muscle	Myositis ossificans (in the brachialis muscle)	Lesions of the biceps brachii muscle	Muscle or musculotendinous junction	Insertion tendopathy
10 Resisted elbow flexion	●●	●○		●●	●●
11 Resisted elbow extension					
12 Resisted forearm pronation					
13 Resisted forearm supination				●	●
14 Resisted dorsal extension of the wrist					
15 Resisted palmar flexion of the wrist					
16 Resisted radial deviation of the wrist					
17 Resisted ulnar deviation of the wrist					
18 Resisted extension of the 2nd and 3rd fingers					
19 Resisted extension of the 4th and 5th fingers					

Lesion of the triceps brachii muscle	Golfer's elbow	Tennis elbow, Types I to IV	Tennis elbow, Type V	Lesion of the supinator muscle	Lesion of the pronator teres muscle	Compression neuropathy: superficial radial nerve	Compression neuropathy: posterior interosseous nerve	Compression neuropathy: recurrent radial nerve	Compression neuropathy: ulnar nerve	Compression neuropathy: median nerve
		○								
●●									○	
	○				●●					●●
		○		●●			●			
		●●	●			●	●	●		
	●●								○	
	○	●								
	○									
		○	●							
			●							

Appendix F

Algorithms for the Diagnosis and Treatment of the Wrist and Hand

INTERPRETATION OF A LIMITATION OF MOTION AND/OR PAIN IN THE DISTAL RADIOULNAR JOINT

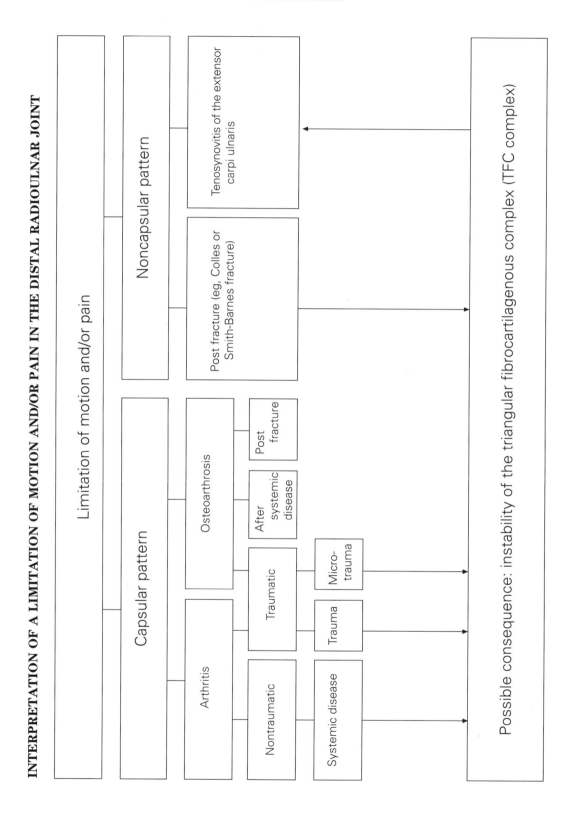

INTERPRETATION OF A LIMITATION OF MOTION IN THE CARPUS

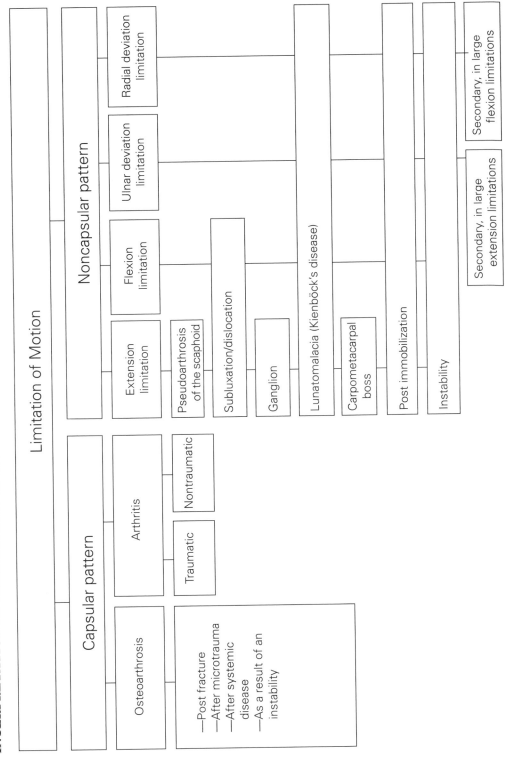

CARPAL HYPERMOBILITY AND INSTABILITY 1

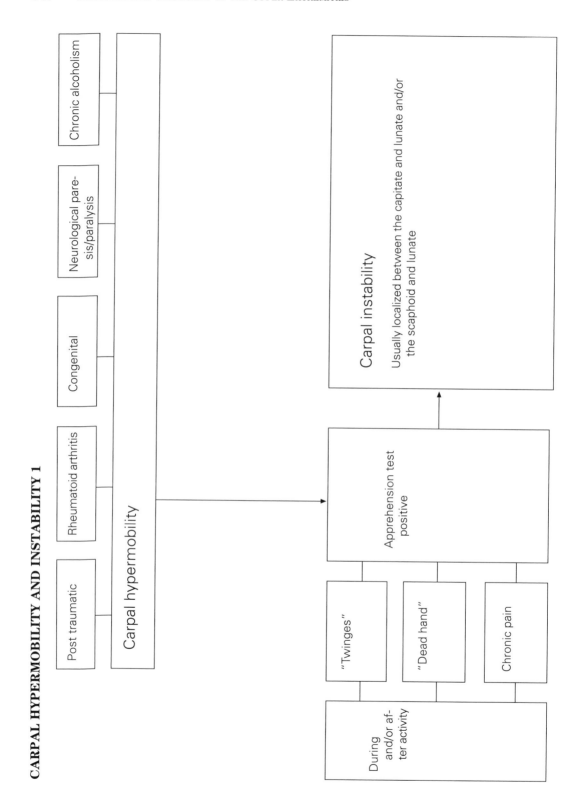

JOINT LESIONS OF THE MIDHAND, THUMB, AND FINGERS

Tests performed	**Lesions** Arthritis of the trapeziometacarpal joint	Arthrosis of the trapeziometacarpal joint	Dislocation of the trapeziometacarpal joint	Dislocation of the metacarpophalangeal joint
Active thumb retroposition	●● ●●●	●(●) ●(●●)	●● ●●●	
Passive thumb retroposition	●● ●●●	●● ●(●●)	●●□ ●●●	
Resisted thumb radial abduction	○		●●	
Resisted thumb palmar abduction	○		●●	
Resisted thumb dorsal adduction	○		●●	
Resisted thumb ulnar adduction	○		●●	
Passive MCP joint extension				●●□ ●●●
Passive MCP joint flexion				●●□ ●●●
Passive PIP joint extension				
Passive PIP joint flexion				
Passive DIP joint extension				
Passive DIP joint flexion				

Note: See Appendix B for legend.

CARPAL HYPERMOBILITY AND INSTABILITY 2: TFC COMPLEX

Triangular fibrocartilagenous complex (TFC complex)

Consists of:
—triangular disc
—ulnar collateral ligament
—dorsal and volar radioulnar ligaments
—ulnolunate ligament
—extensor carpi ulnaris tendon sheath
—ulnocarpal meniscus

Findings in the functional examination of the wrist in a TFC complex instability

Pain and/or locking, possibly with a "paralyzed" feeling in passive pronation and supination of the carpus in relation to the radius and ulna

Passive ulnar deviation is usually painful, especially when combined with slight flexion or extension of the wrist

Passive wrist extension can be painful

Passive compression of the radius against the ulna can be painful

Sometimes the joint play between radius and ulna and/or ulna and triquetrum is greater in a dorsodistal and palmar direction

In palpation: tenderness at the dorsoulnar aspect of the wrist just distal to the ulnar head

Lesion of the MCP I ulnar collateral ligament	Lesion of the MCP I radial collateral ligament	Arthritis of the MCP and IP joints	Arthrosis of the MCP and IP joints	(Sub) dislocation of an MCP II–V joint	Collateral ligament rupture of an MCP II–V joint	Dislocation of an IP joint
●□ / ◐◐	●□ / ◐◐	●● / ◐	● / ◐	●●□ / ◐◐◐	●□ / ◐	
●□ / ◐◐	●□ / ◐◐	●● / ◐◐	●● / ◐◐	●●□ / ◐◐◐	●●□ / ◐◐	
		●● / ◐	● / ◐			
		●● / ◐◐	●● / ◐◐			
		●● / ◐	● / ◐			!
		●● / ◐◐	●● / ◐◐			!

Appendix G

Peripheral Neuropathies of the Upper Extremities

OVERVIEW OF SYMPTOMATOLOGY WITH MECHANICAL IRRITATION (PRESSURE/STRETCH) OF NERVE STRUCTURES

Location of the irritation	Localization of the symptoms	Changes in pain and/or paresthesia
Spinal cord	Extrasegmental electric current feeling without aspect*; possibly extrasegmental pain with ventral compression as a result of pressure on the dura mater	None
Dura mater —ventral	Extrasegmental pain, possibly extrasegmental paresthesia as a result of pressure on the spinal cord	With stretch of the dura mater, an increase in pain can occur (possibly of the paresthesia also)
—dorsal	Here the dura mater has few nociceptors, and therefore causes minimal symptoms	
Dural sleeve and cuff	Segmental radiating pain, without aspect	None
Ventral root	Segmental radiating pain and/or paresthesia, without aspect, as a result of ischemic changes	Rubbing the area manifesting the symptoms can sometimes increase the pain and/or paresthesia
Dorsal root	See ventral root	See ventral root
Spinal nerve	The spinal nerve consists of the union of the ventral and dorsal roots; thus the clinical symptoms from irritation are the same as described above for the roots	
Ventral ramus	Segmental radiation of pain and/or paresthesia without aspect	None
Dorsal ramus	Paravertebral pain. Also pseudoradicular pain from the (medial) facet joint capsule	None
Recurrent nerve (meningeal ramus)	Pseudoradicular pain from the (lateral) facet joint capsule and the posterior longitudinal ligament	None
Trunk Fascicle Division	These are formed from different ventral rami; the clinical symptoms from irritation are the same as with the spinal nerve, with the realization that the symptomatology can extend over different dermatomes	Paresthesia can sometimes increase with movement
Peripheral nerve	Clinical symptoms manifest in a clearly defined skin area (cutaneous innervation) in which the sensation is affected. Motor deficit can occur in muscles innervated by the peripheral nerve.	Initially paresthesia can increase with movement and/or rubbing the area manifesting the symptoms; later they decrease

*Aspect: one affected side, eg, anterior, posterior, medial, or lateral

IRRITATION (PRESSURE/STRETCH) OF NERVE STRUCTURES

Motor changes	Reflex changes	Sensory changes	Release phenomenon*
Ranges from incoordination to spasticity	Hyperreflexia; pathological reflexes (eg, Babinski)	Hypo- to anesthesia; Brown-Sequard syndrome	None
None	None	None	None
None	None	None	None
Dependent on the amount of compassion: deficit of the muscles innervated by that root	Sometimes significant hyperreflexia; later hypo- to areflexia	Less often seen than motoric changes	None
See ventral root	See ventral root	More often seen than motoric changes (segmental)	None
Dependent on the amount of compression: deficit in muscles innervated by that ramus	Hypo- to areflexia	Hyper- to anesthesia	
Dependent on the amount of compression: deficit possible but difficult to objectify	Quite possible but not objectifiable	Paravertebral hyper- to anesthesia	None
In most cases concerns compression of short duration (eg, thoracic outlet compression syndrome) and therefore no motor deficit occurs	None	Usually none	Sometimes present
Dependent on the amount of compression: moderate to severe deficit of the muscles innervated by the peripheral nerve	Hypo- to areflexia	Changes in sensation in the area of cutaneous innervation	Sometimes present

*Release phenomenon: the occurrence of symptoms when the compression is lifted.

CLINICAL REVIEW OF PERIPHERAL MOTOR DEFICITS OF THE UPPER EXTREMITY

The most characteristic nerve root is indicated in **boldface** type.

Temporalis muscle (m.)	CN V
Masseter m.	CN V
Pterygoid muscles (mm.)	CN V
Orbicularis occuli m.	CN VII
Platysma	CN VII
Pharynx	CN IX, X
Sternocleidomastoid m.	CN XI
Trapezius m.	CN XI
Tongue	CN XII
Diaphragm	C3,**4**,(5)
Levator scapulae m.	C**3,4,5**
Rhomboid mm.	C4,**5**
Serratus anterior m.	C**5,6,7**
Supraspinatus m.	C4,**5**,6
Infraspinatus m.	C4,**5**,6
Pectoralis major m.	C**5,6**,7
Subscapularis m.	C**5,6**,7
Latissimus dorsi m.	C6,**7,8**
Teres major m.	C5,**6**,7
Deltoid m.	C**5,6**
Biceps brachii m.	C**5,6**
Brachialis m.	C**5,6**

Radial nerve

Triceps brachii m.	C6,**7,8**
Brachioradialis m.	C5,**6**
Extensor carpi radialis longus and brevis mm.	C**6,7**,8
Supinator m.	C5,**6**,7
Extensor digitorum communis m.	C6,**7,8**

Extensor digiti minimi m.	C**7,8**
Extensor carpi ulnaris m.	C**7,8**
Abductor pollicis longus m.	C**7,8**
Extensor pollicis longus m.	C**7,8**
Extensor pollicis brevis m.	C**7,8**
Extensor indicis m.	C**7,8**

Median nerve

Pronator teres m.	C**6,7**
Flexor carpi radialis m.	C**6,7**
Palmaris longus m.	C7,**8**, T1
Flexor digitorum superficialis m.	C7,**8**
Flexor digitorum profundus II, III m.	C7,**8**
Flexor pollicis longus m.	C7,**8**
Pronator quadratus m.	C7,**8**
Abductor pollicis brevis m.	C**7,8**
Opponens pollicis m.	C**7**,8
Flexor pollicis brevis m., superficial head	C**8**, T1

Ulnar nerve

Flexor carpi ulnaris m.	C7,**8**, T1
Flexor digitorum profundus IV, V m.	C7,**8**, T**1**
Hypothenar mm.	C8, T**1**
Interossei mm.	C8, T**1**
Adductor pollicis m.	C8, T**1**
Flexor pollicis brevis, deep head	C8, T**1**

SHOULDER-ARM PAIN AND/OR PARESTHESIA

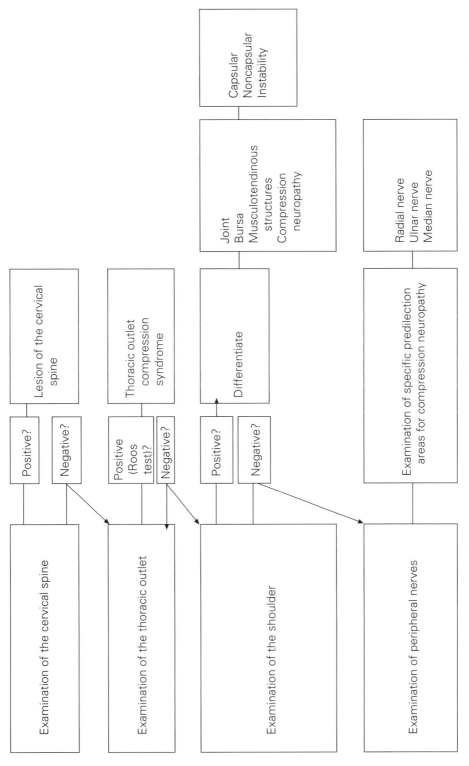

Keep in mind that some neurological diseases such as multiple sclerosis, syringomyelia, paralysis agitans, and chorea can begin with paresthesias in the hand.

THORACIC OUTLET COMPRESSION SYNDROME (TOS)

Cause	Treatment
Long-standing shoulder problem with or without a limitation of motion	Primarily treat the shoulder problem
Limitation of motion in the acromioclavicular joint	Mobilization of the acromioclavicular joint
Limitation of motion in the cervical spine, particularly the cervicothoracic junction	Mobilization of the cervicothoracic junction; sometimes mobilization of the first rib
Poor posture with shortening of the scalene muscles, pectoralis minor, and pectoralis major	—Stretch shortened muscles —Strengthening of thoracic extensors and scapulae stabilizers —Instruction in proper posture
Scheurmann's disease (see above for poor posture)	See above for poor posture
Hypertrophy of the scalene muscles, eg, with —weight lifters* —with chronic obstructive pulmonary disease**	*Stretch scalene muscles **1 Teach diaphragmatic breathing 2 Stretch scalene muscles 3 Mobilize first rib
Congenital bands and/or cervical ribs	—When appropriate, mobilize limitation of motion in cervicothoracic junction —Stretch scaleni muscles —Mobilize first rib —If necessary, instruction in proper posture
Unilateral muscle development, eg, with athletes participating in racket or throwing sports	Muscle strengthening of the nondominant side
Heavy bosom (release phenomenon = symptoms occur after the pressure is released, ie, mostly at night)	—Wider bra straps —Before going to bed in the evening, attempt to bring on the paresthesia by positioning the shoulder girdle, passively, in elevation (eg, resting the elbows on the arms of a chair)

Index